Consumed in the City

Thanks for your
dedication & TB control

Chris Caudill

PAUL DRAUS is a research scientist at the Center for Interventions, Treatment and Addictions Research in the Department of Community Health at the Wright State University School of Medicine. He worked in the field of tuberculosis control in New York City and Chicago from 1992 to 2000.

Consumed in the City

Observing Tuberculosis at Century's End

PAUL DRAUS

TEMPLE UNIVERSITY PRESS
Philadelphia

Temple University Press, Philadelphia 19122
Copyright © 2004 by Temple University
All rights reserved
Published 2004
Printed in the United States of America

Library of Congress Cataloging-in-Publication Data

Draus, Paul Joseph.
Consumed in the city : observing tuberculosis at century's end / Paul Draus.
    p. cm.
  Includes bibliographical references and index.
  ISBN 1-59213-248-0 (cloth: alk. paper) — ISBN 1-59213-249-9 (pbk : alk. paper)
    1. Tuberculosis—New York—Epidemiology   2. Tuberculosis—Illinois—Chicago—
    Epidemiology   3. Urban health—New York   4. Urban health—Illinois—Chicago.
  I. Title.

RA644.T7D738 2004
362.196′995′009747109049—dc22

                                                                        2003063402

2 4 6 8 9 7 5 3 1

Contents

Acknowledgments

MORE THAN a decade of my life was consumed in the process of producing this manuscript, from beginning to end, so naturally there are a few people to thank. At Loyola University of Chicago, Professors Anne Figert, Emily Ignacio, Peter Whalley, Judith Wittner, and Talmadge Wright all offered valuable criticism and advice concerning both the research and the writing process. At the hospital, Robert Cohen, Shirin Muzaffar, Debra Rudder, and William Traynor all supported my attempt to bring sociological insight to the practice of TB control, and I could not have completed the project otherwise. My coworkers and friends in New York and Chicago also deserve mention: Roberto Acevedo, Linda Agulefo, Caterina Barone, Peter Braithwaite, Rita Cameron, Larry Fleming, Michael Lewis, Nikos Mitropoulos, Charlie Monsanto, Relda Pious, Maria Retana, Delia Saucedo, Freddie Tolbert, Annie Williams, and others too numerous to name. At Temple University Press, Micah Kleit and Michael Parker believed in the manuscript from the beginning and guided me through the process of publication.

I owe my gratitude to all the patients, and their families, who let me into their homes and shared their lives and wisdom with me, and without whom this book would have been impossible. On the West Side, Jerome Cole, Cornelius Howard, Robert Ramseur, Timothy Robinson, Willie Williams, and many others served as my professors in the university of the streets. Special thanks are owed to Chris Caudill, who helped whip the text into shape. Eternal gratitude is owed to my mother, Geraldine Draus, who always inspired me with her model of unconditional care, and my father, Walter Draus, who always wondered when I was going to write a book. And finally, I must give credit to my wife and companion in life, Carla Gonzalez: your radiant smile provided endless inspiration, and your strong shoulders offered unflinching support.

I apologize for leaving anyone out, and for the possible failings of the work itself. And to Solomon, happy birthday.

Prologue

A Day in the Life, Chicago, 1998

THE FIRST question to answer: What am I doing here?

It is the last day of September, two years before the end of the twentieth century. I am sitting on a milk crate cushioned by a dirty old jacket, under a tree in an empty lot at the corner of First Street and Jefferson Avenue on the West Side of Chicago (these are disguised names, so don't try to find them). I have been stopping by here every morning lately, usually between 8 and 8:30. This morning there are four guys out here, not including myself and Hank, who sits in his old red Chevy a few yards away, sipping wine from a plastic cup and listening to dusties on the radio. Lewie, KJ, Montgomery, and a guy named Fred whom I have never met before, are sitting in a circle on plastic barrels and milk crates, splitting a bottle of malt liquor in a paper bag between them. Lewie gives up his seat for me and shows me a car stereo that he is trying to sell; it is an AC Delco with auto reverse cassette, a big blocky thing that wouldn't even fit in my Toyota's dashboard. They say they found it stashed somewhere and ask if I want to buy it. I find it interesting, would actually like to have a big fat car stereo like that, but I have no place for it, and besides, I have no money on me. "Sorry," I say, though I am not really sorry.

Later a guy with a shaved head and a gold bracelet walks up and shakes my hand; he looks familiar, but I wait a moment and he reminds me who he is: "I'm Duck," he says, "we met over by Billy."

Yes, Billy. Billy is an acquaintance of mine, and a true neighborhood character. We were just discussing him, as a matter of fact, perched on the barrels and crates, before Duck walked up. I told them that Billy was in a nursing home in Joliet, some fifty miles south of the city, where I stopped to see him last Friday and brought him some hot sauce as a belated birthday present. The guys on the corner had been wondering where he's been ever since the hot August day when the ambulance took him away. He had a seizure in the parking lot across Jefferson Street. "How is he doing?" they want to know, and I tell them he can walk, but not very well, he tends to run into walls, so he uses a wheelchair which he pulls along with his feet.

"He scoots himself around, huh?" asks Lewie, imagining the sight.

I tell them that Billy wanted me to drive him back up to Chicago but I refused. He wanted me to drop him off in the neighborhood. "You did the right thing not to bring him back," says Lewie, "let him stay there for awhile. There ain't nothing out here no-way. He'd be back on the corner drinkin' by the end of the day. Fallin' asleep. Pretty soon it'll be fittin' to get cold anyway. Let him stay in there until the winter breaks." Montgomery chimes in, "You tell him that Monty says he should stay there."

They all agree, as they sip their beer, that Billy is better off where he's at.

Fred says that if Billy had a good woman he might be all right. I ask, "Didn't he used to have a woman?" Fred laughs, saying, "maybe, a long time ago. Women and men tend to go their separate ways after awhile. You see women around here, pushing they babies in they strollers, ain't no man around, and the men, they be sittin' around, drinkin' wine." He pauses. "It's kind of fucked up, really."

Then he says that people around here are too poor to afford blood tests—unlike the suburbs, where anybody can get one—so a guy might never know if a baby is actually his. If a woman likes him, says Fred, she'll tell him that the child is his, and she might have been pregnant two months before she met him. The kid'll be born, it'll be his, for all he knows, then a couple years later, she'll tell him it ain't his, when she wants to get rid of him.

A guy pulls up in his pickup truck, they wave to him, and a few minutes later he drives off. A crowd of pigeons descends and feeds on the seed he has left behind. "Does he come out here every morning?" I ask.

"Yep," says Fred.

"You know what Billy said to me once?" I ask Sam, and then I continue: "He said, 'We feed our pigeons on the West Side of Chicago.' He said, 'This ain't no residential area: this is a neighborhood.'"

Sam laughs, and says, "That's Billy."

KJ, Monty, and Lewie take some smoke bombs (which they also tried to sell to me) and go to the other side of Hank's car and light them off, watching like kids as they emit feeble streams of blue and yellow smoke. When the guys come back, I ask them, "So, how long have you guys been in this neighborhood?"

"Shoot," says Lewie, "I've been in this neighborhood for like thirty-four years." Monty says he's been there forty. Lewie says that KJ has been there since 1949, but KJ denies it.

"You guys remember Lord Tiny?" I ask, and they say yes, but don't elaborate. Lord Tiny is somewhat of a legend around there, a long-dead street gang leader, but I am curious about him. Most of what I know about him I heard from Billy.

Fred stretches and says, "Well, I better try and go make some money today."

I look at my watch: almost 8:30, time to get going. "Me too," I say, and wave at all the guys. Monty wants to know if he can get thirty cents. I told him I don't have anything, but I get in the car and look around and find two dimes. He comes over to the window even before I signal and says, "How about twenty cents?" and I say, "here, it's the best I can do." KJ says he will bring out a boom box tomorrow to sell to me for seven dollars.

Then I drive down the road toward my next stop.

Later that same day, I go to see Homer White on Ward 33 at County General Hospital. Yesterday he had two guys in his room playing cards while I was there. Today he is by himself. I ask if he won the card game, and he said they were just playing for fun. I asked where those guys came from. He said they were his brothers and they had come all the way from Michigan to see him. He said that his Momma raised her kids to stick together and stand by one another. He says when he sees kids today he can tell that they ain't been raised right; it all starts in the home, and that's the truth. Listening to him I hear echoes of other older men I have talked to, and I think how valuable these guys are, and how rare: the old-timers, with roots going back to the soil somewhere, with a solid sense of what's right and wrong, outside the brittle law of the convict code that prevails in the streets.

"If you have kids, you don't have no picks," he says. "You don't have no favorites."

"You love 'em all the same," I say.

"That's right," he says, "and if they fight, you say, 'don't fight.' Love one another. Stand by one another. Your people is all you got."

He tells me about his brother's ex-wife, who has several kids, some of whom are his blood nephews, some of whom aren't. When he goes down to Mississippi, he says, he treats them all as his nephews. And they all treat him as an uncle. If he needed a ride from the train station, they would be there, he says, in twenty or thirty minutes.

"Treat them with respect, and they'll treat you with respect," I say.

"That's right," he says. "Don't have no picks."

I shake his hand before I go. I say, "We'll talk again."

"Is this what your job is?" he asks.

"This is part of it," I say. "I'll tell you about it later, if you want to know."

But I had to ask myself: How do I explain what it is I do? Why *am* I here? Perhaps that is the best place to start. How was I to make sense of what I saw and heard?

I was led into the hospital and onto the street corner because I was following the trail of *mycobacterium tuberculosis*, the germ that causes the disease commonly known as TB. I met these men, and many other women and men, through my role as a public health worker attempting to control the spread of the disease. I started out doing public health in the ghetto and ended up doing sociology of the ghetto.

Some might argue that the last thing the ghetto needs is more sociology, and what it actually needs is more public health. I couldn't argue with this. Being a sociologist in the ghetto is sort of like being the anthropologist on an Indian reservation—every ghetto has one, and has nothing to show for it.

To answer the question, "Why sociology?" it is necessary to return to the street corners and hospital rooms themselves. That's where it all comes together.

Consumed in the City

Introduction

TB and Sociology

THE MAN was 54 years old, short and slight of build, a heavy smoker, and a habitual drinker. One day in early winter, while working in the detached garage outside his small home, he slipped and smashed his chest against the side of the car. When the pain in his chest did not go away, he went to the doctor. He was told that he had a tumor, that it was most likely cancer, and that he needed surgery. It was almost Christmas, so they told him to wait until after the holidays. The impending event hung over the family. The surgery was scheduled at a large private hospital in downtown Chicago, twenty miles from his working-class neighborhood, on the far South Side. The last time he was hospitalized was for an emergency appendectomy more than twenty years earlier.

Following the surgery, he was placed in a postoperative recovery room with another patient. Then, suddenly, he was moved to an isolation room. Nobody explained why. His son's fiancé was a nursing student and had rotations in another hospital on the North Side. She was the first to visit him after the room change. In her presence he cried, not knowing what was happening to him. He didn't understand why he had been shut away in a room by himself, or why people were walking in and out with masks on. He was confused, alienated, and afraid.

When they cut him open they found something in his lung, but it wasn't cancer after all. It was an old colony of disease which he had contracted when young, a disease that had killed many thousands, a disease which had once been considered incurable. It was tuberculosis, or TB, and for many it was a disease of the past, a disease of tenements and factories, of crowded ships and sweatshops. Like others who suffered from TB in the days before antibiotics, the man had recovered his health after a stay in a residential sanatorium. His immune system had contained the deadly bacteria, encasing them in thick scar tissue. But age and stress can weaken these internal defenses, and he now had "consumption" once again.

This was the reason why he had been suddenly switched from an open bed to an isolation room. It was a standard precaution in possible cases of infectious TB, one that is still followed to this day. Unfortunately, no one had bothered to explain. The large modern hospital, with its multitude of personnel and procedures, was overwhelming to this simple and mild-mannered man. If not for the familiar presence of the student nurse, who investigated and explained the situation to him, he might have remained in the dark, unsure of his own fate, scared and alone.

The year was 1962. The man was my grandfather. The young nursing student was my mother, and she related this story to me in the mid-1990s. At the time I was a health worker specializing in tuberculosis control, working for a large public hospital in downtown Chicago. I recount the tale here for several reasons, not only to show my own family's connection to the long and tragic history of this disease, but also to demonstrate that the issues discussed in the following pages are nothing new: the alienating experience of the hospital, the fear of a deadly diagnosis, the cultural distance between the neighborhood and the medical institution, the impact of poverty, addiction, and social class, and the persistent problem of compliance. I did not know my grandfather—he died when I was only four years old—but after many years of working with TB patients in the field, his story seemed familiar enough.

My own involvement with the disease began when I was in my twenties. In 1992, I was one of many individuals hired by the city of New York to aid in the struggle against a resurgent wave of urban tuberculosis. I was a field-worker, and my duties included interviewing patients with active, infectious TB, tracking "delinquent" tuberculosis patients, returning them to clinical care, and threatening "noncompliant" patients with involuntary detention, or quarantine. In late 1993, I accepted a job working with tuberculosis patients back in Chicago, the city where I was born. From November 1993 until July 2000, I went out every day to meet TB patients and to watch them swallow their pills, ensuring their successful treatment and thereby limiting the spread of the disease. After hearing that story from my mother, I wondered what it would have been like to attempt to do this job with my own grandfather. According to my mother, he was a nice man, but he was a lousy patient. He was the unschooled son of Polish immigrants, a steel worker for more than three decades, a shot-and-a-beer kind of guy. In later years, he was diagnosed with advanced emphysema, but still kept up his old ways, smoking and drinking with his buddies in the neighborhood. If not for the strong hand of my grandmother, who was also known to drag him out of corner taverns on occasion, he might have been "just another skid row bum." I had dealt with homeless, alcoholic Polish men in both New York and Chicago, and I knew how difficult and stubborn they could be. When I saw these guys on the street, I couldn't help but imagine that they were fathers, uncles, brothers, husbands, that they were also a part of a family and community, as my grandpa had been.

Seeing TB patients as members of families and communities was not always easy. As a public health worker, I was conditioned to see them in terms of their infectiousness, their treatment regimen, and their willingness to cooperate. I was not a doctor, but I was working out of a medically defined paradigm. In the standard medical interview, the practice of taking social history is an accessory to the doctor's main goal of isolating the condition or infectious agent, and treating it through direct intervention, either chemical or surgical (Waitzkin 1989, 231). Social context and personal biography are considered seriously only insofar as they affect the likelihood of successful medical treatment. Addressing social conditions takes a back seat to the more immediate task of isolating and eliminating the germ within the body. This is especially true when the practices of medicine and public health take place within institutional domains, such as offices, clinics, or hospital rooms.

However, when you leave these controlled settings and enter "the field," you can no longer ignore the other factors involved, because they stare you in the face wherever you go. You see babies sleeping on blankets on wooden floors, wearing nothing but soiled diapers, and playing with their siblings, cousins, and neighbors in fenced-in yards of dirt. You see boarded-up windows and gang graffiti layered like scabs and scars on once-resplendent houses and buildings. You see neighborhoods with no grocery stores or bookstores, but liquor stores and currency exchanges on nearly every corner. And, in my case, you can't help but notice that you are often the only white person there.

At the same time, you also notice that the vast majority of people treat you with the same respect that you treat them. You see that they are honestly trying to deal with their lives and get through each day in the best way they know how. But you also come to understand, through the evidence before your eyes, that the circumstances they face are worlds apart from those taken for granted by people who reside just miles, or even blocks, away. In another time, another place, another society, the person sitting before you, sick with TB, infected with HIV, addicted to drugs, saddled with a felony conviction and hard memories of years behind bars, the shadows of poverty, violence, and racial or ethnic exclusion following them wherever they go, could have been your brother, sister, father, or mother, and could one day still be your own child.

As a public health field-worker, employed first in New York City and subsequently in Chicago, I tracked the disease of tuberculosis across the urban terrain for more than seven years, treating it in the social soil where it grew. From this perspective, I saw that tuberculosis was only a small part of a larger problem for many individuals, and that medical treatment, while effectively curing the disease, often failed to address the conditions that actively undermined their health. Due to the duration of tuberculosis treatment, ranging from at least six months to as long as three years, field-workers charged with administering medications for tuberculosis enter into long-term relationships with TB patients. Lacking the expertise and the authority of physicians and nurses, these workers are nonetheless confronted with the personalities and daily physical troubles of patients in ways that many medical professionals are not. Within the more medicalized environment of the hospital or clinic, it is relatively easy to ignore or overpower patient concerns, and poor patients in particular may have few means for contesting the ways in which they are treated. Patients who are truly upset may simply leave the hospital or clinic (proving to some that they were not "really" sick to begin with), and patients who are acutely ill will stay because they have little choice. But the TB field-worker must adapt to the patient's environment, and this poses a different set of problems.

Success in the field was often a by-product of intangible negotiations, social relations that determined whether or not a person would be trusted, even if an institution was not. Accomplishing this required some degree of empathy, some willingness to see things from the point of view of the other person. To borrow a phrase from one of my supervisors at the Health Department in New York City, patience and persuasion were our only tools. Concerns of patients that might have seemed trivial from the standpoint of the hospital took on more weight when one entered the neighborhood or home where a person might be existing in extremely delicate circumstances: sleeping on a friend's couch, for example, worried about being kicked out on the street if the nature of the illness is known, or existing on a daily basis within a street environment dominated by illegal activities, where discretion and respect are fundamental values, and the threat of violence is a constant.

Seeing the disease within this socially embedded context was what finally led me into another field—that of sociology. I entered a doctoral program in 1994, while continuing to work the streets, treating tuberculosis. As a sociologist by night, analyzing my day job in public health, I traversed much theoretical terrain, ranging from the sociology of health and illness to the sociology of poverty and inequality, from urban sociology to the sociology of occupations. I discovered that the theoretical perspectives found in sociology were quite comparable to those employed by individual patients, health workers, and the media. Beyond this, sociology provided a means of addressing questions that were not even raised by a purely biomedical account of tuberculosis.

Biomedicine is commonly defined by sociologists as the reductionist analytical mode which views "health" as the absence of disease or pathology in the individual human body. Through its use of technology, modern medicine provides a means of identifying, isolating, and eliminating the sources of disease within the biological body, in the same way that a mechanic removes a faulty part or system from a malfunctioning machine. Specific illnesses or syndromes are caused by specific agents such as germs, viruses, or toxins and modern medicine spends much of its time and energy developing chemical or surgical weapons specifically designed to destroy or remove these agents. The diagnostic microscope of the medical eye tends to systematically cut away all but the specific targets of those weapons. In the process, human beings may be neglected, even when their own bodies are under the gun.[1]

The sociological critique of medicine usually takes one of two forms. The first might be called the *social forces* position, because it focuses on large-scale, structural factors, such as poverty, racism, economic depression, or environmental degradation, examining their impact on the health of whole communities rather than individuals. Some of the best examples of the social forces position relate directly to tuberculosis. Medical sociologists McKeown (1979) and McKinlay and McKinlay (1986) have demonstrated through historical studies that dramatic decreases in rates of tuberculosis in the United Kingdom and United States occurred prior to the development of effective medical treatment. They attributed these decreases to improvements in material well-being and public hygiene rather than improvements in medicine. The "heresy" thus advocated by medical sociologists like McKinlay strongly asserts that medicine as a professional practice actually has very little to do with the health of populations as a whole (McKinlay and McKinlay 10). Rather, the most important improvements have come as a result of social or political movements or environmental improvements which have addressed basic inequities in the distribution of resources and services.

The second critique, which I shall call the *illness experience* position, considers the subjective accounts of individuals who are coping with disease, disability or death, placing emphasis on the meanings of illness within specific contexts, and how these are mediated through interactions with institutions, communities, and others. Social histories of tuberculosis, such as those by Bates (1992) and Rothman (1994), examine the specific experiences of tuberculosis patients and their physicians in social and historical context, demonstrating how the patterns of both disease and treatment were shaped by the society in which they occurred. These works provide ample evidence that medical care never takes place in a vacuum, as much as it might aspire to do so. Many sociologists see the practice of medicine as containing an implicit ideology which, by focusing exclusively on individual symptoms, treatments, and behaviors, actively inhibits a more expansive social definition of health. Problems defined as "medical" are assumed to be properly addressed by medical means and medical expertise, which effectively removes them from contestation within the social domain. Occupational injuries, for example, may be treated medically as individual ailments, through physical therapies, behavioral interventions, surgery, or drugs. In the process, the cultural or class dimensions of these conditions may be obscured.[2] Like the social forces position, the illness experience position highlights dimensions of health and illness that fall outside the purview of standard medical practice, and lie instead in the realm of the social. This book is informed by both critiques, as I consider historical and economic forces, the intervening influences of hospitals, neighborhoods and public health agencies, and the accounts and experiences of individuals afflicted with tuberculosis in the urban United States in the 1990s.

After years of working in the field, I concluded that tuberculosis necessitates sociology in order to be understood. It cannot be separated from its social trappings. Like many other afflictions, TB primarily affects the poor. What makes TB different is the fact that it is infectious and airborne. In general, people do not worry that schizophrenia or alcoholism will be passed along to them on a subway train. But the fear of lower-class contagion in public places profoundly affected the response to resurgent TB in the 1990s. Such fears, informed by deep social divisions, were reflected in disease control practices at both the institutional and state level. As a disease that is only "a breath away," TB carries a fear component potentially greater than that of HIV/AIDS. This fear is easily transferable from the germ to those individuals (or classes) most commonly associated with it. In fact, as a high proportion of both TB and AIDS patients are from similar demographic groups, attitudes towards them have often been conflated. TB and AIDS, like other high-profile social problems associated with "the underclass"—homelessness, street crime, drug addiction—have in their time been both causes for public alarm and targets of public policy. Because TB cases are directly monitored by government agencies, the relationship between medicine and the state is also an important part of the picture. Seeing tuberculosis sociologically, therefore, requires not only a consideration of large social forces such as race, poverty, and inequality, but an analysis of the discourse and practices of institutions such as medicine and public health, which are empowered by the state.[3]

All of these forces play out dynamically within the contexts of actual human lives. To catch them in active interaction, I have used narrative and ethnographic methods. By focusing on the level of lived experience and seeking to capture relations in vivo, within a concrete chunk of geographic or experiential turf, ethnography provides an array of means for locating and illustrating the multiple overlapping linkages between individuals, the immediate social contexts that surround them, and the larger social landscape (Dyck 244). Though theoretically informed, this approach can sometimes yield results that complicate rather than confirm the expectations of social theory. In a 1980 interview, Robert Coles quoted Flannery O'Connor, who stated that "The task of the novelist is not to resolve mystery, but to deepen it!" Coles then went on to say: "The danger with social science, the danger with any kind of intellectual process, is that we take ourselves too seriously, and that we forget the difference between products of our own thinking and the world itself. We impose our own notion of reality on the world and see only our notion of reality rather than the defiant complexity of the world—and of course the mystery of the world" (Coles 66). As both a writer and a social scientist, like Coles, I wish to explain social reality and to describe complex human situations. I employ ethnography and narrative as tools to express, however imperfectly, the ways I related to and documented these human situations.

In a sense, the view of disease revealed by the tools of ethnography is both broader and more fragmentary than that provided by biomedicine. Seeing people as complex human beings, living within meaningful social worlds, grants us a greater appreciation of their creativity and individuality. Narrative accounts show people as nuanced and complicated individuals, both fascinating and frustrating in their idiosyncrasies. At the same time, narrative returns illness and suffering to its "natural" environment: embodied, social, and embedded in daily life. Through them we can see the specific ways in which social forces impact people. As Brody (1987), Kleinman (1988), Frank (1995), and others have extensively argued, stories constitute the stuff of which everyday life is made. They are not optional, but necessary components of human life (Frank 1998a, 330). Narrative can help to return to people some of their power and their agency, which may be marginalized by professional discourse. According to Foucault: "The chronicle of a man, the account of his life, his historiography, written as he lived his life formed part of the rituals of his power. The disciplinary methods reversed this relation, lowered the threshold of describable individuality and made of this description a means of control and a method of domination" (Foucault 1977, 191). The restoration of the human chronicle, then, can potentially counteract those very forces of domination that Foucault so meticulously describes in all his writings on power and knowledge.

For evidence of this, those working in the field of health and illness need only listen to patients themselves. Wherever they encounter the health system, people tend to use their own experience as a critical measure of the efficacy of medicine. As one TB patient said to me, "I live in this body twenty-four hours a day. I know everything that goes on here." He was using his own bodily awareness as both a counterweight to medical expertise and as a yardstick for its success. The social concept of "health"—as it is defined subjectively and contextually—therefore provides a means of criticizing "legitimate" or "official" medical knowledge (W. Wright 13). Sociology can be a vehicle for such protests, voiced by individuals in dialogue with institutions, professions, and other organs of organized expertise on a daily basis, to gain legitimacy of their own.

In *The Alchemy of Illness,* Kat Duff compares the experience of being ill to that of occupying some subterranean land—an underworld: "There is, perhaps rightly so, an invisible rope that separates the sick from the well, so that each is repelled by the other, like magnets reversed. The well venture forth to accomplish great deeds in the world, while the sick turn back onto themselves and commune with the dead; neither can face the other very comfortably, without intrusions of envy, resentment, fear or horror" (Duff 11). On the social level, poverty, especially when intertwined with race, has a similar alienating effect, on both the people who suffer from it and those who don't. The ghetto, in particular, has a relation to "mainstream" American culture which mirrors the underground world of illness. It turns inward, sharply conscious of its own exclusion, while those who venture into the ghetto from outside its unguarded but very real borders are always conscious of their intrusion.

Health and wealth are often accompanied by an unspoken arrogance. Those who have look down on those who don't, often without realizing it. We don't identify our own daily lives with the struggles of poor and sick people, we tend to morally judge them for their failure to conform to the norm. Such an uneven relationship can be unwittingly replicated by the research process. Prescriptions—both medical and social—are usually made from the high ground of relative health and wealth, from which position it is quite easy to believe that one possesses the right answers. "After all," the logic goes, "this problem that we are studying is not a problem for *us*. It is a problem for *them*." In the same sense that the opinions of the poor and the sick regarding their own condition are relegated to a category of "subjective" knowledge, so does the *stigmatization of subjectivity itself* contribute to the continued subjection of the poor and the sick. In a study such as this, which deals primarily with the stories of poor, sick people, it is doubly important that the actual words of subjects share space with those of the author.

In addition to providing a context for suffering, narrative is a mode of conveying sociological information which allows the sick, the poor, and the otherwise excluded to determine at least some of the terms by which they will be known. This is in direct contrast to the usual modes of biomedicine and positivist sociology, which routinely place individuals—or their words—within categories or typologies, as though an entire complex and contradictory existence could thus be collapsed into a ready receptacle. The same argument might be made concerning the academic or professional treatment of the colloquial spaces where many people spend their time. Again, this is especially true in poor urban communities, where physical decay of the built environment, economic devastation, cultural identity and spiritual despair go hand in hand, and where the stigmas placed on individuals, groups and places often become interchangeable. Such entangled processes of deterioration and adaptation, over time, have profound consequences for health.[4] This complex set of relationships comes together within the context of the local life-world as revealed in individual experiences and accounts of illness.

For this study I conducted more than twenty semiformal audiotaped interviews, ranging in length from forty minutes to three hours, and countless more informal interviews in all manner of locations and situations. My interviews dealt directly with the tuberculosis experience: how the disease was first diagnosed, what the symptoms were like, the experience of treatment, and so on. In the process of examining these issues, however, I also asked about the social circumstances that surrounded the emergence of the disease. Oftentimes, I would pursue these other threads. As I did so, I saw certain themes emerging repeatedly: the omnipresence of violence, the interaction with institutions and bureaucracies of various kinds, the influence, both positive and negative, of local social ties and networks, including the presence and absence of family, gender roles and sexual relations, and the all-pervasive influence of race, poverty, and economic struggle.

In my interviews, I sought to probe the connections between neighborhood social characteristics, and individual lives and fortunes. I paid close attention to references to violence, stories of family stability and disruption, daily dramas of microeconomics (jobs, hustling, welfare benefits, and so on), influence of local social relations, and regular interaction with local and state institutions and bureaucracies: police, hospitals, prisons, jails, welfare offices, schools, and so on. As a field-worker, I also observed these interactions first-hand, both in the institution and in the street, and I took extensive notes during more than seven years of fieldwork in the area of tuberculosis control. Some of these notes were written before I officially began my dissertation project, but remained relevant nonetheless. In the end, my shelves contained more than twelve hand-written journals, in addition to copious notes made on my home computer.

Organizing this amount and variety of data was a potentially daunting task. In the end, I used the disease as a guide and the role of the public health field-worker as a lens. I saw the data falling into discrete, yet organically linked, domains. As a TB control specialist, I learned the "facts" about the disease before I ever saw any patients. I met TB patients in the hospital initially, and then followed them into the community, where I saw the raw conditions of their lives revealed more clearly than I otherwise would have. This study follows the same path, from facts to experiences, from social theory to direct observation and back again. Important concepts are discussed as they arise, and tied to the general themes that persist throughout. The theme of observation runs throughout the book, linking the use of ethnographic method to the practice of Directly Observed Therapy, or DOT, which was central to the TB control efforts of the 1990s. In both ethnography and public health, observation is an activity that is charged with issues of social power. By placing an emphasis on the active role of the observer, I wish to highlight the crucial importance of vantage point as a component of interpretation: where we stand affects what we see and how we see it. This is true of doctors, patients, and sociologists.

In putting the book together, I was concerned with telling stories of individual humans and their thoughts and struggles, and of a more general predicament, faced by millions living within impoverished conditions. In the end, it is hoped that this study will achieve several ends. By taking the reader on a sort of sociological journey through the world of tuberculosis control in the United States in the 1990s, it may provide a view of an epidemic as seen from the ground floor, through the eyes of a public health worker engaged in daily interaction with the patients who suffered from it. In doing so, it offers insight into the sociological aspects of that epidemic, which was so powerfully shaped by prevalent conditions of political, social, and economic inequality. It demonstrates that there is an important role to be played by workers who traverse the borders between medical institutions and the communities where people live. Finally, this work argues that an ethnographic perspective, based on principles of respect and reflexivity, may inform and improve the methods currently employed by medicine, epidemiology, and public health.

I am not interested in disputing the benefits of modern medical technology, or the fine work of trained professionals who are engaged in both clinical and social struggles for health. Doctors and nurses, while identified here as part of a larger system, are not necessarily in control of it, any more than I was as a TB field-worker. They all labor within the same paradigm, just as plant managers and assembly line workers both serve the dictates of the market and the clock. Visionary physicians, from Rudolph

Virchow and Alice Hamilton, to Norman Bethune and Paul Farmer, like Hippocrates himself, have all sought to include the society as well as the individual in their diagnoses and prescriptions. No one can question the urgency of helping those individual human beings who are already sick, and seeking to relieve their most immediate afflictions. But if, after doing so, we fail to look up from the bottom of the cliff where the bodies pile up, we will continue to place Band-Aids on broken bones. This, I believe, is one of the lessons that TB has to teach: look up the cliff, follow the causal stream to its source, and question what brings people to the edge, where illness pulls them under. TB must be seen not only as a problem in and of itself, but as an index of graver social ills. Though we may treat the disease in isolation, we must recognize that it has its roots in soil we all share.

1 Bugs in the Big Apple

Chasing TB in NYC

I REMEMBER several works of popular culture distinctly influencing my decision to move from Laramie, Wyoming to New York City in the summer of 1992. First was the 1991 Terry Gilliam film *The Fisher King*, a surreal story about a radio disc jockey who is suddenly plunged from the heights to the depths of life in 1990s Manhattan, where the streets were haunted by living specters of AIDS, homelessness, and mental illness. That film captured the growing chasm between the privileged and the disenfranchised, even in an environment where they could reach out and touch each other at any moment. Mario van Peeble's *New Jack City* and Spike Lee's *Jungle Fever* also painted nightmarish portraits of 1990s New York. In these films, the devastating impact of crack cocaine on the inner city was depicted as a logical, if awful, consequence of the wholesale isolation and abandonment of communities afflicted by poverty. Such images might not make the big city seem inviting to most, but to me at age 24 they exerted a fascinating pull. If there was a gulf between races and classes I wanted to cross it. I remember repeatedly listening to U2's *Achtung Baby* album, and the lyrics to the song "Zoo Station," which said something about being ready to take it to the street.

After four years of college and two years of graduate school, I decided I was ready for a full immersion in urban reality. I had just completed a master's degree in American Studies, and now I wanted to study America up close. In New York, I thought, I could find the best and worst of everything. I hoped to find work in the Big Apple's social service sector, hopefully doing some sort of outreach with the homeless population. I had spent the previous summer working at a small homeless shelter in Santa Fe, New Mexico. After that I journeyed to San Diego, where I volunteered at a much larger shelter, and spent one night sleeping on the street with some homeless guys, whom I had met at a food line. These experiences were my sole preparation for doing social work in America's biggest city.

Before my departure from Laramie, my thesis advisor cautioned me about the "wicked cases of TB" that were going around New York at that time, and which had already received some attention in the major media. I promised not to catch any nasty bugs. Several months later, I sat on a bench in Battery Park, at the southern tip of the island of Manhattan, eating a bagel and staring over the spangled water at the Statue of Liberty. I had just urinated in a cup and presented the product to a nurse for drug testing. It was the last hurdle to clear before I started in my new position as a fieldworker in the Bureau of Tuberculosis Control.

As it happened, a series of articles was then running in the *New York Times*. It was called "Tuberculosis: A Killer Returns," and detailed the resurgence of TB in New York City. The first installment of the series announced: "Neglected for Years, TB Is Back with Strains That Are Deadlier." Another article, with the similar title "The Return of the Big Killer," appeared in the October 10, 1992 issue of *New Scientist*. It quoted Tom Frieden, then Director of New York's TB Control Bureau, concerning the resurgence of TB disease in New York: "This was a time bomb constructed by social and economic inequality and ignited by the HIV epidemic" (Phyllida Brown 31). In the same article, Frieden also declared that the number of health workers employed by the city would increase dramatically in the following months. According to these reliable sources, I was entering New York in the midst of a public health crisis. Despite my degree in an apparently unrelated field, my lack of health-care experience, and my shaggy, shoulder-length hair, I was headed to the front lines in the latest campaign against this deadly disease.

As dangerous and exciting as all of that might sound, the reality of my daily routine—like that of most soldiers, I suppose—was much more banal. My first weeks working as a New York City Public Health Advisor (PHA) were spent in three activities: learning the textbook facts of tuberculosis, "shadowing" more experienced PHA's, and sitting around a cramped office at our base hospital in lower Manhattan. The last activity was the dominant one—or at least it seemed so to me. We had textbook training downtown each morning, after which we were supposed to return to our field offices, where we spent the rest of the day studying the Core Curriculum on Tuberculosis, a series of instructional modules developed by the Centers for Disease Control (CDC). These covered every aspect of our work, from the diagnosis, treatment, and epidemiology of TB to the techniques of conducting patient interviews and field investigations. Before we ever saw any actual sick people, we learned the difference between tuberculosis infection and tuberculosis (one is symptomatic and contagious, the other is not), and we learned to categorize all of humanity into one of six classes, based on their TB status. These classes were:

Class 0: No tuberculosis exposure, not infected.
Class 1: Tuberculosis exposure, no evidence of infection.
Class 2: Tuberculosis infection, no disease.
Class 3: Tuberculosis: current disease.
Class 4: Tuberculosis: no current disease.
Class 5: Tuberculosis suspect.

The category of patient determined what the Health Department's role was in regulating and monitoring them. Class 3s had the highest priority and demanded the most attention. These were the public health risks, and our job was to ensure that they were converted from a harmful category to a harmless one through the supervised administration of medical therapy. Though one of our primary goals was that of *helping* patients with TB, our work was everywhere infused with the suspicion of transgression. Our job was to prevent it if we could, record it if we saw it, and to carry with us always the warning of potential punishment—the shadowy arm of the state, policing the irresponsibly ill.

Once in a while, we were allowed to accompany another PHA "into the field." This was what we waited for, because it meant escaping the confines of the office and actually seeing TB patients in the flesh. We did home visits in the community when it was necessary, and ventured into hospitals to see patients and review medical charts. As I made my way through the formal classroom training and worked my way into the field, it was these latter activities which came to predominate. There, in the medical records department (usually located in the basement of the hospital), we spent days turning the pages, piecing together the fragments into something resembling a cohesive narrative, describing a human life. I remember thinking to myself: behind all of this chicken scratch there breathed a real person. One man I watched, through the daily progress notes, creeping closer and closer to death: more and more medications were administered with fewer and fewer results, the drama of his demise obscured by the dry notation. The medical notations were full of arcane abbreviations: DNR—do not resuscitate, SOB—shortness of breath, IVDU—intravenous drug user, ETOH—alcohol abuser. Through the gauzy web of records we peered at the evidence of others' suffering, translated into medical code.

We learned how to pick out and record relevant symptoms, medications, and test results, as well as notes on social history, drug abuse, sexual habits, and so on. We were engaged in the practice of observing others, albeit indirectly, and of enmeshing them within yet another layer of documentation. The goal of this observation was the direct or indirect medical monitoring of every single case of tuberculosis diagnosed and treated within the political boundaries of the city. It was done through a variety of methods, most of them enacted by "foot soldiers" such as myself and reported back in writing to a central surveillance authority. In this manner the TB surveillance system aspired to be a sort of Panopticon. One of the central concepts in the work of French social theorist Michel Foucault, the Panopticon is defined by him as: "a generalizable model of functioning; a way of defining power relations in terms of the everyday life of men . . . It is polyvalent in its applications; it serves to reform prisoners, but also to treat patients, to instruct schoolchildren, to confine the insane, to supervise workers, to put beggars and idlers to work. . . . *Whenever one is dealing with a multiplicity of individuals on whom a task or a particular form of behavior must be imposed, the panoptic schema may be used*" (Foucault 1977, 205, emphasis added).

The first manifestation of a panoptic mentality, according to Foucault, was the plague-stricken town of the seventeenth century. In *Discipline and Punish,* Foucault recounts at length the process by which the population of such a town was segmented and systematically observed by town officials. This process, this system, is paradigmatic for Foucault: "The plague-stricken town, traversed throughout with hierarchy, surveillance, observation, writing: the town immobilized by the functioning of an extensive power that bears in a distinct way over all individual bodies—this is the utopia of the perfectly governed city" (Foucault 1977, 198). It is no coincidence, therefore, that the practice of urban infectious disease control would resemble, at some level, Foucault's description of Panopticism.

At the time of my public health training, I had not read Foucault, although I was learning his ideas all the same. In doing our chart reviews, for example, we were implicitly guided by the medical gaze, seeing people as systems and symptoms to be tested, rated, and recorded. In Foucault's words, "The examination leaves behind it a whole meticulous archive constituted in terms of bodies and days. The examination that places individuals in a field of surveillance also situates them in a network of writing; it engages them in a whole mass of documents that capture and fix them" (Foucault 1977, 189). The process usually begins when the physician is confronted by a suffering human being, seeking help for something that they can't address on their own. The doctor forms a diagnosis, a medical judgment, which is further legitimated by appropriate medical technology.[1] This new "fact" is then recorded on a piece of paper, in a chart, in computers, and so on. If that diagnosis is TB or another communicable disease, it may fall within the domain of the public health surveillance system. The agents of that system start not from the patient, but from the paper, the received knowledge, the diagnosis—which is the first thing they see and the first thing they know. At that time it is the *only* thing that is real to them. Yet the diagnosis itself may not tell you very much, as the following field notes illustrate:

11/14/92

I've been working for a month and a half and have yet met only two patients in person, one Marvin Jackson and one Manuel Hernandez. Marvin Jackson lay shivering and suffering like Christ in his bed, brown body bare except for a sheet covering his groin. He was coughing and had a hard time talking. Manuel Hernandez, on the other hand, was watching movies and looked like he was ready to go home. He's being held in respiratory isolation because he has MDR TB, and his sputum smear results are still slightly positive, despite months of therapy.

1/3/93

Diana Green had almost an air of elegance when we picked her up in front of her apartment on 11th Street on New Year's Eve. She is tall and byzantinely thin and was wearing a long coat and a beret type of winter hat. It wasn't until after she got in the car that the true cheapness of her clothing became apparent—the thin canvas tennis shoes, the scarf knit out of furry pink yarn. Under her coat she wore a plastic rosary and some olive drab pants and a sweatshirt, all of which somehow hung on her ethereal body. She talked to us with a deceptive familiarity, considering that she had only met me once (in the hospital) and hadn't met Isabel at all. She freely called us by our first names and described her problems with Medicaid, methadone, and the medications in an unremitting stream.

1/8/93

Today I met Emilio Moreno, a man with green hair who recently went crazy. His wife gave me a long list of friends with odd names, saying, "All these people are poor, they're all artists, they live on the Lower East Side." I assured her that there would be no cost for any TB medical care if she received it through the city clinics. She seemed reassured. She wasn't wearing any mask in the room, even though her husband was in respiratory isolation with infectious TB. She said she didn't want to alienate him in his last moments. She held his hands and he trembled, and when I left he actually said good-bye.

In these narrative snapshots, one can detect traces of human volition, as one might glimpse the movement of a deer in the woods. From the silent suffering of the man imprisoned in his bed, to the woman who refuses to comply with infection control recommendations, to the friendly cooperation exhibited by a patient toward people whom she has barely met, all these brief instances indicate the presence of real, individual people, and not simply cases or categories. In each case, we see a public health worker, empowered by the state, entering into the private world of another's suffering, and attempting to grapple with it, not as a medically trained professional armed with diagnostic knowledge and potent pharmaceuticals, but as an ambiguous intermediary. The popular image of medicine usually involves two basic parties: the sick, and the doctors and nurses who treat them. In actuality, in the modern medical system there are a range of other people involved in carrying out the "doctor's orders." As public health workers, we were situated between the individual patients and the large institutions of medicine and government, and were accountable to all of them. We were entrusted with the task of controlling a deadly disease, and we had been well trained in the basic facts of that particular affliction. But that did not necessarily prepare us for the complex array of people and situations that we would confront.

Around this time in my training, a doctor at a public methadone clinic told me, "I didn't go into the field of addiction control to become an infectious disease doctor." He said that twenty years earlier he would have seen three or four people die in a given year at a given clinic; now it was more like thirty or forty each year. He said that it was a different world now, and he got to spend the twilight of his career "watching young people die." On Emilio Moreno's ward the next day, I was struck by the thought that he might have died since I last saw him. His name plate was still up there next to his door, signaling that some life yet throbbed on inside. If he had indeed "expired," the name on the door would have changed. From my perspective, the difference between life and death was made manifest in such superficial details. The whole reality of the thing had not, at this time, hit me. TB still seemed to be a sort of phantom that stalked behind the walls and under the beds, pulling people down, leaving only their names and medical records floating on the surface like the flotsam of a ship. It all remained abstract somehow.

One day, after work, while sitting in a café in the East Village and reading *Moby Dick,* I saw a flyer tacked to the wall. It was a homemade missing poster, and the young man pictured on it was somebody I knew. I had met him only a couple times, through an old friend of mine. He was a very polite and friendly guy, about my age, who had moved to New York to begin an acting career. Then one day, after leaving a New Year's Eve party, he disappeared and was never seen again. As I sat there in that café, I was suddenly struck with both the inevitability and the unpredictability of death. A passage from *Moby Dick* expressed this beautifully, as the narrator Ishmael discusses the ropes that encircle the crew of a whale-boat: "All men live enveloped in whale-lines. All are born with halters around their necks; but it is only when caught in the swift, sudden turn of death that mortals realize the silent, subtle, everpresent perils of life. And if you be a philosopher, though seated in the whale-boat, you would not at heart feel one more whit of terror, than though seated before your evening fire with a poker, not a harpoon, by your side."[2] In a similar way, public health workers employed in the control of a fatal disease had to be aware of the dangers posed by hidden microbes, and the thin lines between health, disease, and death. It was only a mask or a shaft of sunlight or an open window that prevented bacteria from leaping from another's lungs into our own. Given the proximity of our work to these hazards—or perhaps because of that very proximity—we were also to some extent oblivious to their very real impact on our patients' lives. I remember asking my supervisor, when I first started, about the frequency of death among our TB patients. He just said, "Oh, yeah, a lot of our patients die." This was simply a fact, and did not in itself mean that we had failed. The Health Department's primary concern was with the TB, not the TB patient.

Later I learned that most of these deaths were not directly caused by TB. This explained the apparent nonchalance exhibited by public health workers when informed that a patient was, in fact, dead. My first assigned case illustrates this. I was given a file for Miguel Ochoa, which had several phone numbers on it. Calling these in succession, I was able to learn that the individual in question had recently been incarcerated. I then called the jail at Rikers Island and talked to an employee there, who told me that Miguel had "expired" while in jail and while receiving treatment. This seemed a very strange term to use. When I relayed it to my fellow health workers, they simply congratulated me on having tracked him down and told me I could close the case, since there could be no more sure end to the trail of TB than death in a jail that had decent infection control practices and clinical facilities. So, without ever meeting this guy, I could take credit for having tracked him down and "completed" him; thereby generating more proof that the system worked. A lot of tuberculosis surveillance was done in exactly this way, working the phones, nailing people down to a location or condition that could be verified and recorded, so that the criteria for treatment could be satisfied, and cases slid down the scale of urgency, from class 3 to class 4.

When Foucault speaks of the "petty machinations of discipline," he is referring to this kind of snooping, intrusive power (Foucault 1977, 170). I became more aware of this particular function of public health, in February of 1993, when I was given a new position. The Bureau was being reorganized and all PHA's were assigned to one of three units: the hospital-based Interview Unit, who saw patients in the hospitals and maintained relations with social workers and discharge planners; the office-based Patient Monitoring Unit, who were responsible for keeping track of all patients currently on TB therapy, and the field-based Return to Supervision (RTS) Unit, who would spend the majority of their time tracking down "delinquent" cases of TB and bringing them back "into the system" (which usually meant reconnecting them with some form of clinical care). I was named to this unit, the so-called TB "SWAT Team." As such I became an agent of both discipline and surveillance. I was not quite twenty-five years old, and assigned to police New York City for disease. Out of the forty-seven PHA's assigned to Lower Manhattan, there were only eight in the RTS unit. Meanwhile, there were 3,811 cases of TB diagnosed in New York in 1992, and 1,296 of these were in Manhattan, which also had the highest concentration of multi-drug-resistant (MDR) TB in the country. We were given use of city-owned vehicles to help us accomplish the task of finding and retrieving people. We were also assigned the responsibility of documenting noncompliance and delivering legal orders of quarantine or detention, signed by the Commissioner of Health.

To be considered officially cured of TB required a professional examination and judgment. A previously diagnosed person, with no evidence of active disease, with no symptoms or positive bacteriology, was nonetheless considered an *active case* until a physician declared otherwise. There are sound reasons, of course, for allowing this final authority to rest with a physician, but it also reveals how the authority of biomedicine extends itself through the public health system to scattered human bodies. As an agent of this discipline, I was made very aware of the close relationship between care and coercion, and what seemed a straightforward task was repeatedly complicated by both social and environmental forces and the vagaries of human will. In the case of TB control, the target population consisted of individuals who had to be physically located, then examined in the form of an interview and processed through the medical system if possible, then placed in a category: living, dead, TB, not TB, cured, compliant, noncompliant, or UTL—Unable to Locate. Until they were officially cured, and as long as they resided within the boundaries of the defined political body, their business was ours: where they lived, where they worked, what they did in their daily lives.

In *Moby Dick*, the narrator Ishmael declares, "No, when I go to sea, I go as a simple sailor, right before the mast, plumb down into the forecastle, aloft there to the royal mast-head." As a young field-worker in New York City, this statement struck a chord. I was out there, in the midst of the vast metropolis, just trying to do my part in the mission. Like the sailor on the whaling ship, or the soldier on the line, the field-worker has only a narrow set of skills and a small degree of power, while faced with forces much larger than him or herself. As whales lurk unseen in the sea, so did the disease lie below the visible surface, enfolded in the layers of a dense and sprawling city, then folded again into layers of fluid and skin. And the city, like the sea, exerted a power all its own. The following selections from my journals illustrate some of the circumstances that we faced:

3/30/93

I finally busted out and flew solo to the Bronx today. It was some housing project way up there off the Major Deegan Expressway, and I wasn't sure what to expect. Turns out it was harmless enough. But the guy wasn't there, the one I was looking for. It was his brother's place, and of course they hadn't seen him in over a month.

Next stop was back in Harlem, where I seem to be spending a lot of time these days. I found an older man on West 140th Street, in a main floor apartment at the rear of the building. It took him quite a while to get to the door; I was about ready to leave when these guys outside told me the old man could barely walk. So I went back and sure enough when I knocked again the lock started to turn. He opened up and let me in.

Now I know the definition of roach-infested. Bugs were crawling across the floor, the walls, and the furniture as I sat there and talked to this sloppy old guy in stained gray long-johns and dull dirty black jeans with silver jewelry looped around his scrawny wrists and fingers. His hair was pushed up straight from his forehead in a mini-Don King, more a result of untidiness than style. Half-eaten dishes of food rested on the coffee table, in the kitchen the sink was piled full.

The roaches were having a field day. And it was dark and there was the feeling that the air had not shifted position in ages. Surprisingly enough there was no stench, at least not that I could detect. He said he would go to the clinic if he had a ride. I told him he had a deal and beat it out of there.

On the street was a younger guy with a missing tooth and a baseball cap. When I approached the building he had ceased his conversation and stared at me, but he turned out to be helpful. I asked him if Mr. McDonald had anyone to help him out in his apartment and he said, "Yeah, he's all right." I said, "the place is a mess," and he said, "he won't let anyone in to clean it, he likes it like that."

I shrugged and said, "What can you do?"

The suspicion one earns just by being white in some places is still startling even after you get used to it. I haven't seen those kinds of slit-eyed tough guy looks since walking into the john at the wrong time in the wrong part of the building in high school.

4/1/93

I woke up to steadily falling rain turning the world to grey. It was quite a change from yesterday. I got up early to make it in to clinic in time to meet a patient. She didn't show. Later she told me she had overslept. "First thing Monday I'll make it Mr. Paul." Uh-huh.

Around noon I got a call for "Dr. Paul." They had my man down at the methadone clinic. When I arrived he was sitting on his plastic window-washing bucket still waiting to be medicated. Apparently they wouldn't let him get his stuff until I got there. I don't think he was too pleased about that, but it was hard to tell.

This was the guy I spent most of the afternoon with, though we hardly exchanged half a dozen sentences. After we got in the car he said, "Can I ask you where you're taking me?" I told him and he said okay, but as far as I knew he hadn't been there before. I went through the trouble of getting him a clinic card which we then brought to the billing window but it turned out he already had one, bent and battered in his billfold. That was the closest I saw him come to cracking a smile. He showed the few teeth he had left (clinging to his gums like tree trunks on a wind swept plain, twisted and brown). I said, "Why didn't you tell me you already had one?"

"I forgot," he replied.

Shortage of teeth didn't prevent him from diving into the pizza slice I bought him, though. When I dropped him off at the subway he said, "thanks for everything."

4/3/93

... I've been spending my afternoons driving around Harlem. I almost found this guy named Grover who hangs around in front of Lenox Liquors. When I got there he had just left and this West Indian guy named Francis walked me up and down the street trying to find him. "He was just here, sitting on the stoop." But he was nowhere to be seen when I arrived. These guys must have a talent, a certain sense of how to avoid what's good for them.

Each day I'm thankful when I roll into the garage safe.

4/6/93

A woman walked up to me on the corner of 127th Street and Malcolm X Boulevard. "Are you new around here?" she asked. "Yes . . . no . . . not exactly," I replied, "I'm looking for somebody."

"Maybe you're looking for me," she said. She was a clean-cut looking black woman who was holding a potato chip bag that was smoothed out so flat it looked like a Jehovah's Witness pamphlet.

"No, I'm looking for a guy named Grover. A tall, older man with a cane." Actually, he's only forty-three, but I was betting he looked wise beyond his years. She said she didn't know him but would check around, and less than five minutes later as I was getting in the car, I saw her coming running up the sidewalk, saying "Mister . . . Mister, I found him." And sure enough, along came Grover, wearing a jacket with a name patch that read "Ralph" and a sweatshirt hood pulled tight over his head. He walked slowly and unsteadily. His gaze was weak with liquor and he was decked out in dirty faded shades of gray and blue. But he turned out to be a gentleman.

We sat in the car to discuss his health. The woman came up to the door and asked if I'd buy her lunch. I said no and she went away. Grover said he never finished his TB treatment. I asked him if he'd be willing to go to the doctor. He said "let's go now." So off we went to Washington Heights to see if I could squeeze him in the clinic. Along the way he talked about the cat he used to love because it killed his rats and greeted him when he came home and how he was locked out of his room one day and there was a sign posted on it that said NO SQUATTERS. After living there ten years, he said. I circled down Riverside Drive and he said how he liked to be near water—"you just look across and there's New Jersey." We pulled up outside and went up the stairs but Grover didn't make it to the john in time and left a trail of pee on the floor of the clinic. He felt so bad he insisted on mopping it up and wouldn't get back in the car while he was still wet. It turned out that it wasn't necessary—I took him to the ER and waited until he [was admitted]. He had his hood down by the time I left; his hair was wispy and wild and I think he was a little bit sober. He didn't want to just be abandoned but when I took off he said, "Thanks for your time, Paul." Grover was a man with true Southern manners it seemed. He came from South Carolina, he said, and grew up pickin' cotton and sloppin' mules. Now living in hallways and roaming all day, every day, up and down a three block area in central Harlem, drinking himself closer and closer to death.

Tonight my dreams were full of Grover it seemed. When I left he was changing his blood-soaked mask for a fresh one. The last thing I saw when I woke from my after work nap was a white wall as in a hospital spattered with someone's blood. Somehow I knew it was Grover.

4/7/93

. . . Today my supervisors sat me down and asked me how I'm managing to bring all these people in. "It's unreal," said Carmela. What could I do but thank them? Today Tina showed up; her chest hurt, she said, and she looked like hell. She was there at the clinic all day almost, getting X-rays, giving up sputum, the whole rigamarole. But she got free lunch and coffee and carfare and I think she liked that. Hell, maybe she even made some new friends.

It was sunny and sixty degrees, a beautiful day to be tooling around the city, listening to cool jazz with the window down, like a cat straight out of Mickey Spillane.

4/10/93

. . . Spanner and I brought Silas McDonald into Bellevue from his roach-infested, ground-floor apartment on West 140th Street. All week leading up to this I was joking about this dirty, filthy, ornery old man, but it turns out he's probably just another one beaten down by being alone. I think he was genuinely happy to get out of the house and I think he enjoyed riding with me and Spanner. He didn't whine or plead about his situation but he simply and with dignity submitted himself to our unprofessional aid. The cockroaches must have sensed that we were all right because they let us leave safely.

4/13/93

Gliding into Chinatown like a lazy ray of sun
looping like a stone flung low over the East River

falling like a ball into backyards of tenements hung with wash
like a hundred years past, ancient clocks, faces unchanged
through the arch into the swarming hive of Manhattan
spring stands unchallenged now
life leaps up on the sidewalk like grass through the cracks
color is back and swings in cool dances—
tinkling jazz is my music of choice as I cruise quiet and low
along the jumping boulevards of old Harlem
ghost rider in a kaleidoscopic kingdom
hood up head down eyes open

I went and saw Grover today, back in the streets. He was sitting on the stoop soaking up the sun on the corner of 127th and Lenox, where I knew he would be. I approached him and his glazed eyes settled on me with shielded recognition and when I took a seat beside him he just drawled "Hi Paul," as though he were expecting me. He wanted to play basketball with some kids across the street, but they wouldn't pass him the ball and an old woman with glasses and grey dreads told him to leave them alone.

"I don't want them playing with big people," she said, "I want them to learn respect."

He thanked her and she thanked him. Grover is a gentle and perceptive soul. He said he'll be on those streets until he's a hundred and forty. Enjoying the day. I told him on Thursday I'd bring him a doggy bag from Sylvia's and he laughed and told me my car needed a washing, which it does. It's bleached with dirt and dappled with bird shit and Spanner scrawled "Wash me" and "Screw you" on the passenger side panel. I can't bring myself to drop five bucks on a wash job that I'd rather do myself for free. But one of these days I will.

4/15/93

I sit next to Grover in the scooped plastic chairs at the clinic, listening to him drawl on slow about his childhood in Greenville, South Carolina. He used to play tight end and busted Jesse Jackson's head a few times on the football field. I quietly endure the few whiffs I get of his sweet, rotting wine-breath, hoping that it's not hopping with bugs. Grover is finally called in after sitting two hours or so and a few minutes later the doctor calls me after him. I said I'm deeply concerned that he could relapse and so I wanted a second opinion from someone who knows TB. According to the printout, Grover's treatment was bare minimum if it was adequate at all, and his X-ray remains abnormal. Grover agrees to return to the clinic tomorrow morning. As I leave him alone with the doctor again, the ripple in my spine tells me I'm doing something right, at least by the measure of my heart. This clinic gives me a better feeling than that medical condo by the Hudson.

I'll drop him back on the corner he calls home. This morning when I got him up there a man in a rainbow hat walked by, touched all our fists to his and said, "one love, brother," like a benediction.

4/17/93

I went to pick up Grover yesterday at 8:30 A.M. I didn't find him in the usual place so I walked up and down the blocks between 128 and 125 to see if I could spot him. I caught sight of him, finally, making his way up the west side of Malcolm X Boulevard, past the empty tables where the African merchants were just beginning to set up their wares. I came up behind him and he said, "Hi Paul, I was just coming back from the park." He spent the night there, sleeping beneath the trees.

And so began another day with Grover, shuckin' and jivin', as he said. From Bellevue we went to Chelsea, where we picked up Spanner, and then headed up to Harlem again. Spanner and I ate at Sylvia's and brought Grover a doggy bag just as I had joked about. He asked us if we would have enough money or if we wanted him to write us a check. I told him I would let him know on Monday what the results of his tests were, all around.

. . . After that, more home visits, and I almost found another one, this guy named Elmo. I found his sister, Lucy, and I asked if he stayed with her and she said "sometimes—he comes over when he wants to eat." I've been after this guy for about a month and was about to write him off as UTL (Unable to Locate).

4/20/93

Today Grover spotted me first. I was about to stroll down Lenox to 125th Street when I heard him calling my name from the west side of the street. I saw him down the last of his bottle and drop it in the trash before hobbling into the traffic like a cripple crossing a river. His right pant leg was cut off at the knee and his sock and tennis shoe were soaked with day-old blood. Apparently someone had tagged him in the shin with a bottle; he asked me if the police had called me. I said no, but then again I was out in the field all afternoon. He showed me the antibiotic the doc at Harlem Hospital gave him before sending him back to the street. Someone called another ambulance and we sent him back. This time I told the ambulance drivers that he was an old TB case who could relapse. I thought maybe that would help get him in but when I called around 4 P.M. he was still waiting. Bet your bottom blood-soaked sock he's back on the street this time tomorrow, sucking 'em down and limping closer to death. At least I can bring him some new clothes, maybe.

4/22/93

Today I was in the Bronx and I found this guy Elmo living on the top floor landing of a six-story apartment building. I'd been looking for him for six weeks and so, on the verge of seeing the face that matched the name, and thereby solving the mystery, my anticipation increased with each succeeding flight I mounted. And the higher I went the more light there was, because as it turned out the stairwell was capped by a massive domed skylight of white glass and iron. And in the middle of this sea of light where the stairs ended there floated a little form on a mattress like a raft, surrounded by the flotsam of a rag-tag shattered life—bottles, shoes, bags.

When I called his name he pulled down the blanket that covered him from head to toe and showed his shiny brown skull. And I felt like I had just found Christ or the Buddha (I was a little short of breath, partly from fatigue from climbing the stairs, partly from nerves) lying there like a mummy bathed in white light atop an apartment building in the Bronx. And he's been up there the whole time, wearing a plastic rosary and cursing Uncle Sam.

4/24/93

Grover put his arm around Victor and I, hugged us close and pronounced us blessed in the name of our Lord Jesus. We brought him two pairs of pants, handed down from Carmela's son. I told him we had to go but he limped in front of the car and came over to the driver's side window. He asked me if he'd done the right thing by leaving the emergency room without being seen. I said, "I don't know, you did what you wanted to do, right?" He said, "Yes, but what do *you* think I need to do?" I said, "You need to get off the street before you end up . . ."

I was going to say "dead," but he cut me off: "Don't say it, if you say it I'll put this cane around your neck and rip your head right off."

"All right, Grover, you wanted to know what I thought. It's up to you."

As he walked away like a cardboard cut-out receding from a flat field of vision I turned on the radio and the sad sound of a saxophone curled up and followed his back as it moved out of sight and became one with the dirty gray sky.

4/27/93

This day it was my sworn duty to bring Elmo in alive to the city chest clinic. I risked my life on the Cross Bronx Expressway, swerving in and out of the path of a careening white van while trying to merge with the traffic. I had to brake to a halt to avoid an accident. Spanner, who I forced to come with me in case Elmo couldn't walk, curled up in the passenger seat with his head in his hands to avoid sight of the impact which luckily didn't occur. All of which only made me more flustered; my nerves jangly as loose guitar strings as I circled about the Bronx looking for Elmo's building.

[After picking up Elmo] While we were waiting to get on the FDR at 125th Street, a black man in a wheelchair rolled by, collecting donations for his own personal relief fund. In the back seat Elmo growled, "This guy's a con man. He can walk as good as I can." Later on the way home he let me in on little bits of his life. To wit: his finger was cut off by the fan blade of an automobile; Lincoln Hospital is a slaughterhouse, you should go up there if you want to die fast; he can't live with his sister anymore because the landlady used to be his girlfriend and she can't stand him anymore. I asked "Did you break her heart?" He answered, "I don't know. I should have broken her neck."

Thursday I'm bringing him back in, which means he'll be sharing a car with Grover. This promises to be an afternoon to remember. These two are a match made in heaven; two South Carolina boys sleeping in hallways in NYC.

4/28/93

Yesterday I rode with Elmo and Grover down to Bellevue, a winding odyssey from the Bronx through Harlem down the island and back up again. Grover as usual generated his share of laughs. As we were riding the elevator up to the clinic he remarked to a man holding a pizza in a box, "I wish this elevator would get stuck so we could all have a slice." Everybody laughed except the guy with the pizza and the woman with the headphones who couldn't wait for the door to open.

Today I was supposed to take a very prominent physician out for a ride with me to shovel a 6'4" drunk off the sidewalk in the Bowery but the guy canceled out without telling anyone. I went back to the Bowery to apologize and they were loading the bum in an ambulance. He was drunk as shit with shit in his pants and all over his face and pale blue eyes peering out like a beaten child. Bets are on that he'll be back on that sidewalk come Monday.

My back hurts from all those hours in the car. That's it. Next week I slow down.

Looking back at these entries almost ten years later, I couldn't help but see them as a preview of my life in the 1990s, and Grover and Elmo were the spitting images of the lost, ornery, incorrigible, and admirable souls I was to encounter, endure, and learn from. Beyond that, the sociologist in me couldn't help but notice that there was a familiar background to their personal dramas: the histories of marginal employment in low-skilled or manual jobs, the estranged yet faithful families, the stubborn addiction and excruciating self-knowledge, the everpresent dangers and the simple, reliable pleasures of life on the streets, all set against the bleak backdrop of poverty, evidenced in roaches, evictions, homelessness, and tuberculosis. (And I was to become no stranger to automobile-induced backaches either.)

The last excerpt above deals with a particular case in New York that deserves further discussion. He was an alcoholic white man who had carried a TB diagnosis for years. He sometimes lived in a flophouse on the Bowery, and sometimes slept on the street. He came and went from local hospitals with frustrating regularity. In the early days of May, 1993, Spanner and I were sent to once again find him and convince him to return for his necessary therapy. We found him all right—he wasn't usually hard to find—but we were not able to convince him of the necessity of more medications. This guy had been defined as a long-term noncompliant patient, and he had already been targeted for involuntary detention. This required that a case be built against him, and for this to happen we had to demonstrate that we had made every effort to offer him an alternative to medical imprisonment and document each contact. So we tried to talk to him about the importance of following the doctor's orders, and so on, but we had no visible effect. Those blue eyes seemed to stare right through us; his brain was wrapped around a bottle. "Look," he said, after we made our pitch about the importance of protecting his health, "I wasn't born yesterday. I've seen guys through the years who have passed away, and right now I want to get a bottle."

"Yeah, and that's your right," I said. What else could I do? After spending an hour that day trying to talk this guy into staying in the hospital, for his own health, I was exhausted. On the street corner, in the Bowery, in the warm spring sun, he treated us like ghosts momentarily interfering in his reality. Those eyes flickered over us and never settled, and we stood there as though on the other side of a screen. I tried to joke with him, saying that one day, after his TB was treated, he could write a book about all his experiences. He responded to this. "I ain't writing no fucking book!" he snapped. The anger with which he pronounced those words, it occurred to me, might indicate that I had somehow struck a chord. He wasn't writing any book. Perhaps he was simply saying that it made no difference, that he could kill himself slowly if he desired, and maybe that was in fact his desire. He wanted to die. The human yearning to choose one's own course in life had taken that turn. That we couldn't take away, at least not yet.

We said to him, "You're going to end up locked up without any drinks, without any checks waiting at the welfare hotel, without anything but TB meds and meals for six months or as long as it takes to cure you." That didn't faze him, either. He had the bottle in his hand already at this point. He drifted back to the sunny corner of Bowery and Grand, paying no more attention to us at all, like a balloon rising out of our reach.

"Should we try again?" asked Spanner, as we watched him cross the street. "No," I said, "What are we going to do?" We had no real power over him, and to tell the truth, I was just plain tired of the guy. He wasn't going to give anybody TB while coughing on the sidewalk, I thought. The sunlight would kill all the bugs, and who would go near him anyway? His fish-eyed friend sitting on the sidewalk babbled occasional semicoherent phrases. Once he said to us, "You're in the right," which he followed with, "You got guts." He held up his fingers in the sign of peace.

To anyone watching the situation unfold on that sidewalk in the Bowery, it must have appeared ridiculous. This encounter could not constitute an ideal example of either discipline or resistance. I didn't feel like a very effective disciplinarian, and his resistance was short on dignity. The pettiness exhibited by each side, with his thirst for booze and my fatigue and frustration reducing each of us to anger and retreat, belied the struggle over power that was taking place. But that is the form that resistance took in this instance. He was indeed a body in need of discipline, from the standpoint of the medical and public health institutions, as the interest of the above-mentioned physician would suggest. In the end, however, it must be stated that this man's will won out, in a small way, over the forces aligned against him. The city eventually tried to detain him in the facility which had recently been constructed for that very purpose. Detention, once called quarantine, was a legalistic solution to the problem of long-term noncompliance with appropriate TB therapy, with strong overtones of law-and-order politics: discipline made naked and overt. I will not go into the details here, but suffice it to say that this Bowery-dwelling man managed to beat the rap. In spite of his addiction, he was able to prove the health department's tuberculosis diagnosis faulty, and thus escaped the consequences of his medical defiance. He was the first one to do so since the brand-new detention facility had opened. Perhaps Foucault would have been proud.[3]

BEFORE LEAVING New York City in the fall of 1993, I had moved from tracking patients in the field with the RTS unit to the Regulatory Affairs unit, housed in the TB Bureau's central office in Lower Manhattan. There I assembled case histories and wrote orders of compliance and detention, which were reviewed by legal counsel and signed by the physician who directed the Bureau as well as the Commissioner of Health.[4] These orders varied in their power; the compliance orders essentially told people that they had to cooperate with a program of supervised medical therapy, take all their medications, attend clinic visits, and so on. Though technically they were legal orders, these were basically unenforceable; their main purpose was that of either intimidating people into following medical orders or building a foundation for later detaining them against their will. In order to do the latter, the Bureau had to be able to demonstrate that it had diligently pursued every other alternative to detention, and that the person in question was persistently noncompliant: unwilling or unable to complete a course of therapy required for them to be cured of tuberculosis. Once detained, patients had a right to appeal and could be granted a legal hearing, where they would be provided with representation and given the chance to plead their case. As mentioned above, the Bowery alcoholic who gave Spanner and I so much trouble managed to avoid prolonged detention because he requested such a hearing and the Bureau's case against him was found wanting. But in many other cases, patients either did not request hearings or were granted hearings but failed to disprove the claims of the Bureau.

The very first person detained in New York City under the revised health code was also a man whom I had attempted to round up and return to supervision while I was still working in the street. My documentation of his refusal to comply with recommended therapy, in fact, was used in building the case against him, and I was actually called as a witness in his hearing. Because he had multi-drug-resistant TB, he had to sit in a plastic tent during the entire procedure, and by the second day, when I made my brief statement, he had refused to subject himself to that experience again. The hearing went on without him. I spoke my piece to a couple of lawyers, a judge, and an empty tent.

His case was a very sad one; he had worked as a nurse at a New York hospital before contracting his TB. Coinfected with HIV, he found that the extreme side effects produced by his prescribed TB meds seemed to make him sicker than the disease itself. In fact, they made him so nauseated that he was unable to eat, and so he stopped taking almost all of them. In medical terms, of course, it was unacceptable to take only a couple of pills a day when he was supposed to take more than ten, even though he claimed to be staying in his apartment and limiting his contact with all people except his roommate. Thus the needs of his body, as defined by him, were brought into direct conflict with the needs of the public as defined by the Bureau of Tuberculosis Control. He was detained, and asked for a hearing. He lost his case, so he remained a legal prisoner, though not a criminal. He stayed in the detention facility, a rehabbed hospital wing located on Roosevelt Island, until he died. My friend Spanner, who by then had been assigned to work full-time at the detention facility, told me that this man was a favorite patient there, and that the staff was heartbroken when he finally passed away. Though I pursued my tasks with all due diligence, experiences such as these made me doubtful about the prospects of either a purely medical or legalistic solution to tuberculosis. No matter what technology, chemical, or law would be developed, no matter how well-oiled the machine, it seemed that some people would always be caught between the gears.

Five years later, I stood in the Medical Records Department of County General Hospital in Chicago (also located in the basement), requesting charts to review. I was now an Epidemiologist in the hospital's tuberculosis control program, and needed to see what background and contact information I could glean from the official record. As I waited for my charts to arrive, I looked at the piles of papers behind the counter, all the people walking in and out of the small office, the obvious systemic imperfections popping like loose threads at every seam. I reflected that this Panopticon, like that in New York, was perpetually out of focus. When I actually received the charts that I requested, this hunch was supported by written evidence. The medical surveillance that could be garnered from this flimsy web of barely legible writing captured only fragments of persons, as though plucked out of a stream. One day a guy was in one clinic, one day he was in another, and it was as though the doctors in each place were just scribbling the same exact stuff, with little or no coordination between them. The only consistency was that generated by the patients' persistent physical troubles.

This system, faulty as it was, nonetheless lent support to Foucault's principles. Not so much because the patients were under constant scrutiny or "discursive domination," but because they were reduced by systems of knowledge and language to objects of scrutiny, subject to the power of the professional gaze. I had the power to review charts because of my position within a medical institution. I could draw information from them, make judgments about people, categorize them, and actually exert influence over their lives. In a sense, as Foucault well realized, we are all subject to this type of scrutiny, to this snooping, intrusive power: be it medical, legal, educational, professional, or correctional. We are all numbers, charts, records, resumes. The more we contest these categories, the tighter they seem to hold us, because we have lost the ability to define our roles in life without them. The ultimate Panopticon, as Foucault insisted, is that which is internalized, and takes on its own life inside our minds. Educated, professional people, granted status by institutions, are as subject to "discursive domination" as those over whom they hold power, because their very existence, their purpose, their importance, is constituted through words, documents, diplomas, and titles. However, because they usually perceive themselves as benefiting rather than suffering from the allocation of powers, it is relatively easy for them to ignore the system of domination in which they participate. The whale-lines are not visible, and death is a nightmare to be avoided.

Tuberculosis in urban America, on the other hand, often affects people who have no status that is not considered negative. Their position in institutions is normally one of subjugation, as "clients," "inmates," "residents," or "patients." Few of them own property or possess degrees. Many have no cars or telephones. They lead precarious lives, and death is an everyday danger. Their resistance to institutions, when it occurs, reveals the inability of the system to achieve its aims, to extend power over bodies in an absolute manner. This is inevitably demonstrated by the occasional patient, student, or prisoner who refuses to be confined, detained, or defined. The tuberculosis field-worker stands at the juncture of resistance and submission, charged with the task of either overcoming that resistance, or else interpreting it back to the physician or the public health authority, serving both as an advocate for the patient and as an agent of institutional control. The mixed role of enforcement and aid, which exists in most professions in one form or another, is clearly revealed in the daily work of disease control agents, precisely because they have so little power to either aid or to control. They rely on the cooperation and consent of the patients to do their jobs. From this perspective, the power of individuals to resist, to assert their own agency, is made manifest, and is certainly real. The cases of "problem patients" therefore merit some prolonged discussion. Regardless of their stature as individuals, their resistance is often compelling in itself, like that of Cool Hand Luke, or R. P. McMurphy in *One Flew Over the Cuckoo's Nest*. Before proceeding to these stories, however, it is necessary to provide some background on the history of tuberculosis disease and its treatment, to explain its "return" to urban America in the late twentieth century, and to explore the institutional and community settings commonly associated with its spread as well as its control.

2 Slow Motion Disaster
Postindustrial Poverty and the Return of TB

TUBERCULOSIS IN the 1990s was like a fire burning in the wrong part of town, a flood in Bangladesh, a famine in Sudan. It was something to be driven past, to be seen on TV or perhaps in a movie. For the average American, it was somewhat exotic because it was so segregated, so walled off from the mainstream middle-class majority. It was a Third World disease, and in the United States of the 1990s the Third World existed on the South and West Sides of Chicago, on the Lower East and Upper West Sides of New York, in the Bronx and Uptown, Brownsville and Englewood. In spite of trade and transportation systems shrinking the world, and the end of legal segregation brought about by the Civil Rights Movement, tuberculosis in 1990s America remained a disease of poor people, black people, immigrant people, the addicted, the overcrowded, the unemployed, and the underfed.[1] The patterns of tuberculosis affliction in the United States of the late twentieth century reflected the fragmentation of life experience across boundaries of class and race and the growing social inequalities in the postindustrial era.

"Postindustrial poverty," according to William DiFazio, is characterized by "nihilism with permanently declining occupational opportunities for the lower classes" (DiFazio 57). He argues that a "vocabulary shift" in the post-1960s period transformed "the language of possibility" and the "language of advocacy" into the "language of individual achievement" (DiFazio 42). Poor people, rather than being viewed as agents of change, or even helpless victims, were recast as defective objects in need of fixing, and whole categories of humanity were defined as "problems" to be managed and administered. By the time I started working in TB control, tuberculosis had become entangled with many of these categories. Just as "homeless" became synonymous with "bum" (in spite of the common sentiment that it can "happen to anybody") so did tuberculosis become identified with its so-called "risk factors." The category of "TB patient" and those of homeless, alcoholic, drug addicted, unemployed, and HIV positive became nearly interchangeable. Like homelessness and addiction, tuberculosis is most threatening when it is visible, and the drama of tuberculosis in the 1990s was all about visibility. The much-publicized "resurgence" of TB in the early nineties managed to break the surface of mass consciousness for a few media moments, and this media exposure definitely helped convince people that TB was a problem. The numerous articles produced in this time, however, bear some scrutiny, and some application of historical perspective.

In November 1992, a group of young public health workers, myself among them, were sent into the field to control the resurgence of tuberculosis that purportedly held New York City under siege. We had just completed three days of intensive training in contact investigation techniques, conducted by representatives from the Centers for Disease Control (CDC). Before letting us go, they told us: "You people are like the soldiers going into Somalia. This is a war, and you are on the front lines. Good luck." This was during the time of the United Nations' attempted intervention in that small African nation, a military-led mission which had ambiguous goals and mixed results. At the time, however, it was portrayed as a humanitarian endeavor with the noble purpose of saving innocent suffering people from malevolent forces. The statement above, comparing soldiers with public health workers, well illustrates a brand of rhetoric that posits disease as a sort of hostile entity, a "killer" that preys on humanity.

In this perspective, the medical and public health systems are envisioned as national defenses against a dangerous microbial invasion. In the case of tuberculosis, this can be particularly misleading, because the disease, although deadly and infectious, actually poses relatively little danger to most middle-class Americans. This is not to say that the threat of tuberculosis, to individual and public health, is not real. The disease was certainly alive and well in the inner city in the 1990s, and in spite of greatly improved control efforts, it has not gone away. I would like to argue, however, that the "war in Somalia" metaphor of modern tuberculosis control, while attempting to serve a greater good, also helps to perpetuate myths and to obscure some of the most basic facts about the illness—most significantly, its intimate connection to persistent poverty and social inequality.

At the same time, however, this particular metaphor reveals something which it did *not* necessarily intend. TB is, in fact, a disease that threatens impoverished places like Somalia, the Philippines, and India, places which rank alongside Harlem, the Bronx, and Chicago's South and West Sides in terms of their morbidity and mortality statistics. It affects people in these places much more than those who live in small towns, insulated suburbs, or upscale neighborhoods such as the Upper West Side in New York or the Gold Coast in Chicago, despite their geographic proximity to those high-prevalence, high-poverty areas. And like the unrest in Somalia, the "epidemic" of TB in the United States of the 1990s was not just the work of some rotten germs or "bad guys": it had its roots in the history of the society. It could not simply be attacked and defeated without wrestling with that history, too. Those who were sent to control it faced the dilemma of carrying out a targeted intervention within a degraded environment. In Somalia, soldiers had to contend with a hostile social environment, the inner city of Mogadishu, which could charitably be described as "unforgiving." The same could be said of the neighborhoods most afflicted by TB. The people truly threatened by those conditions were those living within them, but social divisions made it possible to portray those people *themselves* as the source of danger.

The novelist Nelson Algren was fond of telling a story about a prostitute who was arrested because of her drug addiction. Upon sentencing her to jail, the judge declared: "We have to keep Chicago strong and America mighty! A year and a day! Take her away!" When she was released a year and day later, the girl mused, "I guess it was lucky I done that time. Chicago still looks pretty strong and America looks mighty mighty" (Algren 32). This story illustrated for Algren the absurdity of blaming the poorest of the poor for the problems that they suffer, as though they, sick, addicted, and powerless as they were, somehow posed a threat to the order of the wealthiest industrial nation on the face of the earth. At the time of my TB "initiation," the streets of downtown New York were bustling, and all appearances seemed to indicate that the place was churning right along. When I left the city, about one year after my CDC training, I felt a little like the woman in that story. New York City, despite the threat ostensibly posed by resurgent TB disease, looked "mighty mighty" to me.

Not that we, as health workers, didn't make any difference—I believe that we did, and the statistics support this belief—but our work was carried out almost entirely in the world of the poor, a world which rarely intersected in any meaningful way with the insulated space of the wealthy. These divisions were deep and wide by the early 1990s, and often it was only by spooking the rich that the poor could be helped at all. That was the real truth revealed in the language used by the media and the public health agencies themselves. The threat of tuberculosis was at least partly symbolic in nature, and the "war" was more like a border skirmish. The actual levels of TB during the much-publicized resurgence of the 1990s, and the levels of spending required to control it, were only significant when compared to the low levels with which the society had grown comfortable. In other words, they *became* significant when acceptable levels of illness were surpassed, and when a sense of tangible danger to the general public was communicated to local and federal governments.

Most professionals in the medical and public health fields are very aware of the socioeconomic factors that influence tuberculosis levels.

They are limited in their responses, however, by the demands for immediate results which are always placed on them and by the very nature of those professions themselves. In his 1993 article "The Historical Limits of the War on Consumption," Barron H. Lerner wrote: "New York officials have long recognized the role of the "plague of poverty" in the spread of tuberculosis . . . Nevertheless, as a result of the structure that public health has assumed, tuberculosis control has sought to detect and treat disease in individual persons rather than address larger societal ills" (Lerner 773). My good friend and cohort Spanner and I would often have this discussion while we worked at the TB Bureau. Over lunch at Dojo's in the East Village we would go back and forth, Spanner maintaining that the Health Department needed more power and authority to go after irresponsible people with TB, me stating that the corralling of individuals would make no difference as long as we had inner cities full of people who were poor, people who were systematically exposed to risks that other populations were able to avoid by virtue of their class position, race, or place of residence. Without the means or the analysis necessary to address these larger issues, I claimed, we settled for catching crooks and incarcerating them. In effect, we ended up punishing people for being poor, sick, addicted, uneducated, and perhaps a bit rebellious.

Spanner would come back and say, "But this guy was given every chance to do the right thing, and he still wouldn't do it, so what choice do we have but to lock his ass up?" "That's not the point," I would always reply, "that's just one guy. What about all the people who are called noncompliant because they are homeless, or don't have transportation, or can't speak English?" Eventually we would both give up and go back to our jobs: he ended up working at New York City's designated detention facility, and I ended up writing the orders that put people there.

Our argument, of course, plays itself out in many different forms and forums in American society. It goes round and round because there is no societal consensus that the health and welfare of each is the concern of all, and we therefore settle for the default position, which is to leave individuals, the market, and cash-strapped institutions to sort things out, and when crises emerge, throw lawyers, guns, money, and medicine at them. Meanwhile, the social system that allots such disparate life chances, stacking the decks for some and leaving others perpetually short-changed, remains fundamentally unchanged. It is this structure which must be questioned if one is to arrive at a truly critical analysis of tuberculosis in the 1990s. According to Paul Farmer: "A critical epistemology of emerging infectious disease would explore the boundaries of polite and impolite discussion in science. A trove of complex, affect-laden issues—attribution of blame to perceived vectors of infection, identification of scapegoats and victims, the role of stigma—are rarely discussed in academic medicine, although they are manifestly part and parcel of many epidemics" (Farmer 1996, 266). This was true of the "original" American tuberculosis epidemic as well as the recent resurgence.

The remainder of this chapter examines not only the facts of that resurgence, but also the rhetoric that accompanied it. First, I will provide an overview of tuberculosis as it has been defined and perceived historically. Then, I will discuss the situation in New York in the early 1990s, from both an "objective" (statistics, medical journals, media accounts) and a "subjective" perspective (that of patients and workers such as myself). Finally, I will move on to explore tuberculosis in Chicago in the mid to late 1990s.

TUBERCULOSIS: HISTORY, EPIDEMIOLOGY, AND SOCIOLOGY

Tuberculosis is an ancient disease, possibly as old as humankind itself. Evidence of it has been found in Egyptian mummies and in the remains of pre-Columbian Americans. It has been one of the greatest sources of death throughout human history, and remains a leading cause of mortality worldwide. The infectious nature of TB, however, was not recognized until the late nineteenth century, when the German physician Robert Koch succeeded in isolating the tubercle bacillus, the species of bacteria that causes the disease. Prior to that time TB, then called "consumption," was believed to be hereditary and noncontagious. According to Nancy Tomes, "Its pattern of spread simply did not conform to physicians' experience with epidemic diseases such as smallpox or cholera, which radiated quickly and more or less predictably from a single infected individual or geographical location" (Tomes 276). Consumption was associated with different types of images than was its successor tuberculosis. For example, the "romantic myth" of consumption as an affliction affecting those with sensitive, passionate, or bookish natures, was a common nineteenth-century convention which seems quite strange today (Sontag 26–36).

An 1864 article by Henry Bowditch, entitled "Is Consumption Ever Contagious?" makes it clear that many physicians suspected the disease to be at least potentially infectious even prior to the discovery of the bacterium. In the conclusion of his article, Bowditch writes: "It may be infectious, and to this extent only. By long attendance of the closest kind, by inhaling the breath of the pthisical patient, by living in the pthisical atmosphere, so to speak, and in general by a neglect of hygienic laws during such attendance, the health may be undermined and pthisis set in" (Bowditch 53).

But the overall consensus of medical professionals in the United States was that the disease was the result of heredity and environment, even though it was sometimes attributed to "constitutional anomalies" (Koch 197). By the early 1880s, however, Koch's research had settled the debate in the mind of Western medicine. The disease, Koch determined, was caused by a tiny living organism, spread from one individual to another through the air. The reason why this had not been recognized earlier had something to do with the nature of the bacilli itself. According to Koch: ". . . the conditions of development favorable for tuberculous bacilli, especially the warmth of 30 degrees C. day and night for weeks are found nowhere except in the animal organism, and there is, therefore, no other supposition possible than that they are dependent for their existence wholly upon the animal and human organisms. They are, therefore, genuine parasites, which cannot exist without a body to support them" (Koch 211). Reenvisioned as an infectious, and therefore preventable, disease, the leading cause of death in the United States suddenly seemed vulnerable to social and medical intervention. What's more, as Koch's writing indicates, the bacterium was not capable of sustaining itself outside the human body, a fact which had clear implications for its control. Controlling TB meant controlling tuberculosis-ridden human bodies. This new perspective contributed to the creation of departments of public health devoted to ridding society of contagion (Trattner 142). It also gave physicians and scientists a new source of authority as they were empowered by the government to do what was necessary to eliminate the plague. Great resources were poured into the public health mission, and it became tied to other platforms of progressive reform.

In the United States at that time, consumption was a burden much more broadly shared across classes. It killed large numbers of people, most of them poor, but many of them not. The romantic notion of TB, alluded to above, was usually associated with the upper classes. The discovery of the infectious nature of TB in 1880, however, changed the image of the disease irrevocably. Rothman (1994) demonstrates how this shift in the sphere of scientific knowledge essentially created a new disease, "tuberculosis," which was viewed in a markedly different way than "consumption" had been. "First and foremost," she writes, "tuberculosis, in contradistinction to consumption, was understood to be a contagious disease; second, it was defined as a disease of only some, not all, people, essentially the immigrant and the poor, not the middle or the upper classes" (Rothman 1994, 181). Consumption, of course, had also disproportionately affected the lower socioeconomic classes, but this was not an issue of primary concern until it was determined that the disease could be passed from one person to another.

As the disease of the poet became the disease of the poor, however, new fears and new hopes arose together. In *La Traviata*, Verdi's opera from 1853, the tuberculous woman, Violetta, is ". . . at once the fallen woman and the pthisic beauty" (M. Morse 11). At that time, consumption was believed to selectively strike those people whose characters or personalities were inherently predisposed to it. For women, this had particular implications: consumption was an outward sign of their sexual natures, of their being "desired, desiring, and desirable" (M. Morse 11). By the time of Puccini's *La Boheme* (1895), Koch's discovery of the tuberculosis bacilli had penetrated the culture, and TB took on a new set of stigmas. According to Morse: "The setting of La Boheme is also significant—Paris, the 1830s, hobohemia, a place where students, poor factory workers, and other 'dregs' of society coalesced and coexisted. This setting corresponds with the increasing awareness that . . . tuberculosis was a disease of poverty, close living quarters, poor nutrition, and poor working conditions" (M. Morse 13). The link between poverty and disease made issues of housing, hunger, and work into public health issues, while at the same time it generated new stigmas concerning the infected (Lerner 773). This era is a very significant one in the history of public health, for not only did it bring about the formation of many of the same institutions which confront TB today; it also originated much of the rhetoric and methods which the media and public health authorities revived in the anti-tuberculosis campaigns of the 1990s.

According to Nancy Tomes, the "socialism of the microbe," its ability to cross social boundaries by literally flying from one person to another through the air, made the disease everyone's worry (Tomes 283). The emphasis of the anti-tuberculosis movement, however, was on personal hygiene and behavior, and the middle-class nature of the "TB crusade" virtually guaranteed that the poor would be singled out for their lack of proper health habits.[2] Nurses of the late nineteenth and early twentieth centuries approached their jobs with an attitude similar to that of missionaries, dedicated to improving health through combating disease (Bates 231). Though some Progressives sought to connect the anti-tuberculosis campaign to a broader critique of social inequality, many efforts to treat TB in these populations were accompanied by lessons in middle-class values of cleanliness and work: "For all TB workers' criticism of irresponsible landlords and factory owners, when it came time to personify the causes of tuberculosis, they almost always chose the homes and habits of the consumptives themselves" (Tomes 288).

This was especially true of African Americans and immigrants (Tomes 286; Ott 100). Katherine Ott argues that "By 1900 the 'contagious consumptive' was a highly politicized entity, most often pictured as a menial laborer or domestic servant, usually a recent immigrant or African American migrant newly arrived in a city" (Ott 101). Contagion was associated with mixing of classes and races. Fears about disease thus became conflated with existing fears of invasion by morally deficient races and classes, who increasingly made their homes in the rapidly growing cities. Feldberg (1995) explores the ways in which ". . . the control of tuberculosis formed part of a larger material, institutional, and ideological effort to shape the middle-class state" (Feldberg 9). In the days of consumption, treatment was informed by a profound fear of all things urban: "If consumption evoked fears about the demise of agriculture, it also raised the specter of another threat to the American order—the rise of industry . . . Consumption thus became associated with men who lived in cities, indulged in frivolous pastimes, and worked at indoor occupations or otherwise shunned the outdoors, but it also came to be constructed as a disease of women, who departed by definition from the male norm" (Feldberg 31). Both women and lazy men, in other words, spent too much time away from the beneficial effects of nature and physical exercise.

Accordingly, nineteenth-century physicians such as Edward Trudeau, himself a consumptive, developed treatment regimens based on the ingestion of good food, clean air, and rugged outdoor living: "Certain that tuberculous disease was caused by poor living conditions and urban life—by both moral and physical contamination—they advocated regimens that would strengthen both body and soul" (Feldberg 35). This fusion of medical and social factors in physicians' ideas about tuberculosis etiology was not easily undone, even after Koch's discoveries were made widely known. Many did not accept the germ theory as a sufficient explanation for the illnesses that they experienced clinically. And, in fact, clinical, experimental, and epidemiological evidence supported the claim that environment was at least as significant a contributing factor in the development of tuberculosis as the presence of the bacteria (Feldberg 48). Throughout most of the twentieth century, in fact, environmental regimens—involving improvement of overall health, diet, hygiene, and exercise habits—remained the dominant mode for treatment of tuberculosis, though these were far from uniform. Patients who could afford private physicians were not subject to the direct supervision of public health departments; they also tended to be treated in private facilities (Abel 1809). When we talk about public health and TB, therefore, we are necessarily talking mainly about the poor.

Abel's sympathetic history of New York City's Tuberculosis Program in the late nineteenth and early twentieth centuries describes how poor patients often resisted the efforts of public health and charity workers to alter their behaviors. According to Abel, many patients were "noncompliant" for very good reasons: "Despite the directive to sleep alone, very sick patients were unwilling to forgo the comfort of sharing beds with others. A woman who kept her windows shut at night in violation of a nurse's decree explained that she did not want to 'freeze to death.' Recommended foods, especially raw eggs, revolted many people" (Abel 1812). It is easy to sympathize with the patient's point of view in these cases, especially since many of the recommendations described above would seem ludicrous today. Yet the central problem of miscommunication, complicated by issues of class, race, gender, and culture, remains today, even though raw eggs are no longer a recommended treatment for TB. When patients revolt, they may find themselves punished by a system which is designed to help them.

The issue of involuntary detention provides a good illustration. The practice of forcibly confining potentially dangerous TB patients was pioneered in the early days of the public health campaign, and was revived in the 1990s. In New York City, again leading the way for the rest of the nation, the health code was revamped in 1993 and a secure hospital wing was opened on an island in the East River. It was especially designed for holding and treating TB patients until the time that they were judged to be medically cured—anywhere from several months to several years—or until they "expired." Detention has its appeal, especially when it comes to the public and the politicians, who like to see tangible evidence that "something is being done" about the impending deadly epidemic. Placing a few rogues behind walls satisfies this need. There are good reasons, however, to doubt the effectiveness of this measure as a long-term solution.

The rationale for detention of chronically noncompliant TB patients is similar to that which motivates the incarceration of repeat criminal offenders. According to this argument, a few people are out there doing most of the damage, and if those people are removed from society, the problem, or a good part of it, will cease. This approach focuses primarily on the behavior of individuals. While it might be claimed that some people have demonstrated themselves to be beyond society's reach, and therefore need to be forcibly controlled or isolated from society, such an approach neglects the fact that certain sets of social conditions—poverty, malnutrition, inadequate housing, addiction—persistently tend to foster the existence and spread of TB. If left unaddressed, these conditions inevitably produce more individuals that need to be isolated. Reviews of the history of detention and other compulsory public health measures find the record to be mixed at best (Rothman 1992, 72; Lerner 1999).

People both inside and outside of the health care system continue to believe that medical intervention on the one hand, and enforcement on the other, have been and remain the keys to successful control of infectious disease, even though in the history of tuberculosis this has been shown to be untrue. The medical and public health measures have certainly played a great part in the control of TB, but these are usually somewhat expedient, targeted at the disease *after* it has emerged as a full-fledged problem. An analogy might be made to the control of fires. The department that extinguishes the most blazes may have much to be proud of, but the city would surely prefer to have fewer fires to put out. Just because prevention is preferable and ultimately more effective, however, it doesn't necessarily follow that effective, high-quality services shouldn't be available when crises such as fires or epidemics do arise. Unfortunately, those neighborhoods that have the most fires often also have the worst fire services, as Rodrick Wallace's (1990) work has shown. The same is essentially true of health care, education, and various other vital services: those who need them the most have the least quality and variety to choose from. In an economically equitable society, where all people had adequate housing, nutrition, education, and employment, it is unlikely that there would be a great need for either TB medicine or health codes that force people to take it. In prosperous sectors of the United States and Europe, this is in fact the case.

TUBERCULOSIS IN THE 1990S: THE OFFICIAL STORY

There was a surge of media attention for TB in the early 1990s, not only in the New York press but in many other publications, from *Commonweal* to *Good Housekeeping* (Bhavaraju 1999). Though the actual rates of TB were nowhere near as high as they had been even two decades earlier, a confluence of factors contributed to a sudden sense of alarm about TB. This alarm was successfully communicated to the political structure and the public at large via professional journals and the mainstream news media, and resulted in increased funding for tuberculosis control efforts across the country.

On the professional end, an influential article entitled "Resurgent Tuberculosis in New York City" was published in the spring of 1991, and sounded the alarm on an impending public health crisis. The authors, Karen Brudney and Jay Dobkin, had studied the first 224 TB patients consecutively diagnosed at Harlem Hospital in 1988, assessing their medical and social histories upon admission and then tracking them after discharge to determine the success of their treatments. Of 178 patients discharged with tuberculosis medications, 89 percent were lost to follow-up and failed to complete therapy, and 27 percent were readmitted within twelve months with confirmed active tuberculosis (Brudney and Dobkin 745). The same problem existed citywide. The city of New York reported

3,811 new cases in 1992, and the case rate of 52 per 100,000 was the highest in two decades; this rate was nearly five times the national case rate of 10.5 per 100,000 (New York City Bureau of Tuberculosis Control 1992, 1). Also in 1992, 14 percent of all tuberculosis cultures in NYC were found to be resistant to the two most effective drugs, isoniazid and rifampin (New York City Bureau of Tuberculosis Control 1992, 10). The spread of TB and the possibility of its incurability made for a potent combination that the media quickly seized upon, and in 1992 media coverage of TB also reached its peak (Bhavaraju 1999).

Among the primary factors contributing to the resurgence were the spread of the Human Immunodeficiency Virus (HIV), marked increases in the homeless population, and the decline of tuberculosis control programs. But much attention was also focused on the problem of patient noncompliance. Brudney and Dobkin argued that ". . . compliance has remained the major obstacle to eliminating what is essentially a curable disease" (Brudney and Dobkin 748). They concluded that ". . . long abandoned strategies will need to be reinstituted for homeless and noncompliant patients: prolonged initial hospitalization, residential TB treatment facilities, and aggressive community-based supervision" (Dobkin 749). In response to the threat of a deadly airborne epidemic, the Commissioner of Health of the City of New York increased funding for TB control from $4 million in 1988 to more than $40 million in 1994 (Dievler 177). Under the leadership of Tom Frieden, a physician with a public health background assigned by the CDC, the City followed Dobkin and Brudney's recommendations and mounted an aggressive campaign against TB, hiring thousands of outreach workers (such as myself) to hit the streets, locate patients in the community, track progress, and even personally administer tuberculosis treatment.

By 1995, the New York City Bureau of Tuberculosis Control was ready to claim some success. In an article entitled "Tuberculosis in New York City—Turning the Tide," Frieden declared that the efforts of the public health system in New York had resulted in a marked reduction of new cases. Among the most significant changes were the widespread implementation of directly observed therapy and involuntary confinement of TB patients on the one hand, and improved infection control measures and medical regimens on the other (Frieden et al. 229). Frieden concluded that maintenance of substantial TB control efforts is necessary to ensure that the decline in TB becomes ". . . not simply a blip on the curve, but the resumption of a consistent drive to eliminate tuberculosis as a serious threat to health in the United States" (Frieden et al. 233). Even more encouraging, for those concerned about rampaging new strains of super-TB, was the decrease in rates of multi-drug-resistant TB in New York City. Multi-drug resistance, or MDR, had become the phantom menace of the TB resurgence. Even though multi-drug-resistant bacteria were not necessarily more virulent than plain old TB germs, the fact that they could result in a case of tuberculosis that modern medicine couldn't cure made them a frightening prospect for health professionals.

This was a big difference from just three years earlier, when the *New York Times* published "Tuberculosis: A Killer Returns," a series of articles that ominously proclaimed: "The United States has stumbled into its first preventable epidemic, a wave of tuberculosis with strains so virulent they threaten to return pockets of American society to a time when antibiotics were unknown" (Specter 1). Other articles appearing around that time had similar titles "The Return of the Big Killer" *(New Scientist)*, "A Looming Public Health Nightmare" *(Lungs at Work)*, "Breeding a Killer: The High Cost of Neglect" *(Commonweal)*, and "A Breath Away" *(Los Angeles Times)*. Though many of these presented balanced accounts of the multiple factors contributing to the resurgence of TB, all of them highlighted the increasing danger of TB, especially the drug-resistant varieties. Many of the articles emphasized the role of patient noncompliance and "homeless, mentally ill people" as sources of TB spread (Bhavaraju 1999). They commonly dramatized their subject matter by raising the specter of poor, infectious, and ignorant patients, spreading TB throughout the city.

For example, consider this passage, also taken from the *New York Times* article:

> "This guy is sick and infectious," said Dr. Karen Brudney, director of the Bronx TB control program, as she strode through the Morrisania Chest Clinic, looking for a particular man she had wanted to see. "He walked 30 blocks to the clinic today because he didn't have a subway token. He shouldn't be here. It's the worst possible place for him—and for everyone around him." Quickly, she gave him a new week's worth of medicine, a subway token and sent him home. But he was one in a seemingly endless stream of poor people to appear that day. None had insurance, and few spoke English. (Specter 44)

In addition to the central image of the "tubercular poor," this account is illustrative of the medico-centric depiction of health problems, with the doctor and other professionals placed in an active role, and everyone else being judged in accordance with their ability to follow the doctor's orders. It is reminiscent of the rhetoric of the nineteenth century. A few lines later in the same article, Dr. Brudney states, about a Dominican woman who passed TB on to her children, "I doubt that they have seen a doctor twice in their lives" (Specter 44). Dr. Brudney may not have meant it this way, but such an account would seem to imply that seeing more doctors would somehow have prevented this woman from getting TB. That implication is faulty on a couple different levels: first, it overestimates the efficacy of clinical medicine in terms of disease prevention; second, it overlooks the role that poverty plays in determining who gets sick. Many people who avoid physicians are perfectly healthy, but most of them probably do not live in Harlem or Haiti or the Dominican Republic.

VILLAINS OR VICTIMS? MEDIA CHARACTERIZATION OF TB PATIENTS

Laurie Garrett's *The Coming Plague: Newly Emerging Diseases in a World Out of Balance* (1994) offers a sweeping overview of many "scary" diseases, new and old, and the threats they pose. The chapter that deals with AIDS and TB is called "Thirdworldization," and it also features an appearance by Dr. Karen Brudney. Again, she shows frustration at her patient's inability to follow appropriate TB therapy. Concerning a man named Vernon, she says, "Everything this man says is a lie. It's amazing. Every single word . . . For months he's been checking in and out of homeless shelters, using false names so the Health Department couldn't find him . . ." (Garrett 519). Finally, Brudney turns to the author and says "That's what we're up against" (Garrett 519). Vernon, according to Brudney, is a totally incorrigible patient. The implied equation is that such irresponsible patients are the problem to be overcome by the public health system.

I do not mean to disparage the work of tuberculosis doctors here, because ministering to the population most affected by this disease is often a thankless and unglamorous task. I encountered Dr. Brudney several times while working in New York and I always found her to be extremely competent and committed to her work. But I do wish to question depictions of disease which imply that exceptionally stubborn or deviant TB patients are the "source" of the tuberculosis problem. The issue of "compliance" is itself misleading, because it is by definition an unstable category. As soon as someone starts taking their medicine as directed by a physician, they are no longer "noncompliant," they are no longer a "problem." Thus the same patients may be compliant one day and noncompliant the next, depending on who is monitoring them and making that judgment. One particular story comes to mind which illustrates the human side of TB epidemiology, from the point of view of both the patient and the worker. Here I will defer to my journal notes from 1993, the height of the recent TB epidemic in New York.

3/22/93

Spanner and I brought a guy in today. Brought him in quite literally, carried him like a sack of potatoes. The man couldn't walk and we listened outside the front door of his apartment in Harlem as he crawled the entire painful way from the back bedroom to unlock the front door, using only the force of his arms, moaning like a dog in a trap as he went. It was painful just to listen to it. We sat on the stairs, outside the door. A couple of times I laughed. In the proper context it would be comedy. As it was it was close. Spanner sat there and winced, probably wishing he had brought my Walkman to drown out the cries.

After he finally managed to open the door we carried him down the stairs, one of us on each side, put him in our vehicle, and transported him to the clinic, hauling him inside the same way. In the office at the clinic I asked him, in the little French I could remember, "Tu as peur?" "You are afraid?"

"Oui, j'ai peur," he replied. I am afraid.

"If he doesn't go to the hospital, he's going to die," said the doctor, not thinking he understood. But out of the corner of my eye I could see him jump just a little, and his eyes grew wide.

So I sat in the ER at St. Luke's Hospital with this man, Mr. Indigo, and a puddle of puke reclining shiny on the floor before the next row of plastic chairs. I didn't even notice it until Spanner pointed it out and then I hardly even cared. We had to wait until he was called for triage. I asked him how long he had been here, in the United States. He said three years. I said, "It's a crazy place, huh?" He said, "Yeah. There's too much freedom. People are too free. They think they can just do whatever." He nodded toward the central reference point, the orange puddle of vomit. "This would not happen over there," he said, meaning in his country of Senegal. "They would throw the person out."

The person in question had puked and subsequently sat down next to us and spat on the floor. Apparently she had been sitting there for three days without even going to see the triage nurse, just sitting around, watching TV. The security guard finally strongarmed her into leaving. I sat there with this polite, petite representative of Africa and I was ashamed for us.

At one point he started trying to get up. "Where are you going?" I asked. "I need to pee," he said. "What, are you going to walk?" Of course, he couldn't walk, his legs simply wouldn't work, and he didn't know why. I put his arms over my shoulder and started helping him to walk—Spanner was outside buying smokes—and then I simply picked him up and carried him to the door that said CABALLEROS, like a man carrying his bride across the threshold. I stood him up at the stall and then stood there as he drained himself with audible relief.

"How long have you been holding it?" I asked.

"All day," he said.

This little man amazed me.

The doctor was fluent in French, and she conversed easily with this man. I remember Mr. Indigo very well; he was wearing a camouflage hat and was very thin, dark-skinned, with a beard on his chin, and soft, sensitive eyes. I remember, too, that he seemed like an educated man. The reason we knocked on his door in the first place was because his name had turned up on a list of TB patients who had not returned to the clinic for proper follow-up. Once we found him, of course, we knew why.

If he had continued to neglect his tuberculosis treatment without explanation, Mr. Indigo would no doubt have been considered a noncompliant patient and a potential public health threat. But the reasons why patients miss clinic appointments are numerous, significant, and complex. For doctors and health officials, the most important thing in the TB patient's life is the treatment and clinical follow-up. The patients, however, often have competing interests. For this reason, the public health effort in New York in the 1990s sought to both better accommodate TB patients and to pursue them more aggressively. This was the approach that worked with Mr. Indigo, who would have remained "noncompliant" if Spanner and I had not gone out to find him, if he had not been able to drag himself all the way down the hallway to open the door for us, if we had not been able to get him admitted to a hospital. Incidentally, I ran into Mr. Indigo months later at the Chest Clinic in Washington Heights— he was walking and looked in good health and good spirits, one of those gratifying cases where one could feel that a well-timed intervention made a difference.

A story such as this would play well in the media, because it rewards our faith in the ability of human beings to overcome obstacles and persevere over adversity, albeit with a little help here and there. Once the details were known, Mr. Indigo easily fit the image of a deserving patient, an "innocent victim" of TB in need of assistance or rescue. Unfortunately, depictions of irresponsible contagion-carriers or "undeserving" TB patients also translate easily into a preexisting moral vocabulary that the media loves to manipulate. Tuberculosis, no longer linked to any strong symbolic stigmas of its own, nonetheless remains a stigmatized illness because of its association with other strongly stigmatized groups or conditions. In the health fields, everyone knows about "risk groups" and what they signify (Fee and Krieger 337–338). It is a phrase so common as to be banal. Yet how often is this "common sense" category criticized in public health practice? Risk groups may be seen alternately as groups which need extra protection, or groups that the rest of society needs protection from. Sontag calls the risk group ". . . that neutral-sounding bureaucratic category which also revives the archaic idea of a tainted community that illness has judged" (Sontag 134). The public health and medical communities use such language in order to mobilize financial support from a political structure that responds to its imagery. As Farmer has written, ". . . the World Health Organization uses the threat of contagion to motivate wealthy nations to invest in disease surveillance and control out of self-interest" (Farmer 1996, 266). But like an antibiotic, this language has side effects, and breeds resistance of its own. The fact that the risk group for TB includes, not coincidentally, poor African Americans, prisoners, AIDS patients, and immigrants can lend ammunition to those who might seek to discriminate against such groups. In a sense, this amounts to a reversal of reality, where the most vulnerable and least powerful are posed as a threat, a "persecutor of the social normal . . . " (Butler 27).

Similar semantic problems surrounded two other "emerging epidemics" of the 1980s and 1990s, both of which were closely related—actually and symbolically—to the resurgence of tuberculosis: homelessness and AIDS. To see tuberculosis clearly, one must view it alongside these other media-magnified developments. There is, of course, a wealth of literature on both of these subjects. What I wish to briefly discuss here is the public rhetoric and the response which shaped most peoples' knowledge of these issues; the process by which they became defined. In fact, the rise of AIDS in the 1980s may be seen as a symbolic signpost, similar in a sense to the wholesale abandonment of the War on Poverty, of which homelessness was but one consequence. In *Inventing AIDS,* Cindy Patton dissects the discourse surrounding the rise of AIDS, and the way the disease was eventually portrayed by both the media and the scientific establishment.[3] Scientists, according to Patton, experience illness indirectly, using macro- or micro-technologies, statistical modeling on the one hand, and electron microscopes on the other. In the beginning of the AIDS epidemic—indeed, before such a thing as "AIDS" existed—most discourse was controlled by those who had direct experience with the disease. These were primarily people in the gay community and their close associates; people who were suffering from an as-yet unrecognized disorder. It was only later, when AIDS became recognized as a scientific "fact," that professionals and "experts" stepped in. When that transition occurred, the lay voices of Persons Living With AIDS (PLWA's) were necessarily marginalized. Suddenly, the mere fact of having AIDS no longer meant that you actually knew anything about it. In the same manner that Foucault describes the establishment of the clinic removing illness from its social context in the home, AIDS as an area of scientific expertise was removed from living communities and resituated in hospitals and research labs.

Of course, the fact that the groups most affected by AIDS were both socially stigmatized and (with the exception of the organized gay community in large cities such as San Francisco and New York) politically disempowered facilitated this transition of knowledge and power. As AIDS was "mainstreamed" (to borrow Patton's phrase) the social and structural dimensions of the disease were deemphasized in favor of behavioral explanations and remedies, and the populations who suffered with AIDS broke down into "deserving" and "undeserving," a moralistic division already long-established in governmental policy directed at the poor (Katz 1989). Ryan White, the little boy from Indiana, was one of the former, along with the occasional heterosexual reportedly infected by an irresponsible dentist, while the bulk of gay and poor AIDS patients, presumably doomed by their own sinful behavior, fell into the latter category. According to Patton, "the 'risky behaviors' for which testing is essentially a confirmatory exercise are already connected in the public mind with gay men, prostitutes, drug dealers, and people of color" (Patton 41).

The problem of homelessness also rose to the surface of public consciousness in the early 1980s. Like AIDS, homelessness was originally articulated as an issue by a mobilized activist community (Stern 293). Also like AIDS, the issue of homelessness, once legitimated as a public problem, was later professionalized, and structural arguments about the sources of homelessness were shelved in favor of behavioral or individualistic solutions such as shelters and training programs (Stern 295). At the same time, the "mainstreaming" of homelessness removed the issue from the domain of the homeless themselves. Their moral authority, which was converted into a small amount of political capital, had stemmed not from their poverty itself, but from their visibility in public areas. Eventually, however, they came to be accepted as features of the urban landscape, to be managed in the same way as rats or cars—especially if they did not have the wherewithal to "correct" themselves. Homeless people, originally depicted by their advocates as "deserving," came to be perceived as a de facto category of "undeserving" simply by virtue of their persistent homelessness. If they really wanted help, why didn't they go into the shelters that the government had provided? Why did they not take advantage of programs that were offered? In the same manner, people with AIDS became less and less sympathetic as the epidemic wore on and their own culpability—by virtue of their "unsafe" behavior—was presumed.

Concerning homelessness, Hoch and Slayton have argued that the "politics of compassion" inevitably backfires, because it overlooks and obscures social and economic pressures which erode the availability of housing for poor people generally. This sort of politics favors emotional individual narratives of downward mobility because they pack more "emotional punch" (Hoch and Slayton 199). At the same time, by emphasizing vulnerabilities and deficiencies of the homeless, the politics of compassion also negates the agency of poor people, assigning the role of advocate instead to qualified professionals (Hoch and Slayton 208). Most homeless people, however, do not suddenly "fall" into the streets or shelters from lofty positions of wealth or prestige, or even of financial security. Most homeless persons come, predictably, from the ranks of the working poor (Hoch and Slayton 201). Addressing homelessness as a separate category, without addressing issues of poverty and housing in general, only serves to sever social services from social structure (Katz 91).

These issues are crucial to an understanding of tuberculosis in the 1990s. HIV/AIDS and homelessness were cited by many scientists as two of the primary factors, along with immigration and a decaying public health infrastructure, that contributed to the resurgence of TB in urban areas. Both were reflective of fissures in American society that had been growing since the 1960s. Standard epidemiology notes the geographic, socioeconomic, and racial specificity of risk for HIV/AIDS, even within an urban environment as densely populated as New York City (Drucker 45). But rarely does it question the structural forces underlying these separations. When social factors are considered in epidemiological research, they usually relate to specific behaviors such as intravenous drug use or sexual promiscuity, which make certain people more susceptible to illness and disease. Such research, maintains Farmer, makes the dangerous error of ". . . conflating cultural (and psychological) difference with structural violence" (Farmer 1997, 353). According to Freund and McGuire, "The effects of social inequality are aggravated in America by the myth that everyone can succeed, and if they fail it is their own fault" (Freund and McGuire 109). The structural violence inflicted by systemic social inequality is thus translated as deficiency on the part of individuals.

The policy which results from such analyses is also predictable: rather than correcting inequities in resource distribution, health authorities seek to correct individual behavior through "educational" programs targeted at specific "cultures." Social network theory, for example, is employed as a means of better predicting and preventing disease outbreaks by targeting specific groups of people who are at risk, rather than entire populations or demographic categories. It provides a more nuanced approach to the idea of risk groups. This approach began in academic departments, but has since been adapted to epidemiological and public health purposes. "Networks," an abstracted way of talking about sets of meaningful human relations, are seen in public health as either "barriers" or "aids" to the task of implementing plans devised by public health bureaucracies. "Networks" can then fill in for "behaviors" or "cultures" as the proximate cause of illness and disease. This can potentially slide into a "culture of poverty" cul-de-sac, where groups of people are seen as endlessly reproducing their own misfortune. Disconnected from an analysis of structures on the one hand, and a sensitive exploration of their contents on the other, networks can simply become self-fulfilling prophecies. The network becomes both the mechanism and the cause of deviance and disease: people who use drugs belong to drug-using networks. Why do they belong to this network? Because they use drugs. Why do they use drugs? Because the people in their network use drugs.

As tuberculosis is suffered most by the same populations which suffer from drug addiction, homelessness, AIDS, and just about everything else, it makes sense that a similar, circular argument would be made to explain the prevalence of the disease. TB patients coming from particular risk groups are often "presumed noncompliant" until proven otherwise. "Noncompliance," as Donovan and Blake (1992) have argued, is a value-laden term which serves to implicate disease sufferers rather than doctors. The phenomenon of noncompliance, with all its local trappings of environment, belief, and behavior, will be discussed in the chapters that follow. For this discussion of tuberculosis epidemiology, it is sufficient to question the categories which are normally employed. To do so, we must first consider some of the structural factors which standard epidemiology often implies, but seldom discusses, as issues in and of themselves.

Rodrick Wallace's work provides an example of epidemiology that considers some of the broader forces that influence both behavior and illness patterns, linking violence, substance abuse, and AIDS with the process of urban decay.[4] The maps used by Wallace to illustrate the rates of intentional violent death, cirrhosis deaths, and low birth weight babies in blighted neighborhoods of the Bronx in 1980 are very similar to those depicting TB rates in the same borough ten years later. Wallace wrote in 1990 that he expected ". . . subsequent rounds of contagious building abandonment and community burnout to occur in regions with a large percentage of poor people living in overcrowded conditions . . ." (Wallace 802). Given these inner-city conditions, it would not be surprising that tuberculosis, an airborne disease to which malnourished people are unusually susceptible, had taken root there. Merrill Singer has suggested that these afflictions might best be seen as components of a broader "syndemic," which he defines as "the set of synergistic or intertwined and mutually enhancing health and social problems facing the urban poor" (Singer 933). From this broader perspective, homelessness, drug addiction, AIDS, and tuberculosis might all be seen as specific manifestations of a much larger, ongoing process in urban America: a slow-motion disaster that resulted in the increasing isolation and desolation of the same urban poor who were later to become commonly known as "the underclass."

This term, originally used by Gunnar Myrdal in the 1960s as a strictly economic designation, was imbued in the 1980s with behavioral characteristics, so that those of the very poor who did not adhere to middle class standards of behavior came to be seen as responsible for their own lack of middle class status and resources—including health. Public health approaches which specifically target individual behavior as the source of health and illness have reinforced this idea, despite the fact that health behaviors in themselves cannot account for the glaring statistical differences in health outcomes between rich and poor (Lantz et al. 1708). The role of economic class has been further complicated by the persistence of race as a valuable predictor of health outcomes, a persistence which may result in the substitution of cultural or even genetic factors as explanations for unequal patterns of health and disease (Muntaner et al. 265). To what extent "race" is actually a proxy for "class" is a question that is not often raised.

Meanwhile, the myopia of the public health system causes researchers to express the overall economic devastation of the inner city one-dimensionally. For example, many referred to a dismantling of health infrastructure as a primary cause of TB resurgence. But this dismantling in itself might be just another symptom of what was occurring throughout the 1970s and 1980s. According to Dr. Stephen Joseph, "We chipped away at, and in some cases nearly dismantled, our public health preventive systems . . . even as we watched in our large cities the increase in social conditions reminiscent of those in the nineteenth century, when tuberculosis flourished" (Joseph 647). This use of the collective "we" is deceptive, and conceals the class implications of this dismantling. The dominant political mode of the post–Reagan era was a reaction against so-called "big government." This provided ideological cover for a systematic agenda of dismantling the welfare state, an effort which was not entirely successful, but was nonetheless devastating for poor and working people (Piven and Cloward 1982, 128).

Health itself, remolded as a commodity rather than a public resource, became more segregated and privatized as a result of these cuts. According to Friedman, the "Yuppie Ethic" superseded the older ethic of community service and responsibility, and the American public bought into what she calls "The Big Lie": "that because it would make it easier for some entrepreneurs, venture capitalists, and big purchasers of care to garner huge profits and savings in the face of massive unfunded need, health care can be remolded into a consumer commodity" (Friedman 341). The widespread fear of a health resource shortage and the adoption of private market models contributed directly to severe cutbacks for health services to the poor, including those agencies responsible for tracking and treating tuberculosis. As the income gap between the very rich and the very poor widened after the 1960s, the middle class found itself in a precarious class position. The characterization of the TB resurgence as a form of encroaching Third World contagion revealed the reality of conditions within American cities—especially the growing chasm between rich and poor—as well as a general fear of lower class contamination. This fear was also evident in the "underclass" literature of the 1980s. The rhetoric of both the media and public health departments, while at times acknowledging the broader societal roots of the "epidemic," also played upon a symbolic language of shadow and light, sin and salvation, civilization and savagery. Tuberculosis, depicted as either the revenge of the slums or the bitter harvest of medical hubris, played the role of grim messenger: a lethal reminder of "our" collective sins and failures, which now threatened not only "those people" (poor, colored, immigrants) but "us" (the white middle class) as well. Social responsibility, then, was communicated through the fear and threat of retaliation. Images of innocent victims alternated with those of evil villains, either people or microbes, and military metaphors were often employed (Herzlich and Pierret 26). Just below the surface of this rhetoric was a deep reservoir of class and race anxiety.[5]

Most empirical research on the experience of people struggling with TB has been based on personal letters or the official writings of patients and doctors (Bates 1992; Rothman 1994). However, these excellent studies are inevitably limited by the nature of their sources, and because of their dependence on the literacy of patients. When the levels of disease dropped, they dropped fastest amongst the classes best positioned to take advantage of improvements in both medical measures and social conditions and most likely to advocate for resources. This contributed to the illusion that the disease had been "eliminated" in industrialized countries such as the United States. The development of successful antibiotics in the post–World War II era ushered in a whole new era of TB treatment and control. The ability to consistently cure TB in individuals made ingestion of drugs the single most important measure in controlling TB, more important than housing, nutrition, or income. Whereas medical practitioners had previously sought to improve health in TB patients—or else to remove them from society—they now concentrated solely on eliminating disease through biomedical means. Although tuberculosis rates had been falling since the late nineteenth century, the advent of antibiotics made many people believe that medicine had solved the age-old problem of TB for good. In the United States, both morbidity and mortality due to tuberculosis continued to drop precipitously from the sixties into the mid-1980s. The success of modern medicine in curing the world's most deadly scourge made it is easy to believe that TB—and infectious disease in general—was a problem of the past.

When tuberculosis rates began to rise again in the late 1980s, many people throughout American society were shocked. They assumed that TB had been eliminated. In fact, TB among American poor people had never gone away, it had simply sunk below the levels considered significant to the general public. In the developing world, it continued to kill millions yearly. TB's re-emergence on U.S. medical radar was attributed by epidemiologists to primarily social factors, including the rise of AIDS, homelessness, increased immigration from Third World countries, and massive cuts in public funding for TB and other health services which benefited the poor.[6] The charge that the "noncompliance" of TB patients was a primary cause of the resurgence, coupled with the fact that the identified "risk groups" for TB included poor blacks, prisoners, AIDS patients, and immigrants, ensured that TB would retain some of its previous social stigma—which, indeed, it did.

In the nineteenth and early twentieth century, medical researchers were worried about the rates of tuberculosis in the black community, not because they were especially concerned about the black community, but because they feared a "galloping consumption" springing forth from the negro race would run roughshod over the general (white) population (Torchia 501). For many years, tuberculosis among blacks was simply ignored by the medical profession, including anti-tuberculosis societies themselves (Trattner 148). Images of disease-ridden blacks propagated by the medical profession resembled other racist media images of the same era, which often depicted blacks as inherently prone toward drug abuse, crime, or violence. The association of images of illness and contagion with negative stereotypes of racial and cultural minorities is practically inevitable given this history. Those on the bottom of the social heap—black folks in particular—had to wait for the benefits of bourgeois largesse or paranoia to drift down. By the time this happens, of course, many people have already died invisibly.

Nonetheless, it must be acknowledged that a successful public relations campaign based on fear can have beneficial effects (Bates 333–334). As Piven and Cloward have argued concerning riots and other urban unrest, disease outbreaks tend to secure resources in the form of funding for expanded services (Piven and Cloward 1971, 242). Public health agencies thus find themselves in a strange position, at times exaggerating the very problems that they are charged with controlling. So what happens when, as in the case of TB in the United States, renewed efforts at categorical control of a disease actually work? The health of the overall population, vis-à-vis TB, is undoubtedly improved; that is, the case rates go down, as they did in New York City and in Chicago in the late 1990s. By the year 2000, both cities were claiming record low rates of tuberculosis. But in spite of these notable decreases, all the other contributing social factors, both structural and behavioral, remained. When tuberculosis has been successfully managed, the power of its image as a microbial serial killer fades, and with the fear goes the public concern and the funding. This is where the language of fear backfires: when the bourgeois center of society perceives that the losses are once again acceptable, and that the suffering is confined, once again, to the very poor.

CONCLUSION

Although AIDS and tuberculosis both disproportionately affect the poor, TB usually receives less attention because it kills poor people almost exclusively (Farmer et al. 1996, 153). In 1990, tuberculosis was estimated to have killed about 2.5 million people worldwide. AIDS in the same year killed about 200,000. Yet funding for AIDS in that year was about 200 million dollars, while funding for TB was less than 20 million (*The Economist*, 81). In the early 1990s, funding was substantially increased for TB, primarily in New York City, due to high-profile nosocomial outbreaks and the emergent threat of multi-drug resistance. But despite declaring tuberculosis a "global health emergency," the World Health Organization spent only $800,000 of its $1 billion annual budget on tuberculosis control in 1994 (Altman A1). Because most cases of TB occur within developing countries and among poor populations, the development of newer and more effective medical treatments for TB is not seen as a priority for pharmaceutical companies, which are busy chasing more lucrative markets, nor by politicians in wealthy countries, who are likely to declare that their "constituents don't get TB!" (Altman A1). Meanwhile, in India, for example, health officials estimated in 1998 that tuberculosis killed 1,000 people every day (Roy 1998).

Tuberculosis, then, is not only a disease of the ghetto; it is a ghettoized disease. This is true both locally and globally. Examining the dynamics of tuberculosis in Chicago will reveal the same patterns just discussed, albeit on a smaller scale. This book deals primarily with the practice of Directly Observed Therapy, or DOT, which is the current standard of care in the United States and recommended worldwide by the WHO as the cornerstone strategy for TB control worldwide.[7]

I use a critical approach to epidemiology as I try to place Chicago's TB resurgence of the late 1980s and early 1990s into historical and sociological perspective. I also question the logic of attempting to treat tuberculosis in isolation from the structural forces that give birth to it and nourish it. Within the environment of the poor inner city, tuberculosis had always smoldered along, claiming its victims each year. When the fuels accumulated (poverty and inequality), the winds picked up (AIDS, homelessness, immigration), and the fire crews withdrew (cutting of public health and social welfare programs), TB was fanned into a flame, and this drew some attention to the problem, which resulted in expensive but effective control. However, the rise and fall of tuberculosis rates is meaningless without the social context that surrounded it. As argued in the Introduction and Chapter 1, the reductionist mode of biomedicine has a tendency to ignore those factors that lie outside the scope of its knowledge and technology. This tendency is most evident inside the hospital, which is where medical professionals typically encounter tuberculosis and its victims. In Chapter 3, I will consider the hospital as an institution where the dominant culture of biomedicine holds sway, but where human subjects (also known as "patients") nonetheless assert themselves in a variety of ways.

3 The Public Hospital

Battles on the TB Frontier

> One doesn't ask of one who suffers, what is your country and what is your religion? One merely says, you suffer, that is enough for me, you belong to me, and I shall help you.
>
> —Louis Pasteur, quotation written on a statue in front of County General Hospital in Chicago

NO MATTER how noble their intentions, medical institutions are not immune to social prejudice. Just as muscular, skeletal, and nervous systems are intimately bound within the same human body, so is the medical system embedded in a larger social body, and it is afflicted by the same problems that perplex the society as a whole (Freund 283). Among these are the everpresent maladies of poverty, race, and gender discrimination. Eli Ginzberg has written that: ". . . every nation's health care system is embedded in its cultural, political, economic, ideological and social institutions, and . . . these must serve as points of departure for any meaningful exploration of health care reform" (Ginzberg 277). At the same time, medicine may also be seen as an ideologic institution which plays a role in maintaining social relations as they are (Waitzkin 1991, 17). Conflicts within medical institutions, therefore, also mirror those that exist in the surrounding society (Todd 1989).

This chapter considers health care as a socially embedded practice, focusing specifically on the problematic relationship that often exists between medical institutions and poor people. I deliberately approach this relationship from the point of view of the patient, for two main reasons: (1) the dominant view in public discussion of health issues tends to be that of medicine and the doctor, while the patient's point of view is often neglected, and (2) my research was conducted primarily among patients, and not among doctors or nurses. I cannot claim to adequately represent the viewpoint of doctors or other medical staff vis-à-vis these particular patients. Nonetheless, I believe that this is a valuable exercise, and may be helpful to medical professionals as well.

In my role as a public health worker, I occupied a middle terrain between patients and a large public medical institution, and its bureaucratic workings often appeared as mysterious to me as they did to them. For example, I had little grasp of the ways in which doctors in the hospital divided up their time and duties, between interns, residents, fellows, attendings, and all the rest. I apologize for this ignorance, but I believe that in this case it is actually instructive: the comings and goings of different doctors are often a complete enigma to patients as well, and I found myself sharing their confusion, and identifying with it. Here is an example of one fifty-year-old black man's impression of hospital procedure:

> Don't nobody seem to know what they supposed to be doin'; they swoop down on you like vultures. I'm tired of sitting here waiting for them to see me, waiting for the shoe to fall. I can take my medicines if they just tell me when and how many . . . They want to do too much, too quick, they don't have time to talk one-on-one to no patient. Your health is as important to you, as the next person they callin' them to go see . . . Ten or fifteen doctors running around, some of them just listening, you think they your real doctor, but they just emissaries, messengers or something. Then one doctor come up out of twenty-five doctors, they tell me I got a hole in my lung. Why didn't all those others say anything?

This shows just how strange the routine world of the institution can seem. In the same manner, many poor patients bring baggage from the home, neighborhood, or street into the hospital, including expectations, prejudices, and problems that are quite mysterious to the doctors and nurses. Often these are attributed to individual personalities rather than to social factors or cultural differences, and this may alienate the patient. Tuberculosis patients in an urban hospital may suffer a double dislocation. Because they often come from extremely marginalized population, and a high percentage of urban TB cases are poor, homeless, and substance-addicted, they are especially vulnerable to medical neglect and paternalism. Secondly, the alienating and stigmatizing effects of the diagnosis itself can serve to reinforce their marginality, making them feel akin to criminals or outcasts. This chapter takes the vantage point of a sociologically trained public health worker to illustrate the skirmishes that occur within the institution of the hospital, between those who suffer from tuberculosis, and those who seek to treat them.

The public hospital is a sort of outpost on the urban frontier, strategically positioned within the intensely segregated space of the city. "Frontier" is a word which has many connotations in Western culture; although strictly speaking it refers simply to a border between two lands or territories, it has also been used to denote the line separating civilization and barbarism, or the known and the unknown. These latter meanings are politically loaded and are no longer considered appropriate in a postcolonial world. Nonetheless, they inform the conflicts that occur within the city itself, and especially within the public hospital, where doctors and nurses wearing white coats, and often white skin as well, do battle with the disease, trauma, and disaster that is embodied for them daily by mostly brown-skinned people. Often they see these conditions as accompanied by, or even stemming from, a perceived ignorance on the part of the people they serve, and they see themselves as opposing this darkness with the light of medical expertise. Physicians who have trained at County General often refer back to the experience as though they had been through a war. In a sense, they have.

INSIDE THE BLACK BOX

People come to the hospital with widely varying symptoms, and those who fit a certain clinical profile—fever, night sweats, weight loss, suspicious chest X-ray—may find themselves presumptively diagnosed with tuberculosis. Newly diagnosed TB patients are normally isolated within the hospital for several weeks, and sometimes for as long as two or three months. There they are medicated and observed until appropriate bacteriological tests reveal them to be noninfectious. When the microbiology lab is no longer able to spot any TB bacteria in sputum samples collected from the patient, the patient is deemed to be safe to others. The medicine administered for tuberculosis is very effective at reducing infectiousness quickly, but it takes much longer—six to eighteen months—to cure a patient completely. For most of this period the patient will not be hospitalized, and the completion of treatment therefore depends on the patient's compliance with the prescribed regimen after leaving the hospital.

In the modern medical world, tuberculosis is not a difficult condition to treat. Once the disease is diagnosed, all a physician normally has to do is to prescribe the appropriate medicines, monitor progress, and test for adverse side effects. The only time the treatment really varies is in cases of drug resistance, where the bacteria are resistant to one or more of the standard TB medications. In these cases treatment is more difficult and complicated, and thus more interesting to physicians. Multi-drug-resistant (or MDR) TB is the form which has received the most medical and media attention in the recent TB epidemics. Yet most TB is totally treatable, and therefore boring from a medical point of view.

For the physician, then, tuberculosis is usually a problem with a fairly simple solution: medication. If the disease is diagnosed in a timely fashion, the standard regimen is over 90 percent effective in curing TB. This, of course, assumes that the patient actually takes the medicine as prescribed. As a general rule, compliance with medical regimens is almost always spotty once a patient has left the hospital. Tuberculosis treatment tends to falter after a few months precisely because the patient no longer feels ill, even though the disease persists. Many people do not consider themselves ill unless they are actively suffering symptoms. If the symptoms disappear, they may minimize or avoid ingestion of medications altogether. According to the physician's logic, the problems of patients are ranked in order of urgency, and prominent medical conditions demand the most attention, while the social relations which give rise to them are neglected or ignored (Waitzkin 1989, 228). Thus, problems which are social in origin—poverty, homelessness, drug addiction, street violence, hunger—are not ranked at all, unless they are redefined as medical problems. They are excluded because these are seen as being outside the scope of the doctor's expertise. Yet it is these very factors that are most likely to interfere with the ingestion of medications and complicate the treatment's outcome.

Directly Observed Therapy (DOT), which involves watching patients take their medicine each day in their own homes after they have left the hospital, is the primary method used by big city public health programs to ensure completion of TB treatment. In essence, it involves an extension of medical authority, carrying it out of the hospital, and into the street. Ideally, DOT, like the hospital, functions as a kind of "black box" (Latour and Woolgar 242): a sick patient enters one side, and a patient cured of TB comes out the other. This was the purpose of the program that employed me at County General Hospital. We interviewed individual patients at the time of their initial diagnosis, and tracked them out of the hospital, into the community, until their TB treatment was completed. If it works, the details are unimportant. What happens inside the black box remains shrouded in mystery, in the same way that the process of making a sausage is left largely undiscussed.

By venturing into the community in order to treat patients, however, the DOT worker is able to see them as subjects or agents, to a greater extent than is allowed within the hospital, where their identities and autonomy are temporarily stripped away. Sociologically, the practice of DOT was fascinating because it provided the opportunity to observe the collision of cultures, wills, bodies, and ideas, not only within the artificial environment of the hospital where medicine is obviously dominant, but also in the community where the balance shifts, and the social factors that influence health and illness become unavoidable. Peeking inside the black box, one can see the messiness of the process by which social problems are medicalized and vice versa, and one quickly grasps the absurdity of prescribing medicine for one specific ailment when all the forces that produced it are unchecked. Often it is like recommending a raincoat for a flood.

TB lies at the end of a long winding road of causation, with many contributing factors jumping on along the way. These factors usually remain
on board throughout the duration of the treatment. Unlike the doctor, the
field-worker sees first-hand the social forces at work outside the controlled (and controlling) space of the hospital. Even in these encounters,
the patient may present a "public" as opposed to a "private" account,
presenting what he or she perceives that the medical representative wishes
to see or hear (Cornwell 15–16). Just as likely, however, is the patient's
allowing the field-worker to see her "uncensored" in her social environment. In my own experience, this has meant witnessing the buying and
ingesting of illegal drugs, as well as the ubiquitous consumption of cheap
alcohol and countless cigarettes. It also has involved entering into overcrowded homes where sanitary conditions vary widely, or meeting men
and women who had no homes at all, but slept in boxes, empty vehicles,
or overnight shelters. Having seen patients in these circumstances, and
witnessed their everyday lives, I became somewhat attuned to the perspectives that they carried with them into the hospital.

The hospital and the ghetto are two settings that may be seen as containing separate and distinct American subcultures—the world of the medical professional as opposed to that of the urban underclass. To the casual
observer they might seem as socially distant as noble and serf, although
they are often shown in conflict, as on the television show *ER*. They are
usually studied separately, by sociologists working in entirely different
areas. Neither of these "cultures," however, is either static or monolithic,
and within the public hospital they intersect and interact in a variety of
revealing ways. This chapter examines these interactions not solely as individual conflicts, or problems of medical practice, but also as social struggles preserved in vivo. For these purposes, I will often refer directly to
interviews or field notes that were taken at the time of the event described.

By way of comparison, I will consider the experiences of TB patients
in several locations, primarily in Chicago. There are two main hospitals
that I will make reference to: County General Hospital in Chicago, and
Maple Grove Hospital, located just outside of Chicago. Both of these are
publicly funded institutions that serve similar socioeconomic classes.
This consideration of tuberculosis diagnosis and treatment within institutional settings will help to illustrate how health care practices mediate
the social contexts that surround them. I would like to emphasize that
issues of health and medicine in the American inner city are not separate
from issues of race, gender, poverty, and community, and that all of them
may be seen in relation to the larger forces that have shaped modernity.
The hospital lies at a crucial juncture in this respect, both historically and
symbolically.

"I'LL GO TO JAIL OR HELL"

The hospital is not only a site of care, it is also often an arena of conflict. The following notes are from an interview I conducted in September of 1998 at County General Hospital in Chicago, with a woman whom I will call Juanita. Juanita's case illustrates many of the most extreme attitudes of hostility and distrust that one can imagine existing between a patient, a hospital, and its staff.

First I told her I was from the DOT Program and she launched right into a yelling tirade. Martha (my supervisor) had sent me there to give it a try because a coworker of mine had found her "very uncooperative"; he said that she was denying that she had TB. And so she seemed at first. She said that she would not give out any information on her family, that she wasn't "breathing on nobody," that she didn't have TB, and if she did have it, she said, "If I got it anywhere, I got it in these hospitals. They tried to keep me as a guinea pig, and I'll go to jail or hell, but I won't let them pin this on me."

She went on about how she had been in and out of hospitals for the last six years, and how she had a serious case of lupus, and that the last hospital she visited did not know anything about lupus, but tried to keep her there, she said, "as a guinea pig." She used this phrase both as a noun and as a verb; for example, she said "they tryin' to guinea pig me." I did not interrupt, but listened to her, and occasionally would ask a simple question, such as: "Why do you think they are trying to pin something on you?"

At first I was nearly overwhelmed by the emotion she unleashed. But as I sat and listened, the narrative took shape. Her appearance contributed to the power of her story. She was completely bald, and in the dim light her head looked entirely smooth, though later I noticed that there was some stubble. This and her extreme thinness gave her an asexual, childlike, or other-worldly appearance; her eyes were a little askew, the reverse of cross-eyed, but did not appear the least bit clouded or blind. At one point, to illustrate the fact that she had "no more blood to give," she lifted up the sheets and showed me her legs, pencil-thin and flaking. Her foot was wrapped in a bandage and for a moment I thought she was going to pull it off to show me the damaged flesh underneath.

I tried to get her to specify which hospital she blamed the most, and to establish the source of her anger, because it seemed as though TB was rather tangential. She was most upset that she had been tested up and down at all these different places, had never been found to have TB before, but all of a sudden they were saying that she had it, they were appearing at her house, threatening to lock her up, putting her in a cold isolation room for five days, and so on.

She had spent twenty-eight days in St. Christina's Hospital; she was taken there from her home by ambulance—she would have preferred to go to County General, but the ambulance wouldn't take her there. She became convinced that they were experimenting on her because they wouldn't let her go, and later they claimed, in a report faxed to County General, that she had had a heart attack and a blood transfusion, which she didn't remember having. She said, "my daughters will take a lie-detector test" and swear that she did not have any heart attack. And the doctors there didn't know anything about lupus, which she said was her most pressing condition.

She came to County General for a stomach problem, was in the emergency room for three hours with pain in her stomach, and "then they stuck me in that freezing-ass room for five days. This doctor tried to WOOF me so bad." She paused, asked me if I knew what "WOOF" meant. I said no, and she said, "they tried to frighten me." He tried to tell her she had AIDS, he told her that she had this, she had that, but she didn't believe him, and he couldn't look her in the eye.

"I'm all dry, I ain't got no more blood to draw; they going to scrape me up and put me under a microscope. I'll be dead, and they'll find someone else to experiment on." She kept pointing to the bed across the room, where a woman lay, concealed by the drawn curtain. She said they were experimenting on her, too; she woke one day and couldn't walk, either. She said the girl's hands were shaking like a leaf, and she didn't know what was going on. She said they were experimenting; they gave people syphilis as an experiment, "and that's in the record book."

"That's right," I said, acknowledging the truth of Tuskegee. It is a documented fact that the federal government knowingly withheld treatment for syphilis from 399 black men for a period of forty years, (from 1932 to 1972), just so scientists could study the "natural course" of the disease (Jones 220). This infamous experiment, known as the Tuskegee Study, has placed a permanent cloud of suspicion between black communities and American medical institutions. References to it often arise in regards to the motives of health practitioners, in spite of strict laws ensuring informed consent. This is especially true when one is made subject to multiple unexplained tests, or treated as a "guinea pig."

Juanita complained not only about all the tests, but also about the medications. She said they were making her take seventeen pills at one time and that they kept upping her levels of prednisone, the steroid that they use to treat lupus. She said that the prednisone was too much, that it was making her sick, and she was highly upset about the fact that the doctors simply took the word of the other doctors at St. Christina, without consulting her in the least. They received a medical record by fax and they stuck her in an isolation room, in the freezing cold room with the fan blowing all the time. When she first came, Juanita said, there were "fifty or sixty doctors standing around, all saying something different." She continued without interruption. "You take a look at that girl over there, before you leave. They guinea-pigging her, too." There was a bed with a curtain drawn around it, concealing the patient from view. While we were still talking a doctor came in and stepped inside the curtain. He asked the patient how she was doing but didn't say anything to the rest of us.

Juanita told me how, after they had put her in isolation, they had her drink a big thing that looked and tasted like clear water, but which gave her diarrhea for three days. They did this to clean her out so they could do a rectal procedure, but then they changed their minds, and said they didn't need to do the procedure. Meanwhile, she said, she had lost thirty pounds since going into the hospital and she didn't have any more to give.

Before I left, she shook my hand, said that I was a "decent human being," and that she would welcome me or anybody else that wanted to come to her house. "I apologize for my attitude," she said. "Sometimes a black person can only get attention if they curse. I didn't make up those words, they in the dictionary."

This encounter is deserving of some analysis. Juanita was a woman enduring pain that was not only physical. Even more excruciating for her, perhaps, was the neglect that she perceived, and which she translated as outright malevolence. The crucial point to be understood here is that from the perspective of the patient in pain, neglect and malevolence might as well be the same thing. The other woman in the room clearly stated to me, "They won't let me pee pee," as though it were a form of intentional torture. It certainly may have felt that way to her. Whether or not the lack of urgency concerning her needs was premeditated by the medical staff is perhaps irrelevant. It's always easier to ignore suffering when it's not your own, but people who are sick and poor are more likely to have their questions and feelings dismissed in medical encounters than are their middle class, insured counterparts. The medical system reflects the social chasms of the world outside it, and maintains one standard for the economically empowered and another standard for those who are not (Scully 10).

Nonetheless, Juanita's accusations are serious, and should be examined in turn. The first thing she said to me had to do with her TB. "If I got it anywhere," she said, "I got it in these hospitals." This is a comment which could easily be disregarded as an example of projected anger. But if one actually considers the statement as a hypothesis, it is entirely plausible. It is a well-known fact of infection control that many disease transmissions occur in nosocomial settings, that is, within hospitals or other health care institutions. The reason is simple: hospitals are places where sick people are grouped together. Juanita's suspicion that she may have caught TB in the hospital is a genuine possibility. The outbreaks that brought TB back into the media spotlight in the early 1990s, for example, all originated within hospitals. Patients with immune disorders are especially vulnerable, and lupus, though less commonly discussed than AIDS, is also a disease which affects the immune system.

Black people have historically been neglected or ignored by the medical profession, unless they were perceived as a threat to the health of others (Trattner 148). Many studies have shown that black Americans still receive poorer medical care in general than do white Americans (Watson 1993; Brooks et al. 1991). Thus, black Americans have a different set of expectations when it comes to health care, and for very good reasons: they tend to be viewed and treated in qualitatively different ways than white patients (Blendon 1995; Scully 132). Juanita's concern about the misdiagnosis of her lupus, therefore, is not simply a flight of paranoia. Lupus affects black Americans three times as often as white Americans, and most of those who suffer from it are women. Diagnosis of lupus is quite difficult, requiring a complete review of medical history and a series of laboratory tests. It is quite conceivable that, between her movement from hospital to hospital, and the regular rotation of medical staff, important information concerning her case might have been lost. Just because they poke and prod and bleed and tweak patients to no apparent end, and take notes every step of the way, it doesn't mean that hospitals have complete or even accurate information.

The fear of being a "guinea pig" is not without justification, either. Aside from the ugly legacy of the Tuskegee Study, there are other historical instances where poor black folks—especially prisoners—have been used as objects of medical research on diseases such as malaria and leukemia (Abraham 204). The medical profession still uses people for its own purposes. For example, it is a fact of modern medical education that public hospitals serve as a patient pool for the training of student physicians. Attending physicians maintain distinct boundaries between public and private patients, and only the most advanced residents are allowed to touch the latter (Becker 263; Scully 122). Students, however, place a high priority on gaining direct experience, and on exercising "medical responsibility," which can only come from performing procedures and forming diagnoses on actual patients (Becker 254).

Guinea Pigs or Fetal Pigs?

Poor patients in public hospitals commonly serve as fodder for the medical student's learning curve, making them functionally equivalent to fetal pigs (objects of examination), if not guinea pigs (objects of experimentation). They are often reduced, in the daily rush of the hospital routine, to living illustrations of particular medical problems, another factor which contributes to their objectification and depersonalization (Scully 118). As modern medical dramas such as *ER* and *Chicago Hope* vividly demonstrate, the physician is still popularly idealized in American society as an individual "uniquely qualified" to address the crises of disease and injury (Jouellet 1). The corollary of this image of the doctor as active subject, again, is the reduction of the patient to a passive object who awaits the doctor's magical ministrations (Jouellet 2). In his book *Beyond Caring,* Daniel Chambliss depicts the hospital as an institution which maintains its moral order through the "routinization of disaster," minimizing the chaos naturally attendant to sickness and death by establishing practices which become priorities unto themselves, apart from their declared purposes (Chambliss 12). The "routine" is what medical staff rely on when all else seems to be falling apart around them; it allows them to convert the chaos into something they can control: "In accommodating herself to the radically different world of the hospital, the nurse comes to routinize her experience there, learning the techniques and the people, developing methods for coping with emergencies, training herself to survive disaster and keep working in the midst of appalling tragedy" (Chambliss 55).

An ironic, unfortunate, yet nonetheless natural corollary of the routinization of disaster is the degradation of the autonomy and dignity of the patient. According to Chambliss, "Patients are institutionally objectified: detached from their own lives and life stories, physically taken from their home settings, behaviorally managed as a conglomerate of discrete parts to be treated by different specialists" (Chambliss 120). The fact that human beings are converted into "patients" by entering the domain of the hospital is itself revelatory. The very establishment of a Patients' Bill of Rights, which has become common in American hospitals, testifies to the fact that those rights granted to all citizens are often suspended when their lives are dominated by the need for medical care (Chambliss 145). The following excerpt from an interview with Lester, a TB patient, illustrates what it feels like to be at the center of the maelstrom of medical activity that concludes with a diagnosis:

> It got to a point where I couldn't breathe that properly, I couldn't even do that. So . . . I said I think I better go to the hospital. Then it seemed like my feets got numb, every now and then it'd get numb, I'd get a shock wave down through my legs. I say, something wrong, so . . . I got to the hospital, County, emergency part, one day I sit up there and got nauseated and then when I coughed, seemed like some phlegm-water come out of my nose a little bit, reddish water, it wasn't blood, it was reddish water, that was, I found out later, Doctor said that was my lung, I was coughin' the stuff out

my lung, it was overfillin'. So that night, in the emergency room, they did some emergency minor surgery, where I had to take my shirt off, and they got some kind of drawing needles, and, uh, it don't hurt, they stuck it in my skin back there in the back, and down into my lung, it was a long needle, like, like acupuncture in other words, but it got a hole in it where it was drain, and they drained two big, uh, vials they called it, of bloody water out of my lungs, cause they do 'em both sides, I had two of 'em, and so then, after they did that, I started, I could breathe a little better, then they said, "Yeah, well we're gonna have to admit you," I said, "Okay." So they took me upstairs and they put me on some IV medication. Then they say, "You look awful skinny," you know, cause I'd lost a lot of weight, cause I didn't have no appetite. And so they ran tests, blood tests, I had about, for the first three days I was there, every other hour, they were feeding me liquid at first, cause I didn't have no appetite to eat nothin', they used to bring the food in, the other guy in the next room, next to me, that's before they found out I had the 'berkolosis, cause then they put me in quarantine, you know, but before then, I used to smell the food and get sick up the stomach. I wasn't throwin' up nothin', wasn't nothin' down there to throw up. So I'd just get nauseated, and so then, after that, 'nother test, 'nother test, and 'bout, by 'bout the, they made sure by almost a week, they come back and told me, "You got to be moved." I said, "For what?" They said, "The doctor come and tell you," that's what the nurses told me, they wouldn't tell me at first. So they took me to . . . IC (intensive care) unit, in the County, that's what part it was, but they had a big old window there where they could watch, and they put all that stuff up to me, hook up machines where they could look on the monitor, the nurse couldn't even be in there with me, at the time 'less they had a mask on, after I find out, she was like sitting out there in the thing monitoring my vital signs, then a doctor come in with a mask, and told me, say, "You have, uh, high grade tuberculosis."

This account reveals the extent to which a patient's symptoms and conditions become subject to standardized procedure, which the patient witnesses almost as though he were an outsider. He politely waits for an explanation, while his body is stuck, probed, and monitored as though it were an unknown specimen. One can imagine how alienating this could be, and how a less-congenial patient might respond. Another patient, a forty-year-old black woman named Linda, was more vocal in her dislike of such treatment:

The worst thing I ever got in the hospital, was getting shots every day, and drawing blood from me. I couldn't even sleep right. Getting blood and shit from me, damn, every day, they had to have blood and shit. Chemistry and all that type of shit. And the IV, I hate that with a passion. And every time, it was mostly every morning, every other morning, I'd have . . . a room full of doctors. Even down to the Indian doctors. Different kinds, standing over me, waking me up. What?! Are you snapping? I didn't know what all.

Damn! Give me a break. Most I hated was sticking them needles in you every day, getting all that blood and shit, it don't take that damn much to test nothing. Doctors kept coming back and forth to the room, goddam, just that quick, same thing, feel like I'm forgetting something. I never did care about that food neither.

Patients, as human beings with a desire for freedom and autonomy, naturally resist the manipulative mechanics of the hospital at times, the same way they resist the discipline of other systems designed to control them (Chambliss 135). As Juanita so bluntly stated, "Sometimes a black person can only get attention if they curse." Many individuals, like Juanita, recognize that the chaos they cause may be the only bargaining chip they have.

In the late 1960s, Anselm Strauss argued that massive medical institutions have an inherent tendency toward complex, impersonal bureaucracy. "The poor," he wrote, "with their meager experience in organizational life, their insecurity in the middle-class world, and their dependence on personal contacts, are especially vulnerable to this impersonalization" (Strauss 266). One might say that the public hospital is the place where the rationalist, internationalist world view of modern professional medicine encounters the local and insular world of the poor. But the alienation and antipathy so often seen between medicine and poor patients is not merely a matter of scale and complexity, for which the poor are unprepared, as though they were naive primitives. The strained relationship between medicine and poor people is also imbued with power relations and prejudices carried over from the larger society.

According to Doug Glasgow, ". . . notoriously overcrowded, inadequately staffed and managed county and city hospitals" form part of a "bungling, corrupt bureaucracy increasing the hardship and discomfort of the poor who seek health care" (Glasgow 13). For Glasgow, the public health system is merely one in a set of networks which play a prominent role in both monitoring and maintaining the urban underclass, the other main culprits being the welfare system and criminal justice system. Juanita's bitter complaints reflect a heightened sensitivity to the sort of surveillance which takes place in the hospital: not only visual surveillance, but also chemical and invasive surgical surveillance. In a certain sense, doctors take your blood so they don't have to take your word—especially when there is suspicion of drug abuse, pregnancy, or sexual disease.

The objectification of the patient is experienced more nakedly by poor, disempowered, and stigmatized populations, and the public health system in particular plays a role in the societal surveillance of poor populations. But is such treatment unique to these populations? According to Laurie Abraham, "Impoverished black women are not . . . the only people who complain about being befuddled by doctors. All classes and races often perceive doctors as aloof technicians who confuse patients with scientific jargon rather than engage them in meaningful give-and-take about their prognoses and treatments" (Abraham 201). As Timothy Diamond demonstrates in his nursing home ethnography *Making Gray Gold,* even the education of nursing assistants—who themselves are mostly women drawn from racial and ethnic minorities—tends to view patients as the objects of "professional" practices. A nursing assistant instructor, whom Diamond calls "Mr. Store," tells the students in his class: "When you get out on that floor I want to hear some technical terms, some professionalism, like 'ectomy' and 'osomy.' Don't say a patient is 'mean', say he's 'acting inappropriately.' Don't say 'touching', say 'tactile communication'" (Diamond 26). The irony of low-paid nursing assistants being indoctrinated with the language of professionalism without receiving any of its benefits reinforces the idea that there is a basic thrust toward "depersonalization" throughout the health care system.

POOR HISTORIANS

It is revealing that doctors, in their chart notes, refer to certain patients as "poor historians," meaning that their stories cannot be trusted, either because they have muddled memories or because they are unreliable. Not surprisingly, these patients are often literally poor as well. When it comes to the importance of any history—individual, institutional or social—outside that which directly relates to the illness at hand, however, health professional themselves are pretty lousy historians. This is true on both the macro- and the micro-level. As McBride has argued concerning the profession of health history, ". . . current scholarship is so sparse on sociomedical developments and health patterns of urban blacks that it provides virtually no background upon which to assess the current diffusion of AIDS throughout the black community . . ." (McBride 3). If such historical study has not been undertaken, even as spending on AIDS research has soared, it is safe to presume that the average practicing physician has not engaged in it. History is not as important to the profession as hysterectomy.

On a personal level, physicians may actively avoid discussing problems which lie outside their purview, such as economic problems, housing problems, problems of physical or substance abuse, and spiritual issues. According to Arthur Frank, "The immediate conflict is between what the physician believes he can't 'even get into' with his patient and the issues that the patient cannot avoid because they are her life" (Frank 1997, 145). Medicine is concerned with identifying and treating disease as an abstract entity; to do so, it must define disease abstractly, as a set of transferable and identifiable characteristics, outside of human experience and human history. At the same time, however, it conveniently ignores the disruptive effects that result from the imposition of a biomedical world view upon human beings (Frank 1997, 145).

This brings us back to the relationship of medicine to human communities in general. American hospitals in particular have evolved along with an increasingly specialized and technologically oriented medical profession, changing from charitable community-supported institutions to capital-intensive bureaucratic research centers. According to Charles Rosenberg, hospitals became medicalized as medicine became hospitalized (Rosenberg 12). Medical sociologist Eugene Gallagher has asked whether or not such "impersonalization" is part and parcel of capitalist modernity, which takes a greater toll on the poor, but affects everybody: "Is medical dignity simply another aspect of the rootless, anomic individual who has, through the vast changes inherent in urbanization and industrialization, been cast out from the earlier security of belonging within a place, a community and a value habitus? Is medical dignity a byproduct of a civilization that requires more radical communal restructuring than simply making medical care more abundant?" (Gallagher 228). Like the Patient Bill of Rights, the concept of "medical dignity" was probably invented to counter the alienating tendencies endemic to the modern medical system. But the fundamental question posed by Gallagher, which is central to health care, is little asked in our present-day society. People are so accustomed to thinking of technological medicine as a practical necessity that they don't often ask why this is so, and what implications it might have for human beings and their communities. Instead, they engage in heated debates about whether or not the services of modern medicine are better treated as human rights or as negotiable commodities. In either case, the nature of medicine itself, as a defining industrial institution, is left uninterrogated.

What Polanyi claimed concerning the institution of the "free market" might also be argued of modern medicine: to exist, it requires the destruction or marginalization of other ways of living (Polanyi 163). Medicine as an institution is emblematic of an essentially modernist culture, an atomized, individualized, and rationalistic culture. In the same way that the introduction of modern markets into traditional societies introduces new forms of poverty and unemployment, which cannot themselves be resolved through the expansion of those markets, attempting to "fix" communities or cultures through the provision of more modern medicine is an exercise in futility. Instead, it simply maintains them in the state of sickness: each "fix" requires another, in an unending spiral, like a drug addiction. This is the argument taken up by Illich, in typically dramatic fashion: "New sickness was defined and institutionalized; the cost of enabling people to survive in unhealthy cities and in sickening jobs skyrocketed. The monopoly of the medical profession was extended over an increasing range of everyday occurrences in every man's life" (Illich 1973, 2–3). Illich's vision of medicine as an industrial appendage which keeps people in their place is frightening and extreme, but it provides a useful way of framing certain questions.

Though an ancient disease, tuberculosis has piggy-backed on the convulsive processes that accompanied the advent of modernity: industrialization, urbanization, war, and immigration. Traditional, that is, preantibiotic, treatments for TB implicitly recognized the connections between these larger circumstances and individual cases of disease, and sought to address them, albeit on the individual level, through altering culture, lifestyle, or environment. This is why so many young men headed for the hills in pursuit of the "fresh air cure" when diagnosed with consumption: they were seeking to de-industrialize themselves. Prominent physicians of the time, such as Edward Trudeau and William Osler, also embraced the notion that a rural, "out-of-doors" lifestyle was inherently more healthy than a cramped urban existence (Rothman 200–201). Such regimens were notoriously inconsistent at curing tuberculosis, but they did hold the promise of radical change within the lifeworld of the patient, introducing him or her to a new set of habits or experiences. Antibiotic therapy, though remarkably effective at curing disease, often does so while leaving the patient in exactly the same position as before. The modern hospital is designed as a space where "medicine takes place," where pills and injections are delivered, surgeries performed, and results measured, and not as a place where people are healed or transformed in any way beyond the purely physical. It operates (so to speak) not through the social and the cultural worlds of its patients, but in spite of them. And if the two conflict, it is the patients who must comply.

The remainder of this chapter approaches the issue of medicine and its interactions with the poor from this perspective: Rather than simply cataloging the abuses or triumphs of the medical system, and people's frustration or satisfaction with it, this chapter examines these issues with an eye toward the broader issues raised by Illich. It also addresses Gallagher's more speculative question: namely, What role does medicine and its institutional manifestation, the hospital, play in the history and life of larger communities? And, in turn, how does the surrounding culture influence the relations inside the hospital? Using the methods of ethnography, this chapter attempts to come to terms with both the little and big questions contained in these relationships.

THE HOSPITAL AND THE STREET

The facade of County General Hospital at the end of the twentieth century, when I worked there, had a certain faded dignity, somewhat like a Roman ruin. In this case, however, the ruin was still in operation. The interior of the hospital featured a mix of state-of-the art-medical technology and antiquated layout, with many patients lying in open wards or cubicles divided only by cloth partitions. County General's clientele came from all over the city and surrounding suburbs, because only at County General could they find comprehensive care regardless of their ability to pay for it. The poor rode buses long distances to get there, and often they regarded it as their hospital.

In *Bargaining for Life*, Barbara Bates chronicled the social history of TB in the United States from 1876 to 1938. About the treatment of poor TB patients in nineteenth-century North America, she wrote: "Despite hesitations and doubts, by choice or the force of circumstance, on foot, by rail, or by horse-drawn ambulance, poor consumptives came to the few institutions in Philadelphia that would accept them. Although the various places involved in the work differed in important ways, they all offered shelter, food, nursing care, medical attention, congregate living and a certain degree of regimentation" (Bates 63). Similarly, a former medical director has stated that County General Hospital "was always a place where the most recent poverty group was taken care of . . . By the mid-Sixties eighty percent of the Blacks born in the city were born at County; fifty percent of Black deaths were in that one hospital—of the whole city! . . . County was the only one that really absorbed the Blacks and made it possible for breathtaking racial exclusion to be practiced every day in Chicago hospitals" (Lewis 87).

Today County General remains a hospital that serves a predominantly black, Latino and poor population, though there are plenty of other groups represented there as well. For Chicagoans, County General occupies an iconic position; for the poor, it's the place where you can always go, for the better-off, it's the place you don't want to end up. As one housekeeper said, ". . . it's like a dumping zone. County is like a trash catcher—they dump all they trash on us" (Lewis 32). According to one doctor, County is "for the people who fall through all other coverage—who, for a variety of reasons, aren't acceptable to be treated at private facilities: either because of their total inability to pay, or the severity of their illness, or because they're unacceptable for other reasons—which could be drugs, alcohol, tuberculosis, sexually transmitted diseases . . ." (Lewis 133). It is a reservoir for the residuum, a refuge for those whom the private health system by-and-large excludes.

But County General is not only a vitally needed medical facility for the poor, it is also an important social center. For hundreds of homeless men and women, it is a regular stop on the "tramp trail," a place where one can find a degree of warmth and peace during the colder months, though this varies with the level of police repression. County General also supports a small informal economy, where one can find cookies, candy, peanuts, bags of fruit, or even jewelry on sale in the hallways or outside the hospital at various times. At County General, patients in either the emergency room or the day clinics can wait hours at a time before they see anybody other than a clerk. A certain amount of socializing within the hospital, then, is not only possible, but necessary. In many cases, these relations may be carried over directly from the community or the street. The hospital then imposes an artificial and temporary separation.

The following excerpt from my field notes shows a patient having difficulty with the transition from street to hospital, something which he confided in me because I had known him in the street before he came to the hospital.

2/2/98

... Stormy says that at County, nobody does anything on time, and people always come into his room, yelling at him about stuff and then getting mad when he doesn't understand it right away. "This social worker was in here a couple days ago, and I swear, I can't remember a single thing she said to me. The only time they on time is when they want to cut you . . ."

He is still getting nauseous from the smell of his hospital-cooked food and attributes it to the meds he is taking, the big white PZA and EMB pills in particular. "On the street I have no problem eating," he says.

The cultural dislocation that hospitalization entails, here centering on the issue of food choice, is usually unaddressed by the institution. Hospital food is notoriously unpopular, and even nutritious food yields no benefit if it remains uneaten. Many patients ask relatives to bring food in to them, and when these networks of support are active, they can provide a good deal of compensation for the hospital's alienating effects. These effects are often even more severe for TB patients. This is due both to the specifics of TB treatment and to the extreme social marginality of many people who suffer from TB.

ISOLATION AND MEDICALIZATION

Cases of active pulmonary tuberculosis at County General (assuming that they were detected, which they usually were by the mid-1990s) were not placed on the open wards but in isolation rooms, where ventilation systems and ultraviolet lights are employed to prevent any possibility of transmission to other patients or hospital staff. People entering these isolation rooms to visit or treat TB patients are required to don masks which are intended to filter any aerosolized TB bacteria from entering their bodies via the nose or mouth. Warning signs posted outside the door remind one to practice this precaution. This practice of isolation, though it fulfills infection control criteria, also has the unfortunate effect of separating the patient socially from other patients and hospital staff, both of whom tend to minimize the length of their visits due to risk of contagion, however slight. This naturally has a disconcerting effect on the patient. According to one TB patient, whom I will call Tara, being in isolation was: "Really, like, crazy . . . cause they like isolate you, off from people, so all you do is have time left to think, you know? So I was in a depressed stage when I got through that . . . I get depressed, you know? I try not to think about it . . . Best to be strong and not worry about it . . ."

Doctors' focus on diagnosis and treatment of disease may lead them to neglect the patient's own feelings of health or illness. For example, one patient of mine was quite angry when the doctors at County General wanted to lance a cyst over his eye. He had been hospitalized while suffering from acute tuberculosis and pneumonia, and was most concerned with addressing those conditions so he could go back to his job selling newspapers. He was concerned that he might lose his regular spot at a busy intersection if he was away too long. More than anything else, he wanted to be back on the street in time for his birthday, so he could make some money and drink malt liquor on the park bench by himself, as he had planned. The cyst over his eye was not impairing his daily function, and he did not view it as an immediate problem. For him, it was not a pressing illness, whereas for the doctors it represented a form of disease, an abnormality to be eliminated. His job selling papers and his desire to drink malt liquor, one might presume, were not perceived as important matters by the physician, at least not when compared to the cyst. He criticized the doctors for not being more straightforward in their approach to him, and his critique was in some ways quite thorough. I have included some of his comments below. I will call him Ted.

> He . . . he sat down, he came in and said "I need some more blood." Man, you just got my blood day before yesterday. You don't need no blood, man. He got another dude with him, right, another doctor, come here or something, and he said, "let me check it." Get up and let him, you know, he talkin' all this shit, I got up and let him check it and shit . . . . Man I have more trouble with these goddam doctors, man . . . I really think he got pissed off, cause I said: I really think y'all know don't what y'all doing.

On the other hand, he respected those physicians who treated him in a straightforward manner:

> . . . don't get me wrong, I ain't talkin' about all of 'em. Like that damn man downstairs, that damn man good. Doctor Hill? To me. You know, he came in, man, told me exactly what was wrong with me, told me exactly what, hey, you got the tuberculosis, told me, hey, man, you might got pneumonia.

He respected Dr. Hill, he said, because he came right in and told him what he thought was wrong and what he was going to do, and he did it. He had come into the hospital sick and in need of help, and Dr. Hill had addressed his problem in a straightforward way. I asked him to elaborate on the problems he had with the doctors. He then went on to talk about some other doctors whom he did respect: doctors he remembered from his home town in Mississippi:

> I got some doctors in my hometown, they'll look at you and tell you, man, you sick. They'll tell you and then know what's wrong with you—without even touching you . . . they would look at you man, especially if they had seen you, you know, say, Hey something's wrong with you.

In these cases, the doctor's ability to identify a problem is closely tied to his or her personal relationship with the patient. The doctor should be able to ascertain an irregularity through a cursory examination; not with the aid of sophisticated tests, but with the art of observation informed by experience and long-term relations with individuals in the community. These were doctors, he told me, who had known him since he was a child. This ideal image of the doctor is thus tied to an ideal of community as well. This idealized community may not exist, but an image of it, often associated with villages or neighborhoods of the past, remains strong.

The institutionally based doctor, unlike the family doctor, treats the patient as a potential nest of problems, which need to be sampled and analyzed. The insight of the physician into the individual person is absent here. This alienated relationship can then be worsened by feelings of hostility, which became manifest in Ted's case. He was referred to in the charts as being angry and uncooperative, and was recommended for psychiatric consultation. He was a very large and loud man, and came across as being belligerent. I asked Ted—whom I quite liked, by the way—why he had, according to the chart, threatened to kill one of his physicians. I told him I was disappointed in that language and he tried to explain.

> I don't never want to kill nobody, man, but see, hey man, when I'm in a situation that, hey man, that I know I ain't did nothin', and I want my freedom, man, I want to be out there, and he up there, man, bull-jivin', goin' all the way around the situation, then hey, there's somethin' wrong. That's

all I'm sayin' man, I don't ever want to kill nobody, but hey man, if I come straight up to tell you, hey man, I want to be out of here . . . But what I'm sayin' is this: hey, I don't wanna go through . . . the rest of my medical history man, you know: "What's wrong with you, what's wrong with this right here, what's wrong?" Man, look, that ain't none of my problem now. You know, take my problem and handle it.

Ted seems to be saying that he wants his problems treated categorically, as separate diagnoses, rather than sharing all of his medical history. More precisely, he is expressing a desire that the doctor might handle his most urgent problem first, with respect for the freedom and autonomy that he was voluntarily surrendering. This is not necessarily different from the doctor's mentality, except that in this case the doctor and the patient had different ideas about which problem should be addressed, and when. By ignoring the patient's concerns, the doctor makes the patient feel like an object or a child. In the following comments Ted elaborates some more on the ways that his treatment as a patient makes him feel:

When people tell you, when your nurse tell you, "Go to your room!" I don't want that shit, see, that hurts your feelings. And, you know, your doctor, man . . . they should . . . tell you more about this disease than try to jump to another decision on you, another thing about your body system. They should sit up and talk to you about this, you know . . . I told you I needed the support from you, and I found that I got a lot of support from him, with this disease, man, not from no doctor. Not no skeazy-ass doctor. That what I call 'em.

Ted is referring to those people who actually sat and listened to him: one of them was a staff psychiatrist, and the other one was me. I reminded him that a psychiatrist is a doctor, but he wanted to make the distinction anyway. The distinction, therefore, seemed to lie not in the title as much as in the method, the approach. His problems with the "doctors" centered on their failure to recognize that he had a life outside of the hospital, and that he was capable of contributing to the assessment of his own problems. For this recognition to occur, dialogue had to take place: the doctors needed to offer information to the patient, and they needed to show concern for his feelings and respect for his judgment.

Similar criticisms were made by other patients, such as Wendell, not only in regard to doctors, but also concerning nurses:

I was in there about twelve days . . . they keep you nearly a month. But they was giving me thirteen, fourteen, some days I was taking nineteen pills. And they would come in there, I say, I say Miss, I can't take all these pills at once . . . I said I ain't never know nobody to take no nineteen pills all at once. They had me take twelve or thirteen pills, take 'em all down after you eat, and they'd walk out . . . Now I questioned some of them, they had to tell me why I was taking those pills, and what the pills consisted of, I thought they OWED me that, to let me know. Or send a doctor in there, to explain to me what the hell I was taking. That mama would come in there, throw them pills at me, say "Yes, take'em, Take ALL of 'em" when you had your breakfast. And I, I know that's wrong, cause I throw up sometimes, when I take them damn pills . . .

Again, the main issue raised here is one of information and concern: not enough information coming from the doctors and nurses, and not enough concern about the patient's feelings. But the orientation of the provider is, often enough, simply toward the achievement of medical goals: in this case, the ingestion of the pills. In purely technical terms, there is nothing wrong with this approach. The fear, discomfort, and perhaps most importantly, the boredom of the patient is not considered a medical problem, and therefore no steps are taken to address it. Another patient, Claudia, expressed disappointment with the doctors' chosen mode of communication:

. . . some of the doctors I got along with and some of the doctors I didn't get along with. Some of 'em, it was just the way that they talk to you, and they say, like, "well, you got to take this medicine, if you don't take this medicine, you gonna die!" You know, and then I was like, well, damn, they can't say it a better way than that? . . . some of 'em that I got along with, but the part that I didn't get along with them when they made cracks, and they come in the observation room, and they know that it's beautiful outside, sun beaming and everything, I'm looking at this window, okay, and knowing that I could be outside, "Well, it's a beautiful day, I think we're gonna put this shade down cause it's so bright in here," you know, and I would get pissed off, cause you knowing the situation that I'm in, why would you say that? And you know I'm gonna curse if you don't get out of here, that's the type of person I was, you know, so . . . but I had to learn to deal with it, but like I said, some of the doctors I got along with, some of 'em I didn't.

It must be stated that these are not randomly selected cases. I chose them to illustrate problems in communication which arise often, though not necessarily in such extreme form. Many patients report no complaints about their treatment in the hospital. Some, such as Lewis, have almost nothing but good things to say:

Oh they treated me nice. They treated me real nice. You know, I ate good, had a TV in the room, it was real nice, you know. Everybody treated me real nice, you know . . . Mostly. Ninety-nine percent of the people treated me nice. You know, you gonna run into, as we say, bad apple or a pony, you know. I don't expect everybody to agree with things I do, or you know, you're gonna have conflict with different people, so I say basically, it was real nice. They looked after me while I was in the hospital, you know, they treated me real nice, they gave me gowns, gave me soap, stuff to shave with, you know. I felt, felt like at home, you know? It was a nice experience, you know.

Another patient, José, expressed a similar appreciation for the treatment he received:

> Oh, they take care of me pretty good here. They give me my medication, they take care of my temperature; they're always checkin' up on me to see if I'm doin' all right. And they feed me good. And they check on me here at night, see how my temperature . . . my temperature's gettin' better, it was real bad. So far it's been like two days without a temperature. It's been okay. So, I guess I'm, I'm feeling a lot better. I hope, hopefully, maybe, today's Wednesday, maybe by Friday they'll let me go. Hopefully. Cause I'm feeling good. But it's up to them.

The last line in that passage from José is indicative of the sense in which many patients surrender themselves to the presumably benevolent discretion of the medical staff: "It's up to them." But such feelings can waver over time, and may not remain entirely consistent as the duration of a hospital stay stretches on. A few weeks after the above interview was conducted, I spoke to José again, and he expressed a different attitude. He was becoming frustrated after thirty-seven days in the hospital, waiting to be medically cleared. I went to visit him in his isolation room and instead found him sitting out by the payphones with his mask on. I asked if he was waiting for a phone call and he said that he was just getting out of the room. He said the doctor didn't explain anything to him: "he just comes in, listens to my chest, and leaves."

Another patient, John, made even stronger accusations. He was being treated at a long-term care facility where he was shipped after spending several weeks at the county hospital. His comments here relate to the care he received in the second hospital, as compared to his experience at County General:

> This place, here . . . defeats your purpose of getting well . . . They said that I would really enjoy Maple Grove Hospital, that it was a nice place, and this that and blah that and blah-zee this . . . you know, just like it was Wonderland. I had a nurse. You know, TB makes me sweat. So I done sweated the whole bed. I called my night nurse, tell her that I'm wet, that I need my bed changed, she told me she don't do beds, that I'm gonna have to wait til the first shift come to get my bed changed. And I'm saying, you mean I got to lay up here in this wet bed, until the first shift, cause YOU don't do beds? And she had a attitude and told me yeah and hung up. So I had to get up and get me some sheets to put over this wet stuff, and get me a blanket, and

lay on top till the first shift came on. Cause, see, I talked to the supervisor, and uh, I guess she got in her shit, cause if her eyes had been guns, I'd a been dead. (Laughs) Then they start comin' in and, "You need anything John?" and, you know, but that was about a week, and now they back to they same old thing.

The poor, especially the welfare-dependent poor, experience such disregard regularly (Harrison 1983, 257). Such conflicts can breed resentment on both sides of the relationship. Differences in class, gender, or ethnicity can aggravate it further (Lewis 5).

The ethnographic material included here is meant to illustrate the importance of the social environment—inclusive of political, cultural, and economic relations—as a component of health and disease in all of those locations where treatment takes place. Tuberculosis is a disease which disproportionately affects the poor, and in turn, contributes to continuing poverty (Harrison 1979, 288). Even in the most marginal occupations, such as gathering junk or selling papers, a certain minimum of physical stamina is necessary for survival. Only in the art of panhandling is an injury or illness a possible plus, and even then it is a dubious tradeoff. For the poor TB patient in Chicago, the disease may simply be another in a long list of personal problems, and it may not even be the most life-threatening, even if it is medically defined as such. For the hustler, an episode of tuberculosis may provide a respite from the harsh and debilitating social environment of the street. The socioeconomic maladies of poverty and inequality precede and surround the myriad illnesses, including TB, which afflict poor people. This link is not simple and linear, but dynamic and complex, and deserves further attention. The dynamic varies, not only across cultures, but also across history.

"San" Memories

Interestingly enough, two patients whom I interviewed in Chicago had experienced tuberculosis in two different eras. Both of these men had very fond memories of the sanatorium where they spent time in the 1970s. It was a large public facility run by nuns, and was situated on a sizeable piece of land in the northwest part of the city. I had first heard about this place from John, the same man quoted above. Initially he described it in a somewhat critical manner:

> They sent me to the sanatorium, matter of fact, they shot me in my arm, and a big huge knot jumped out on my arm, so they hurried up and sent me to the sanatorium. And this sanatorium was . . . way up north, and it was run by [the mayor's] brother, and a lot of times if they didn't have actual people that had TB, they would go on Skid Row, and get winos, and bring

them in, because they were ran by the state, and so the state paid for a head-count. Now, they had, they weren't even physicians, I think these guys was just in training, up on the third floor, cause they were lookin' to cut on peo-ple. They also had people that were permanent. That permanently lived there. Now, at the time, I was cool, I did what was required, I got my INH shot, I take my little walk, out in the unrestricted area, and find me a tree, and cool out.

When I asked him more about the environment of the sanatorium, he said:

Oh, that place was huge. It was mammoth. You had, they had they own theater, like you go to a theater downtown or something? They had they own theater. They had, uh, they had restricted, they had so much land, they had restricted areas and stuff. Like I said, I personally, I liked it there. I was having a nice time. It was just my stupid old doctor, that I couldn't get along with, cause she thought I was going to get drunk, and I'm telling her, I don't even drink. I just got married, here I am charged up cause I finally got three negatives, I finally got the weekend to go home, and she gonna tell me no. Cause if I go home, I'll get drunk. That kinda made me snap . . .

It is worth noting that it was not the institution that alienated the patient in this case, but the doctor, whose presumptions about the patient's behavior were imposed over his own knowledge of himself. The institu-tion itself was remembered fondly. Donald, a fifty-year-old African Amer-ican quoted earlier in this chapter, had also been to the "san" on the northwest side. He compared it to the contemporary hospital in this way:

I did my time there . . . I didn't like it there, but it wasn't someplace you would really dread. You can't really compare because that was a different place, they didn't take care of but one thing out there . . . and then the time was different. This is a different era. Now they downsizing, they want to use less people to do more work and all. Everybody's loaded down . . . I worked on an assembly line and they did the same thing—more work and no help.

Another man, whom I met a year later, and who was also sent to Maple Grove after a stint at County General, also had some comments to make about both places. Boris was a Serbian immigrant who was sent to the sanatorium shortly after moving to the United States. I wanted to know more about the similarities and differences between the hospitals he had been in recently—County General and Maple Grove—and the sanato-rium where he was in the seventies.

"How do you like this place?" I asked, about Maple Grove.

He said, "They put you here like a dog. They don't even bring you food; I had to call to get my breakfast, and an hour later they brought me something. They lock you in like a dog. At least at County General people come to visit, the doctors come in. Here you could die. You have to call, you know."

I then asked him about the place where he spent some time with TB in 1973.

"It was nice and quiet, the food was good. I gained thirty-five pounds in twenty-one days when I was there. You could do things, make purses, wallets, fix things, learn mechanics, take classes."

"What about this place?" I asked.

"Nobody cares in this place. Employees don't give a shit."

"Can't you walk around outside here?"

"One guy came in and asked me if I wanted to go for a walk. I like to walk, but I don't want to go out in the hall with a mask on and everyone looking at me."

"How was the staff at the hospital in the seventies?"

"It was like a family over there; everything was so nice, so friendly, like a family."

"You were just a young guy, then, right?"

"Yeah, I was young, I didn't speak no English, but it didn't matter. I hang around with the black people, we share things. One guy I remember, his name was William, would jump over the fence, he would go buy liquor. He was a big guy, seven feet tall."

He smiled, remembering his time in the sanatorium.

The language of contrast here is striking. At one place, he says he is treated "like a dog." The other place he remembers being "like a family." Granted, some families are quite close with their dogs, but we can safely presume that he is not equating the two. Instead, he is making a distinction between two very different ways of doing medicine, and two very different cultural environments of care. In one place, the patient feels like he is one of a group. In the other place, he is sectioned off and made to feel like a caged animal. Though he might want to venture forth from his room, the necessity of wearing a mask, marking him as a TB patient, makes him unwilling to do so. He is afraid because he senses that other people are afraid of him. Donald's comparison of the contemporary hospital to an "assembly line" is also relevant. Workers on an assembly line do not have time to spend on individual products.

At the sanatorium, Boris had had no reason to feel singled out and stigmatized: everyone there was in the same situation, though some were better and some were worse cases. Activities were available, not necessarily as a means of "therapy," but as opportunities for recreation, learning, and creativity. Classes were not given to achieve a medical goal, but as something interesting in and of themselves. Seen from this perspective, the sanatorium of the 1970s is the more convivial setting (to borrow a term from Illich). The hospital of the 1990s, though superior in its technical capabilities, is lacking in capability for fulfilling the needs that a social environment—even an impoverished one—might provide. In the same way that the bland but nutritionally "correct" food of the hospital fails to satisfy the patient's hunger as a Polish sausage eaten on the street would do, so does the extension of professionalized "care" fail to satisfy a basic human need for belonging, for acceptance, for sociability.

"QUIET, I'M WRITING . . ."

I would like to give an example of at least one physician whose approach and outlook was markedly different from those described above. She was a senior physician in the Department of Pulmonary Medicine, who had been working at County General for over a decade. Her approach to TB patients was notably nonjudgmental. The patients, in turn, respected her for this. In one case, I brought a patient named Bill in to see her after he had a particularly alienating encounter with a young male physician. Afterward, I asked him about the difference between the two physicians. About the first physician, his main complaint was that the man didn't listen to him:

> When I tried to tell him about how I was doing, he said: "Quiet, I'm writing." I remember those words exactly: "Quiet, I'm writing." Then he asked me: What makes you think you're getting better? But he wouldn't listen to the answer. I told him I was gaining weight, my physical strength was coming back, and my complexion coming back, but it was like he didn't want to hear that. His whole thing was, he wanted me to come back in the hospital.

Bill had been diagnosed with TB a few months earlier. Although he had been faithfully taking his medicine on a daily basis under the DOT program, he was still running a low-grade fever. But he had several children at home (who were also being treated) and he understandably did not want to return to the hospital where he would be unable to care for them or to work around the neighborhood to make the "little bit of money" that helped him pay the rent and feed his kids. His abnormal X-ray and fever, however, had convinced the young doctor that this man belonged back within the medical institution.

I thought perhaps a second opinion was in order, and so did he. I got his care switched over to the more experienced physician mentioned above. She examined him and concluded that his X-rays were in fact improving, but that his TB had been very extensive, and it was simply going to take a while for all the disease in the lung tissue to clear and to heal. His fever, she judged, was also not necessarily serious. In fact, it was lower than it had been when he was previously released from the hospital. More importantly, however, she took the time to explain all of this to him. She sent him for more X-rays and blood tests and sent him home.

When I asked Bill what it was that she had done differently, he replied: "She gave me words of encouragement. She gave me reasons why she needed the tests, a reason to want to have things done. Otherwise I'd a been ticked, having to wait around like that" (to get the tests done). When I spoke to her about it, she said that she was concerned about what the other physician had done. "The patient said that he simply wasn't listening. That's a bad habit for a physician to get into," she said.

Such a problem may not only be a matter of insensitive or inexperienced individuals. To some extent, the apparent arrogance of physicians may be related to their institutional training (Scully 118). It may also have a lot to do with the heavy workload that is typical in public health facilities. Finally, it may reflect the institution of medicine itself, and can be magnified in the context of the public hospital, where patients are often both stigmatized and disempowered. In this case, the young physician's apparent lack of interest in the patient's personal experience, and his desire to put the patient back in the hospital, would seem to indicate that it was exactly the de-personalized aspect of the institutional environment that was seen as ideal. Inside the hospital, tests could be taken and the patient could be monitored abstractly and "objectively," sealed off from the messy facts of his outside life. Such attitudes are indicative of a continuing faith in an exclusively biomedical model.

On another occasion, the same senior physician had expressed to me her concerns about impending changes at County General. A lot of physicians were coming to County General from private hospitals, and they brought their social prejudices with them. She said she was especially struck by the consistent failure of these new physicians to recognize the valid concerns and worries of community members—especially those whom they happened to label as "bad" or "unreliable" patients. The shortcoming of the institutional, medical approach to illness lies, at least in part, in its inability to comprehend the enormous impact of the social environment and its crucial role in the success or failure of treatment. Acknowledging this can possibly lead to another way of conceptualizing what medicine is, and what it should—and should not—do.

SOCIOLOGICAL STORIES

As Waitzkin has noted, folk beliefs concerning health tend to recognize the connections between individual problems and the torn fabric of the larger community, where modern medicine often does not. Such beliefs, according to Waitzkin, ". . . permitted a diversity of explanatory frameworks for health problems as well as a greater openness to holistic and social explanations for processes of disease and death" (Waitzkin 1998, 9). Along the same lines, social epidemiologists such as Bruce Link and Jo Phelan have argued that ". . . our tendency to focus on the connection of social conditions to single diseases via single mechanisms at single points in time neglects the multifaceted and dynamic processes through which social factors may affect health . . ." (Link and Phelan, 81). In poor communities, health and illness are tied to whole arrays of interlocking social forces. This excerpt from an interview with a County General TB patient named Isaiah illustrates some of the various ways that life in a ghetto community impacts one individual's health. I asked him how he usually ended up in the hospital.

> Most of the time it's from the seizures, except for the time that car hit me, and I didn't have no choice but to go, cause I couldn't move the leg, and uh, the other time was when I got cracked in the head with a piece of glass lamp, the other was when I got cracked one night coming down the street, I went to the store for a friend of mine, and on the way back, it was a robbery in the process, and they found a new victim—me. And it was kind of embarrassing. You know, you tryin' to reason with 'em, but they don't want to reason.

These might seem like examples of one individual's extremely bad luck, or very bad judgment, but Isaiah's situation was not atypical in the social environment that he occupied. The alcoholic seizures, accidents, and violence are all social in origin, and all are reflective of Isaiah's local world. Ultimately, issues of health must be addressed not at the level of the individual alone, nor solely at the level of national policy, but at the level of the local community as well.

It is worth noting that when I asked Isaiah what his experience was like his answer to my question came in the form of a story, or rather, a series of stories lumped into one. In African tradition, the griot, or village storyteller, provided a source of shared historical wisdom and reflection for the entire community in which he lived. Similarly, in American history, the autobiography—the individual telling his or her own story—has been the dominant form of literature for African Americans. Oral expression and story-telling are privileged modes of moral communication in many traditional societies, but in our modern, technological, and text-based world, the spoken word is seen as the stuff of entertainment and demagogic politics, or of children and other unsophisticated people. This academic and professional prejudice against colloquial language reinforces a more widespread prejudice toward the lower classes in general, and blacks and other minorities in particular.

Having known Isaiah from the street (his story is discussed more fully in Chapter 6), and having seen the facts of his daily life up close, I was able to visualize the circumstances that he was describing, and his account made sense as part of a larger picture of life in a very poor inner-city neighborhood. For the doctor within the hospital, however, such an account might simply come across as a confusing welter of subjective, anecdotal evidence. The hospital is a fortress of medicalized meanings, and its function depends on its ability to arrive at correct diagnoses in due time. Stories like Isaiah's, then, become something to sift through in search of a single cause, a condition which can be addressed through medical means. This sifting process, however, is itself a subjective one, and allows ample room for stereotypes and prejudices to creep in and influence both judgments and practices. Often this simply means that patients' own stories, accounts, or concerns are neglected or ignored, as some of the examples given above illustrate.

This is easily done, simply because poor patients have few resources with which to challenge the decisions of the medical institution. They may choose to endure alienation, boredom, and painful test procedures, or they may choose to simply leave the hospital. Though the latter decision might remove a burden from the hospital staff, it does not address either pressing health conditions or the social factors that underlie them. Granted, medical professionals do not necessarily have the knowledge or the resources to address social concerns at all. As a consequence, these are often ignored or shoved off onto social workers or field workers such as myself. The myopia of the medical model also enables doctors to freely prescribe medicines and therapies, without ever considering how they will be bought, stored, or ingested. I have seen bags of expensive HIV and TB medicines wasted and squandered because the patient (a) did not understand how they were to be taken, (b) was suspicious of their efficacy, (c) suffered from side effects, or (d) was living in circumstances which made the successful pursuit of any complex regimen unlikely. When such a result occurs, neither the patient, hospital, nor community is well-served.

CONCLUSION

If we envision the public hospital as a site of cultural contestation, where the local colloquial world of the poor patient collides with the rationalist perspective of modern medicine, then it becomes possible to read these encounters in a more complex way, rather than judging them simply by virtue of their success or failure. Qualitative sociology has something to offer here, as both a complement and a corrective to more reductionist modes of thinking. Patient-based narratives, for example, convey much sociological information that is often excluded from the diagnostic, and therefore the prognostic, process. Creating a space for such narratives to be heard allows the sick, the poor, and the otherwise excluded to determine at least some of the terms by which they will be known.

In this chapter, I have used my own position as a public health worker to present particular troublesome interactions as the patients relayed them to me. I have tried to capture some of the essence of their frustrations, and to interpret them sociologically. As a specialist in the area of tuberculosis control, assigned the role of mediating between tuberculosis patients in the community and a large public medical institution, I was able to gain some insight into the opposing sides of this cultural divide. As I stated above, this divide is often reflective of those that exist outside the hospital's walls; interactions within the hospital are laden with conflicts of class, race, gender, and culture that run deep in American life. Chapter 4 follows the tracks of tuberculosis as they radiate out from the hospital and into the surrounding communities. Combining the methods of epidemiology and ethnography, I will place tuberculosis within those neighborhoods and populations where it most often occurs, and to illustrate the ways in which the disease intertwines with the social circumstances of peoples' lives. Once again, I will be using the work of the tuberculosis field-worker as the vantage point from which to make these observations.

4   Cavities of Contagion

Networks and Nodes of TB in Chicago

TUBERCULOSIS, CHICAGO STYLE

IN NEW YORK, my buddy Spanner and I used to joke about "jacking into the matrix" every morning when we hit the streets of the city looking for lost TB cases. We had taken the phrase from William Gibson's cyberpunk novel *Neuromancer*, where it referred to the process of entering the virtual world, a world that was dependent on the "real" world, existing in parallel to it, subordinate and separate, but nonetheless real. For me, what the term also evoked was the sense of the city as a living grid, composed of countless interrelated parts, tied together by the entangled strands of human relationships, yet divided into sectors by history, power, money, steel, cement, bricks, parks, and bridges, as well as space and time. Venturing forth into the social realms of TB patients was mind-altering because of its very reality. In spite of modern transportation and communication technologies, many people in large cities such as New York and Chicago live intensely local lives. This is especially true among those populations most susceptible to TB, many of whom have no addresses or phones, much less cars or computers.

Our health department automobiles gave us quick access to these multiple sectors, which amounted to different local life-worlds. We were urban planet-hoppers, on a mission to arrest disease. To do this, though, we had to understand the rules of the worlds that we entered—we could not simply walk in and unilaterally have our way. Like fire-jumpers, we had to know and respect the landscape. But my experience in New York was more kaleidoscopic than ethnographic. I saw patients there for relatively brief periods of time, and did not spend long periods in particular neighborhoods. When I moved to Chicago in late 1993 and began working in tuberculosis control at a large public hospital, I had a much different experience. In part this was due to the fact that Chicago's social geography differs markedly from that of New York. New York has a densely packed hub in Manhattan, with rich and poor, black, brown, and white peoples often living side by side and on top of each other, passing in the street every day and mingling through an extensive transit system which is widely used on a daily basis by almost everyone. The outer boroughs, though more horizontal than vertical in orientation, are also multicultural patchworks.

Chicago, on the other hand, is a city that is radically segregated into distinct zones or territories, with New York-style diversity being the exception rather than the rule, and confined mainly to the high-density neighborhoods along the northern lake front. Though there are stretches of the South Bronx and Brooklyn in New York which are populated almost entirely by poor people of color, and neighborhoods such as Harlem or Bensonhurst or Washington Heights, which are known by reputation as black, Italian, or Latino-dominated areas, New York is a compressed polyglot mosaic compared to Chicago, where whole swathes of the city are profoundly racialized. There is no doubt that Chicago is ethnically diverse, and that New York is also ethnically divided; but New York is Balkanized, while Chicago is sliced up like a pie. The lines of division in Chicago are as precise as ZIP codes and seem to be accepted within the city itself, as natural and inevitable as the location of Lake Michigan.

The West Side and the South Side of Chicago, for example, are commonly perceived by Chicagoans as "black" areas, even though there are large pockets of white, Latino, and Asian population located within them. My grandmother and my godmother both lived on the far South Side, and we visited them there every holiday when I was a kid, yet as a suburbanite I was always instilled with a fear of the South Side. If you were going to visit downtown Chicago and planned to take the "L," Chicago's subway system, people would always warn you, "Watch out that you don't end up on the South Side." My grandmother didn't help this any when she would talk with reverence of the late local alderman who had "kept the niggers out." My father promptly expressed his disapproval of Grandma's bigotry, but the underlying message was successfully delivered in many subtle and not-so-subtle ways: "we" just don't live around "them." This sentiment, and the reality of racial segregation, persisted thirty years after Martin Luther King endured a rain of bricks while marching in the Windy City.

New York, for all its attitude and local pride, was a place full of people who originally hailed from elsewhere. If you adopted the New York attitude you could be accepted there, the right to remake oneself being respected above all else. Even at their most provincial, New Yorkers seemed savvy about conflict and difference, perhaps because it was such an integral part of daily life. But going into many Chicago neighborhoods was like crossing the Berlin Wall, entering a curtained world where everything was twenty years behind. A stranger stood out on the other side, especially if he was the wrong color. In those long miles of segregated city, in the ghettos full of open bull-dozed spaces, it was easy to feel stranded, with no taxicabs or payphones or restaurants that weren't encased in scarred Plexiglas.

The job was different, too. As a city worker in New York, with colleagues who hailed from Haiti, China, Nigeria, Jamaica, Greece, and Trinidad as well as Carroll Gardens, Co-Op City, Ukrainian Village, and Jamaica, Queens, it was inconceivable that one would try to match the ethnicity of individual workers with that of individual patients. It would simply be too complicated a task. But in Chicago, when I started working at County General, I joined a staff that included just two other field-workers: one was African American, the other was Mexican American. Both were natives of Chicago, and patients were initially distributed to them largely on the basis of ethnicity and neighborhood. This was an attempt to meet the ideal of the "indigenous" field-worker, but given the small size of our staff and the broad breadth of our territory it amounted to a kind of crude color-coding. If it was the South Side or West Side, the case went to Matthew, the black worker, and if it was a Latino, the case went to Gloria, the Latina worker, and the Europeans, North-Siders and leftovers went to me. Over time, as patients got ill with no regard for the availability of appropriately ethnic field-workers, this informal system largely fell by the wayside, but the fact that it was used at all tells you something about the way Chicago was conceptually split into large, mutually exclusive sectors of black, brown, and white.

This racial spatialization was a product of Chicago's segregated history, and it is also reflected in the epidemiology of disease and illness in Chicago.[1] Even in an age of high disease prevalence there were gross disparities in TB rates across neighborhood areas and racial lines in Chicago. According to a 1949 U.S. Health Service report, "The greatest prevalence of tuberculosis is found under conditions of poverty, overcrowding, and lack of proper facilities for cleanliness" (U.S. Health Service 502). For the nonwhite population the death rate in the 1940s was much higher than that of the general population: 250 per 100,000. Even this figure was probably artificially low due to erratic systems of reporting deaths, especially in poor neighborhoods. Historically, the highest rates of tuberculosis were found in those community areas that had the highest percentages of black residents. In fact, low rents were found to correlate strongly with tuberculosis rates, *except* in black neighborhoods, where residents were charged higher rates for inferior housing. Wartime jobs and losses of farm land in the South drew swarms of black settlers to Northern cities. The 1949 study did not attribute the high rates of TB in the black population of Chicago to an influx of sick people from outside the city however, rather to poor distribution of TB services within the city itself (U.S. Health Service 504).

In the post-war era, effective antibiotics, TB control efforts, and increased prosperity all contributed to a four-decades-long plummet in disease levels, a trend that continued into the 1980s.[2] Then, in 1988, there was a jump in the number of TB cases, and from that point they continued to rise yearly, peaking in 1993 at 799 cases. In that same year, Directly Observed Therapy (DOT) was widely instituted across Chicago, both through the Department of Health and through grant-funded programs like the one at County General, where I was employed after I left New York. There was a drop of 82 cases from 1993 to 1994, and with the exception of 1997, the number of cases dropped every year. The number of newly diagnosed cases hit an historic low of 470 in 1998, and continued to decrease thereafter (Chicago Department of Public Health 2001). In retrospect, then, the "resurgent epidemic" looked like a minor upward bump on an otherwise smooth angle of decline. Even so, the resurgence of tuberculosis in Chicago in the late eighties and early nineties (though small compared to that which took place in New York) was significant by local, regional, and national standards.

In a citywide meeting of tuberculosis control workers and professionals held in Chicago in 1998, the keynote speaker was Dr. John Sbarbaro, a leader in the area of tuberculosis control for over twenty years and an advocate of universal DOT. In his talk, Dr. Sbarbaro gave a useful encapsulation of TB in the twentieth-century United States, at least from the point of view of public health. In 1900, he said, nearly everyone had TB—its presence was ubiquitous. In 1905, TB specialists based in sanatoriums handled the bulk of TB cases. By 1950, the advent of effective chemotherapy resulted in the transfer of TB care to general physicians. Rates continued to drop through the 1960s and 1970s, resulting in fewer resources dedicated to TB. In 1971, there were seventy-two hospitals nationwide specializing in TB care. By 1988, there was only one hospital in the entire nation that specialized in TB. Sbarbaro attributed the resurgence of TB in the late 1980s to leadership failure in three key arenas: politics, physicians and public health. I summarize his comments below:

1. There was a failure of political leadership because after the sanatoriums were closed, funds which were supposed to be redirected into TB outpatient care and public health agencies were redirected and sent elsewhere. This was a situation similar to what happened with mental health dollars after many state institutions were closed. No federal dollars were spent on TB between 1970 and 1980.

2. There was a failure of physician leadership because there was no

attempt to transfer skills in TB treatment through the training of new physicians. So, in effect, decades of experience were lost. And, as recently as 1997, surveys showed that significant numbers of private physicians still prescribed incorrect regimens for tuberculosis (Sumartojo 1993).

3. There was a failure of public health leadership because effective TB control programs were not implemented. DOT as a means of TB control was not employed, even though as early as 1965 Sbarbaro himself had stated that patient noncompliance was "the most important issue in TB."

The standard explanation for the decline and rise of TB rates, as illustrated by Sbarbaro's account, focuses primarily on the role of medical and public health interventions. Such accounts allude only indirectly to the economics and politics which drive disease patterns and the social structures which lock entire groups of people into perpetual states of risk. Based on this reasoning, one might assume that tuberculosis is not prevalent in the affluent suburbs because the people there have access to better quality tuberculosis care. In fact, this is probably not the case. There is little or no TB expertise in the suburbs, and the private physicians there are *not* experienced in its treatment, but suburban people do not suffer any risk from TB because they are never exposed to it at all. Certainly it has not been necessary to institute directly observed therapy in the suburbs, and it might be very difficult to do so, due to middle class standards of privacy. People in the suburbs, in addition to being largely unexposed to tuberculosis, are also less susceptible to the germ. When we look at the neighborhood areas in Chicago with the highest rates of tuberculosis in the 1990s there are certain commonalities that immediately stand out.

With a couple exceptions, all the high-prevalence areas were characterized by high rates of poverty, racial and economic homogeneity, and steeply declining population since the 1960s. By 1990 many West and South Side neighborhoods were almost entirely poor and black, and had similarly high rates of residential segregation, poverty, and unemployment. Residential segregation is a factor associated with many health problems, and it impacts tuberculosis transmission in both direct and indirect ways, through a concentration of poverty effects and isolation of high-risk groups (Acevedo-Garcia 2000). Plummeting population density is also a factor that has powerfully shaped the daily lives of these communities. It is commonly attributed to processes of deindustrialization, suburbanization, and "white flight," which accelerated in the wake of the urban riots of the late sixties. Visually, the effects of declining population and deindustrialization are manifest in the landscape of the Chicago ghetto: stretches of open land, strewn with rocks and rubble, burnt-out or abandoned buildings, half-occupied commercial strips, and an overall impression of poverty and desperation: men sitting around, kids hanging on corners, women selling themselves in broad daylight. The presence of behaviors widely perceived as "deviant" becomes all the more obvious in such a vacant and dilapidated environment.

From an epidemiological perspective, loss of population is significant because it is often accompanied by disinvestment and decay or destruction of housing stock. This may result in the "doubling up" of the remaining population, causing multiple individuals and families to occupy apartment units, basements, cars, or other spaces which may in themselves be unfit for healthy habitation. The direct implications for the spread of an infectious airborne disease like tuberculosis are obvious. However, there may be other, more indirect consequences of population decline that also impact TB rates. Poor, low-density neighborhoods often lack easy accessibility to affordable fresh food; instead they are dominated by corner stores which stock low-quality canned goods and junk food at high prices. They are also commonly home to multiple competing markets of liquor and drugs. In these circumstances, individual health behavior cannot be considered separately from local conditions and norms.

Sbarbaro, in his talk, used the phrase "DOT Chicago Style" to describe an approach characterized by discreet, low-key, "tough love." Its real effectiveness, he maintained, was in fact based not on the exertion of authority, but rather on the establishment of a meaningful personal relationship with the TB patient. With the implementation of widespread DOT, TB rates in Chicago fell rather sharply after 1994. The details and dynamics of DOT practice will be discussed in Chapters 6 and 7. What's significant about DOT, from the standpoint of social geography, is that DOT programs took TB control efforts into the community sites where transmission actually occurred. Once in those specific locations it was possible to see the strands of social structure and individual agency endlessly entangled. As a field-worker, trained in both sociology and epidemiology, I discovered over and over again that an understanding of social factors and social barriers is crucial to an understanding of tuberculosis.

Recovering addicts are taught to avoid the triggers—people, places, things—that will lead them back into the vicious cycle of substance abuse. It is no coincidence that the same formula can lead to disease: personal associations, occurring within tightly constrained circumstances, producing similar health outcomes.[3] Poverty plus population loss can create the equivalent of the teeming urban ghettos of a century ago, paradoxically existing within an otherwise barren terrain, without the internal economic diversity that characterized historical ghettos.[4] By examining some of the particular circumstances surrounding disease transmission, I hope to demonstrate how the epidemiology of tuberculosis in Chicago is revealed in the people, places, and things that are encountered in the neighborhoods of the city.

Epidemiology in a Day's Work: TB on the Street

Epidemiology, as discussed earlier, is technically defined as the study of patterns of illness or injury in populations. As such, it depends heavily on the gathering of data, statistical analysis, and keen observation. Its purpose is usually instrumental; that is, it has the explicit goal of either preventing or controlling illness. Though they may embrace a biomedical model, epidemiologists necessarily see health and illness within a social context, and they often employ multifactorial explanations of disease. Health problems, in this perspective, emerge from "causal webs," not from a linear succession of cause and effect. The very notion of public health arises from the practical application of epidemiological knowledge within community contexts, and even a germ-theory pioneer such as Louis Pasteur recognized the importance of "terrain" in contributing to disease causation (Dubos 1960).

Ethnographic methods can augment epidemiology by bringing this "web" or "terrain" into clearer view. The following ethnographic field notes describe some of my first attempts to make contact with an older Polish gentleman, whom I will call Stanley. He had tested positive for TB infection at a mass screening that I conducted at a religious mission in a Latino neighborhood on the Southwest Side in 1997. He was diagnosed with active disease less than a year later at County General, but the bacteriology did not confirm this diagnosis until after he had been discharged from the hospital. Then I had to try to find him.

4/7/98

. . . it was about twelve o'clock, so I figured I might as well try my luck looking for the Polish guy in the mission . . . I went over there and saw Moises, the young guy who runs the place for his father, the pastor. I gave him a note with my phone number on it and told him to page me if the guy showed up. He said he thought he had seen him last night.

As I drove back toward the hospital, crossing Frontier Avenue, I saw two white dudes, one of whom I recognized. I rolled down my window, blew my horn and yelled "Stanley" and sure enough, the guy turned his head. I called him over and told him I was from County General. I told him to wait a second while I parked my car, which he did. As I approached I asked if either of them spoke English. They both said they spoke a little bit.

Our communication deteriorated from there. He showed me his pills, and none of them were for TB, just pain pills for his legs. I tried to tell him he needed to come in to the hospital, that he could get sick and die if he didn't. I offered them a ride to the mission, which they accepted, but then they had to stop to sell some aluminum cans at a recycling station along the way . . . I gave him the appointment form, and again tried to tell him that he needed to go; and this time I said I would send the police after him if he didn't. That was the wrong move; he got pissed.

"No police!" he cried. "What sick? What sick? First sick, then no sick, then sick . . . " He picked up his bag and stormed off quickly down the sidewalk, toward the mission. I asked his friend what was wrong with him, and he said he didn't know. "Maybe nervous," he said.

At first, Stanley seemed like a very hard nut to crack. Even in this brief account, it's apparent that the workings of the medical system were a mystery to him, and that the diagnosis of tuberculosis was less urgent than his immediate concerns: earning some money, getting a drink, and finding a place to sleep. I was discouraged, but persisted, laying off the threats and using a more cooperative approach. He agreed to come in to the clinic when I offered him a ride on his clinic day, and he got along quite well with the doctor who saw him there. I was eventually able to persuade Stanley to meet me once a week to make sure that he had an adequate supply of medications and was taking them properly. He completed a full course of treatment in this way, and his disease was cured.

At the end of the process, however, he remained homeless, living a day-to-day life of survival on the street. This is part of the reason that I continued to meet him when he called me, even after my professional obligation to see him had ceased. I had a good relationship with him, in spite of the rocky beginnings described above, and in fact he was a useful person to know. Some analysis of his situation will be helpful here, for the above-described events are laden with both sociological and epidemiological information.

The most obvious point to make is that my encounters with Stanley and his crew took place not in anyone's home, or in the hospital, but in the street. These men were in the street for the better part of each day, and sometimes all night as well. Most public health-oriented epidemiology focuses on behaviors: the things that people do (or don't do) that place them at increased risk of illness. This can involve sexual activity, diet, substance abuse, or violence, all of which are potentially attributed to "culture" or "lifestyle." For example, one might attribute the risk for tuberculosis to the persistent alcohol abuse and homelessness of these men. Alcoholism tends to suppress immunity and impact nutrition, making one significantly more susceptible to infection. Alcohol abuse can also

impact economic status, even resulting in homelessness, while the fre-
quenting of homeless shelters, in turn, increases the likelihood of exposure to diseases such as TB. All of these factors might be attributed by
some researchers to factors residing within individual psychology. To
borrow Farmer's phrase, "an immodest claim of causality" might link the
economic marginality—and thus susceptibility to illness—of these men to
their "lack of self-esteem" or their "present-day orientation" (Farmer et
al. 1996, 171). Such analyses tend to leave important determining factors
unexamined, however.

The larger structural forces implicated in the physical deterioration of
individuals are numerous.[5] In Stanley's case, one could talk specifically
about the cutting of aid to the poor, in the form of cash, housing, and
medical care, deindustrialization, disinvestment, population loss and
unemployment, and marginal labor markets. As aspects of the larger
social structure, all of these things are beyond the control of any one individual, particularly a poor individual. All of them nonetheless impact
greatly on poor people. Poverty itself might best be examined as it is manifested in the everyday lives of poor people, not only in behaviors, but also
through factors that we might roughly categorize as local institutions and
local networks.[6]

"Institution" and "network" are both terms with distinct connotations
in sociology, but I will use them in a particular way here, based on the
immediate context of these men's lives. Living on the street, they depend
on certain things. Of the things mentioned in the above field notes, local
institutions would include the mission, the recycling station, the labor
pools that provide daily employment, the hospital, the streets, alleys, and
parks where they sleep and walk and work during the day, and the police,
who patrol them in all of these places. Local networks would include the
personal associations that connect them with all of these locations and
institutions: the people they encounter there, and on whom they depend
for social support or material resources. Institutions and networks are
both intermediate forms of social structure, and are not really separate
from the social structure as a whole. However, it is useful to distinguish
between networks and institutions and social structure in the general
sense, because the character of networks may determine the way institutions will be used, or not used, and thereby alter or modify the impact of
social structure on individuals.

Stanley, for example, had a bad history with Moises, the manager of
one of the missions that provided food and shelter. Because of that sour
relationship, he tried to avoid using that mission, even though its services
were valuable to him. Conversely, the impact of structures on individuals
may be mediated and altered by social networks: the cutting of welfare

benefits, for example, may be offset by resource sharing or innovations in strategies of survival. In Russia, a system of social networks and relationships, broadly referred to as *blat,* provided a way of circumventing the rigid structures of Soviet society (Ledeneva 1). Similarly, as Carol Stack (1974) and others have documented, extended family relations have historically been used to spread the burdens of poverty within the black community. Likewise, individuals within institutions may bend rules to benefit the marginalized. There was another mission in the general area, for example, which was run by a minister whom Stanley respected, so he often used that one instead of Moises' mission. The malleability of local networks and local institutions does not completely compensate for larger structural effects, such as systemic unemployment or soaring housing costs, but is significant nonetheless.

Along these same lines, I also served an important role for Stanley. I was capable of connecting him with resources that he might not otherwise be able to access, little things like petty cash, food coupons, or clinic visits. He would still call me once in a while to ask me for small favors, even after his TB treatment was completed, and I would always respond. While I liked him and felt sorry for him, there was another reason why I maintained contact with Stanley. He was friends with other guys who were both Polish and homeless, some of whom had had TB in the past or might have TB in the future. TB moves through just such chains of relation, composed of immune-compromised bodies. Stanley was a valuable link in this chain; first, because he now liked and trusted me; second, because he spoke better English than any of the others. He was my "gatekeeper" to this network, to use some common parlance of the social sciences. Like police work, the practice of epidemiology necessitates such contacts within groups of people who might not otherwise reveal themselves to the well-meaning, street-level bureaucrat.

One day Stanley called me from the convenience store where we used to meet on a weekly basis. He said he needed to see me and I drove over there around noon. He had a brace on his leg and said his kneecap had been shattered and he was unable to work. He wanted to know if I could give him anything to help him get through. After I gave him ten dollars in cash and another ten in fast food coupons, I asked him if he had seen Josef, another homeless Pole afflicted with tuberculosis. Stanley normally worked the same day labor job as Josef, and he said he thought that Josef might be out working. Sure enough, as soon as I left Stanley there on the corner I spotted Josef. I was driving down the road and looked up at a moving truck in front of me. The rear sliding door was up and there were six guys sitting inside on stacks of newspaper. When I pulled up closer to the van, I saw Josef hunched inside.

Naturally, I followed that truck. I trailed it from a distance, as it rounded corners and dropped guys off with stacks of advertising papers, which it was their job to distribute. They crossed Pacific Avenue, turned left, crossed Charles Road, turned right, and finally Josef debarked from the truck on the other side of Carolina Avenue. I got out of my car and called his name as he gathered the papers into his shoulder bag. He looked up and didn't seem the least bit surprised to see me standing there. "Hello, sir," he said. I asked him about his medicine and he said that he ran out of it maybe two weeks ago and hadn't been back to the clinic yet. I asked if he could make it next week and he said he could, on Tuesday, around 11 or 12. I wrote up an appointment for Tuesday, telling him to try to arrive by 10. "Thank you, sir," he said, and hoisted his bag of papers for the afternoon.

In this instance, it was the entree into the social network, provided by Stanley, which enabled me to find Josef. Such an event might be a major breakthrough in a case where one is attempting to locate a man with no address and no known next of kin. Josef did in fact show up for the clinic appointment that I gave him, although he remained a troublesome patient. The reasons why he was troublesome, I would argue, had as much to do with the circumstances of his life as they did with him personally. In particular, the nature of his employment made it almost impossible for me to find him on a daily basis.

The same had been true of Stanley when I first started seeing him. I was able to convince him to go to the clinic the first time only by offering him ten dollars in cash on the spot. This type of trade-off was often necessary to compel individuals to participate in the TB program. Though it might seem that attending a clinic visit would be a logical choice for a TB patient whose life could be in jeopardy from disease, in fact this involved a substantial sacrifice on Stanley's part. It meant losing a day's work, a day's pay, and possibly a couple of meals. By offering him the ten dollars, I sought to offset some of these costs. But ten dollars a week, which was our standard "allowance" per TB patient, was not enough to justify regular participation in the program if it meant his missing out on a job. The leafleting work that Stanley did required him to be in a certain location at a very early hour, and occupied him for most of the day, in a wide variety of locations.

Such flexible employment situations are common among poor and homeless men, and the reasons why are fairly clear. These jobs tend to both facilitate and exploit the economic marginality and substance addiction which are characteristic of many such individuals. Labor market practices, in this manner, both reflect local conditions and help to perpetuate them (Peck 124). In Chicago, where industrial manufacturing jobs hemorrhaged throughout the 1980s, the number of people employed by the temporary-help industry increased by almost 100 percent between 1989 and 1994 (Oehlsen 12). Men such as Stanley and Josef, who had been blue-collar workers in their younger days, naturally found themselves without many other options, due to their age, language limitations, and alcohol problems. Nevertheless, they did work as often as they could, if for no other reason than to feed themselves and their habits. Flexible labor solved a problem, but it created another one: it provided no health insurance, nor hope of any, and it contributed to the continuance of a manifestly unhealthy lifestyle. Groups of alcoholic men, riding in trucks, sleeping together in shelters or perhaps in cars or hallways, provided ripe opportunity for the spread of tuberculosis infection and disease. The regular circuit of locations and resources, referred to by many homeless men as "the tramp trail," also provides a well-trod path for the germ to follow.

Another TB patient, Jerry, a black man in his forties whom I had known years earlier, made these remarks about what he called "the slave market":

> Well, I don't make a lot of money, and I been working eight years, and I feel as though the people at least could show respect and say, here, five-fifteen or something like that, but they going by the rule, cause law say minimum wage is four and a quarter, so [they] don't have to go beyond that, cause law say, I could keep you like this here. It's up to me to give this to you. See, like the five-fifteen, once you get that, the law say, if it weren't for that, you wouldn't even have this here. See that's where I'm talking from. So, in order for me to move on, I had to try to do better for myself, to where I get paid a little bit more change, cause I know, that's what I'm looking at. Four and a quarter. I'm just making it, you understand, but uh, if you been working somewhere for a certain time people should have enough, just enough to say you earned a raise or something like that, you know what I'm saying? But that's the way it is. I ain't got no control over that.

This illustrates the kind of trap some people can get caught in at the low end of the income spectrum, and it feeds into the vicious cycle of poverty and disease (Singer 936). The next episode, based on my field notes from the very same day, presents a different social and epidemiologic situation, also seen from the ground up.

LATER THAT DAY: TB ON THE BLOCK

After my adventure trailing Josef, I met up with Nick, a fellow fieldworker, on West Florida Avenue, in an attempt to read some skin tests that we had placed the previous Monday. I caught up with a couple people and read their results before Nick arrived, and then we sat in the car and waited for the others. It was 5 P.M., and as the sun went lower the activity on the street picked up. Young men started pitching pennies. Some other guys showed up in a Cadillac and stood outside of it, talking about the recent college basketball championships while the heavy bass reverberated around them.

Every so often Nick got up and went to the house across the street to see if anyone else was there yet. All the casual acquaintances of our source case had negative reactions so far. These were the guys who would regularly hang around the house with him, playing dominoes, drinking wine, doing drugs, and whatever else. "Five o'clock, they be getting off work, and then the party starts," is what Curtis, the source case, had told us. Curtis had active pulmonary TB, and we were looking for others who might have been infected by him, or by somebody else, as yet undiscovered. We were waiting for Curtis's friend Reggie, who lived with his mother in the first floor apartment of Curtis's building. Around 5:30, I knocked on his mother's door and she told me he wasn't home yet. We spoke to Curtis, who lived in a small apartment in the basement. He told us that Reggie had said that he was going to be running late. Not long after that Nick said, "the guy with the Caddy just pulled up." I got out of the van and walked over to Reggie. He saw me and pulled up his sleeve to reveal the results of the skin test. He was definitely positive; his forearm was swollen in three different places. I pulled out my ruler and pen and went to measure the size of the reaction right there in the street, and he said, "Come on, let's go in the house."

So we went in to his mom's house and I looked at his arm under the light. I measured the induration, or area of swelling and hardness, at about 21 millimeters, which strongly indicated tuberculosis infection. I started explaining to him the difference between infection and disease, and told him that he would probably have to take a pill for six months to prevent active disease.

"Six months?!" He exclaimed.

"Mmmm-hmmm," said his mother.

"What are you saying 'mmm-hmmm' for?" he asked her.

"I told you not to be hanging around him in that basement like that," she said, referring to Curtis' subterranean hole-in-the-wall.

"I'm a grown man," he said, "What are you going to tell a grown man? If I want to do something, I'm going to do it. Am I right or wrong?" He directed this last question at me.

"You're right," I said, and I told him that Curtis was taking medicine now, and therefore there was no longer any reason to avoid hanging around with him.

"Six months?!" he exclaimed again.

"Yeah," I said, "and no drinking."

"What?" he yelled, though in a good humor. "That does it, I ain't gonna not drink for six months."

"That's up to you," I said.

He also wanted to be sure that I didn't say anything about this to anyone else on the block. "These people be nosy," he said, "and a lot of them would love to hear some gossip about Reginald Loomis."

"I won't say anything," I told him. "I've been watching. I see what goes on, people walking back and forth, talking all day long." His mother nodded. "I won't tell anybody anything."

He and I walked out to the street together and I gave him a written referral to the clinic for a follow-up exam. I told him that my phone number was on there if he needed to call me. Then I went back to the van where Nick was still sitting, watching, waiting. Reggie's relationship with his mother and with the other people on the street reveal two aspects of the local social world: the close, caring family relationship that endures, and the casual, daily interaction with acquaintances whose influence is important, even though the relationships themselves may not be considered meaningful. The epidemiology of tuberculosis in the American inner city of the 1990s is illustrated in these examples: the poverty, first of all, but also the overlapping and intersecting associations, the crowded houses with boarded-up windows and the cramped vans full of men making a few bucks for the next meal, the next drink, or the next fix.

Nick's slow, patient approach to the contact investigation was perhaps the only way to see these relationships without the help of insider information. Nick told me that when he first started this job he tried to be like a cop; staying out late at night, following people around at a distance, seeing where they went. It was only then that he could piece together a story, make a connection between the case of illness and the social situation that produced it. This involved visualizing the intangible tendrils which connected individual predicaments to larger historical and social circumstances. The networks, the associations, the grapevines: these provide the crucial link between the lives of the individuals and the social forces which shape and constrain their lives. Within this environment, Reggie's mother and his associates on the block were connected, even though they may have rarely interacted personally. Sitting in the car, watching the movement from building to building, enabled Nick and me to draw the lines between them.

NETWORKING AT THE ALL-NIGHT CAR WASH

Social network theory was developed in the sixties and seventies as a method of describing the intermediate forms of social structure and the ways in which they influence daily life and life outcomes (Aldrich 281).

Network theory attempts to fill "the middle range" in sociology; to borrow Merton's words, it lies ". . . between the minor but necessary working hypotheses that evolve in abundance during day-to-day research and the all-inclusive systematic efforts to develop a unified theory. . ." (Merton 39). As such, it lends itself well to applications which seek to bridge the gap between social structures, institutions, and disparate individuals. The fields of public health and social work have adapted network theory to augment their attempts to provide services to people who are "at the margins of society" by developing a better understanding of key relationships within the community (Gaitley and Seed 14). These networks are then seen as potential aids or barriers to the purposes of public health programs.

Network theory also has obvious implications for epidemiology. When asked how they think they first got tuberculosis, for example, patients frequently make reference to street networks, especially the act of "drinking behind peoples." For example, one man stated:

> Well, actually, I don't know how I caught it myself. Well, it started off, I'm gonna be honest with ya, I started off by smoking behind peoples. . . . So this girl . . . she told me that she had it, no she didn't tell me she had it, she just told me that, you know, she was sick. . . . So one day she come over with some cigarettes, you know, she had some cigarettes. Then I got to coughing, then I was coughing more, then I started . . . behind other folks . . . in between, I don't know exactly how I got it, but I got it between her and somebody else.

Another man, Lester, attributed his infection to an older man he used to hang out and work with at a garage on the South Side:

> It musta been somebody over there that I was workin' around or somethin' at that other shop over there that probably had it. I know, I take it back, I know there was a guy I was with, there was a old guy, every time he smoke a cigarette, he coughin' all the time. Come to think of it—yeah, over there by the garage, and I know every time we'd be sittin' around, he'd, every time he'd light a cigarette, he coughs. He be coughin', coughin' still be smokin.' And once he throw the cigarette away, and cough a little bit more, then he'll stop. Then, but every time he get ready to light up a cigarette, soon as he light it, he start coughin'. It coulda been from him, cause me and him work together sometimes, on cars, you know, we'd be up, I'd be up under that car with him, we like, puttin' the trans up, I got one side, he got one side, and I'm tightenin' the bolts up on this side, to the bell housing, and he doin' this side, and he'll stop and cough up under there. That could be how I caught it, come to think of it now. Cause other than that, I can't think of nobody else. That girl I was talkin' to at the time, I don't think she, there weren't nothing wrong with her, she was healthy, she wasn't sick, she didn't

even smoke neither. I can't think of the old guy name now, I know we called him, uh, Leon. That ain't his name though.

Street associations often have informal qualities, where people can spend hours and hours together while actually knowing very little about each other. Sometimes, as in the above example, one may not even know these associates by their real names. Mark Granovetter has argued that "weak ties" are often just as influential in one's life as "strong ties," because they connect one to worlds outside one's closest friends, relatives, and acquaintances. According to Granovetter: "The macroscopic side of this communications argument is that social systems lacking in weak ties will be fragmented and incoherent. New ideas will spread slowly, scientific endeavors will be handicapped, and subgroups that are separated by race, ethnicity, and geography, or other characteristics will have difficulty reaching a *modus vivendi*" (Granovetter 106). In the mind of the epidemiologist oriented toward infectious disease, weak ties can serve as messengers of disease, or "vectors," while close-knit "clumps" composed of strong ties may serve as "reservoirs," pockets where germs may hide and grow. In the above example, the acquaintance at the garage, who the informant considered a "weak tie," may actually have been the one who gave him the disease, while those friends with whom he shared lodging every night in a car lot on the West Side remained uninfected. Recent studies documenting that TB can be transmitted through casual contact reinforce the notion that both "weak ties" and "strong ties" are crucial to an understanding of how the disease spreads within communities (Altman A9). One investigation in the rural South, for instance, found that tuberculosis was spread to nine persons over an eighteen-month period through participation in a floating card game. The connections between the individuals were missed by investigators the first time around because initial interviews had focused on households (strong ties) and not on more informal relationships (weak ties) (Bock et al. 1225).

One tool that helps illuminate the role of social networks in such contexts has been the development of "gene fingerprinting" technologies which enable researchers to verify that different cases of TB are produced by the same strain of bacteria. Restriction-fragment-length polymorphism (RFLP) analysis therefore shows relations where none were previously known to exist—at least by epidemiologists. Referring to two RFLP studies of tuberculosis transmission published in *The New England Journal of Medicine,* Frieden and Hamburg concluded ". . . that indigent patients were more likely to have identical isolates and that certain racial and ethnic groups had more clustering, although the particular groups were different in the two studies, suggesting that transmission is related to social and economic factors, rather than to race itself " (Frieden and Hamburg

1750). Such new insights may spur epidemiologists to pay more attention to the nuances of social context.

Meanwhile, researchers in social network analysis have also sought to develop techniques which will shed more light on the subtleties of how disease spreads. Realizing that "factors other than physical distance" can impact the likelihood of disease transmission, they have statistically modeled the "structured diffusion" of disease in an attempt to better understand this process (Morris 29). People's relations with one another, even within a limited environment, are selective. Individuals do not associate with all other persons in a group equally, and statistics must find a way to mimic these patterns. Technical innovation at both the macro and micro ends of epidemiology cannot substitute, however, for the act of actually entering the field and seeing the places and people. Attempts to apply theoretical models to concrete problems without any sense of ethnographic and geographic context can end up reproducing the same inadequacies that they aim to overcome. Descriptive, or ethnographic epidemiology, can fill some of the gaps which inevitably open between theories, imaging technologies, statistical models, and the reality that they attempt to describe.

One example, again drawn from my day-to-day work in Chicago, illustrates how a combination of complementary methods can create a better picture of the ways in which social context (which encompasses behaviors, structures, and networks) influences the spread of disease within communities. In February of 1998, a man was diagnosed with tuberculosis at County General. The man, whom I will call Freddie Valentine, left the hospital prior to being medically discharged, and thus was not interviewed by a member of our TB field team. However, he did return to the hospital for his scheduled appointment in the standard manner, and I was able to interview him at that time.

I asked him about his experience with tuberculosis, how he got it, and how it made him feel. He was a man who was used to being very active, who worked almost every day at two different jobs, and who also split time between several different women. He said that he first realized that something was really wrong with him when he found himself lying in bed with a woman and having absolutely no desire for sex. He came to the hospital emergency room and was admitted and isolated, but before long he was feeling better and signed himself out of the hospital so he could go back to work. I asked him where he might be located if I needed to talk to him, and he told me about a 24-hour hand car wash on Chicago's West Side where he worked on evenings and on weekends. I was familiar with the place, having driven past it many times, and I wrote it down as a possible contact site.

I thought nothing more about the car wash at the time. But when Mr. Valentine did not show up for his next monthly appointment, I went to the car wash to find him. I went there several times with no luck, and I spoke to the man who managed the place. It was then that I realized that this very same car wash had been mentioned by another TB patient, who had also worked there. The connection between the two was initially missed because neither patient was properly interviewed upon diagnosis, and the first guy had been lost to follow-up shortly after his discharge from the hospital in 1997. This excerpt from my journal gives a sense of how I began to suspect the role played by the car wash:

5/30/98

Just as the streets are heating up like frying pans over a slow flame, I am fading. I stopped by the car wash to ask after Mr. Valentine. I left a note with the owner's daughter. Guys sitting around on crates and curbs eyed me suspiciously, and I looked back, seeing diseased lungs inside the wasted bodies and glassy eyes. Not all of them have this appearance, some are burnished with a veneer of vitality, stripped to the waist in the sun, gold chains shining. But I counted at least five within sight, probably ten within a stone's throw. The Car Wash as Nerve Center, a new theory. Another case has emerged from just up the block, and somehow I see Valentine as the key, the man with all the answers.

6/7/98

I visited the car wash again as the sun was waning. I got out of my car and started to walk inside the car wash area, but instead I veered over and knocked on the window of a parked car in the lot. A guy cracked the door and some smoke leaked out and I asked if they had seen Mr. Valentine. One guy I recognized from the last time I was there, the other guy I didn't recognize, so I didn't think it was him. I couldn't recall exactly what he looked like, but I thought a bell would ring if I saw him.

"He hasn't been around yet," said the one guy. Then he turned to the other guy, turned back, and said, "Check inside." I thanked them and began walking to the car wash itself. As I did this I spotted another man approaching, a tall and lean figure heading toward me up the driveway. I saw him wave to me, and then I knew it was him.

He shook my hand and apologized for not calling me, and I said that I was glad to see him. He told me that he was almost out of meds, which I doubted, but didn't question it at this time. I told him I had a bag of meds for him in my car and that I wanted him to come in to the clinic next week if possible. He asked what kind of hours they had, and I told him it had to be in the morning. He said he could make it, and he told me to leave the appointment slip in the office at the car wash, where he would pick it up. I shook his hand again after I handed him the meds in a plain black plastic bag, and he told me he would be in touch. That quickly, the long-awaited encounter was over. As I got in my car, he climbed in with the other two guys in the smoke-filled vehicle . . .

My repeat visits to the car wash intrigued me, and I became determined to dig a little deeper. Chris Caudill, a CDC officer stationed at the Chicago Health Department, was also interested in doing a more extensive investigation of the site. We decided to go over there together with a bunch of TB skin tests and see how many we could get. I was betting that transmission took place mostly in the evening and night time, and probably during the winter, when the doors of the car wash were closed, and when men were hanging out inside the car wash itself, or in the parked cars in the lot. The original documented case of tuberculosis associated with the site, Mr. Greenwood, had been potentially infectious for a good part of the year 1997, having been hospitalized originally in January, and returning to the hospital again in December of that year. At both times sputum tests had shown him to be emitting live bacteria. So it was likely that those who had been working the night shifts consistently over the past two winters had been exposed. Mr. Valentine himself had probably been exposed in this way.

With the cooperation of the night manager, who was also the owner's daughter, we got over forty employees of the car wash to show up on a warm June evening, when they were scheduled to pick up their checks. Without any prompting from us, the owner made their continued employment contingent upon receiving the TB skin test, and they lined up dutifully. We also had some cash to hand out—$5 apiece—and that didn't hurt participation, either. I stuck them one at a time while Chris gathered the demographics. Two days later we returned to read the results. The TB test is an antibody test; it tests for tuberculosis infection by "faking" a new TB infection. Those who have antibodies will react (unless their immune systems are severely depleted); those who don't have them will not. The measurement of the reaction size is indicative of infection; in a relatively high-prevalence area, reactions as small as 5 or 10 mm may be considered positive for TB infection. Reactions of over 15 or 20 millimeter are considered to be strongly positive.

At the car wash, we found an extremely high rate of positivity, even by high-prevalence inner city standards. Of the 42 persons interviewed, 38 were actually skin tested (4 had previously been positive reactors and therefore had no need of a new test). Of these 38 tests, 24 results were read, and of these 24, 17 had positive reactions greater than 5 mm. Many were greater than 20 mm. As a result of the investigation, 16 individuals were placed on preventive therapy (to ensure that they would not develop TB disease in the future), and 3 new active cases of tuberculosis were detected. That made for 6 total cases associated with the car wash, and a case rate estimated at 13,333 per 100,000 (Caudill, Draus, McAuley, and Paul, 1999).

We returned to the car wash following the contact investigation with a short survey that we had prepared as a means of measuring social and behavioral characteristics of the people who worked there. We got twenty people to participate in the survey, which asked simple questions about frequency of drug and alcohol use, work activities, length of employment, and socialization patterns. Characteristics common to all the diagnosed cases included: having worked at the car wash for more than six months, regular use of drugs or alcohol with coworkers, and sleeping overnight at the car wash. These results indicated some of the social and behavioral patterns that probably contributed to the high levels of disease transmission at the car wash. The following excerpt from my footnotes describes the experience that Chris and I had while interviewing some of the car wash employees:

11/29/98

We finished up at the car wash tonight; we found Weasel and Wacko and some old drunk guy who was hanging around in there, and said he had worked there for a couple years, and Chris let him do the survey even though he wasn't on the list. It was probably useless, as the guy was barely coherent, but that was informative in and of itself.

Weasel was sweeping up at the beauty parlor next door when I came over, but it turned out that he had already done the survey . . . He was on the list under his real name, which nobody used. Wacko was staying around the corner on Willis Street. We went over there and knocked on the door; it smelled like weed and a lady's voice answered the knock: "Who's there?" I told her I was from County General and was there to see Wacko; she opened the door and seemed suspicious at first but then Wacko walked up and said, "I ain't goin' to the hospital," but we explained that we wanted to just ask him a few questions and give him five bucks, and then she let us inside and offered us seats on the couch. It was small and dark in there; there was a wooden bar across the door from the inside and pictures of various children from various eras on the walls and a banner which read "Welcome Home" over the door.

Wacko was honest and cooperative and answered all the questions. He said he never hung out at the car wash after work but that he sometimes slept there. He said he sometimes slept on a couch, in a chair, or in a car. He said he would wash a car with just one other guy at the same time. He no longer works at the car wash; he got fired. He was also supposed to have an operation on his back, but was afraid and didn't go when he was supposed to. He had just smoked some weed and that's why he was a little paranoid, he said.

Again, what the epidemiologist would notice here would probably be the congregation of immune-suppressed bodies sharing air over extended periods of time. As a sociologist, I also couldn't help noticing the role that the low-wage, flexible employment of these men played in facilitating the spread of disease.

Another contributing factor was the structure of the car wash itself. Basically a hundred foot tunnel with a sliding garage door at either end, both of which were often closed due to weather or security concerns, the car wash was a site not only of labor but of recreation. The car wash had no air circulation system other than floor fans in the summer. In addition to the half-dozen or more men who were working during a busy hour, there were typically several others sitting on a couch or chairs positioned around a television set in an area immediately adjacent to where the cars were washed. As the car wash was open around the clock, one could imagine that at some hours "hanging out" was a more likely activity than washing cars. There were no set hours of work, either, so the workers could basically come and go at will. The fact that the car wash was always open and the terms of employment were so flexible made the car wash a viable source of both income and shelter for many economically marginalized individuals. We hypothesized that both the structure of the car wash and its function within the neighborhood as an intersection of overlapping social networks contributed to the spread of TB in this case.

Genetic RFLP analysis later showed that all the cases of TB at the car wash did indeed originate from the same genetic strain of the disease. Microbacteriology in this case thus confirmed the epidemiology that we had already done, establishing that this was indeed an intensely localized outbreak. RFLP results also revealed that the car wash strain of TB was associated with at least thirty-five other cases diagnosed within the surrounding communities since 1996. Many of these cases had no previous known connections to one another; some of them were people whom we had known and treated for TB in past years, in separate localities. The results of the study therefore suggested that there were links between cases of TB that were not discovered by prior contact investigations (Caudill, Draus, McAuley, and Paul 1999). The exact nature of these links might never be known, especially if the disease had been transmitted through a "weak tie," such as a street acquaintance, which might be identified only through a nickname or alias. In such situations, statistical models of "structured diffusion" might also be of little help, as the patterns of association are not themselves structured in any predictable way. This example highlights the value of ethnographic investigation of the actual environments where disease transmission occurs. Ethnography is capable of capturing the anomalous nature of relationships which might not fall into any preconceived category. The car wash, as our investigation indicated, was much more than simply a workplace; it was a unique and distinct social space.

Eventually I got Mr. Valentine to agree to participate with our directly observed therapy program, and I began meeting him every morning at his other job, where he worked as a freight handler at a busy warehouse. He would tell me my car was dirty and that I should bring it to the car wash so he could take care of it for me. "It's depressing to look at," he said. So one day, as the following excerpt shows, I tried to take his advice:

2/5/99

Last night I went to the car wash to see if Valentine could clean my vehicle and found the joint in full swing. A car was idling outside the big sliding door waiting to get in and there were four or five more cars inside. I parked and walked around to the front to see if he was in there but it was so crowded and noisy that I just decided to go home instead. But I got to see how the transmission of TB had happened, in all likelihood: guys were packed in there, working, watching TV, hanging out, smoke and steam everywhere, music blasting, a sensory din.

The next day I asked Fred about it, and he said, "It's always like that. This is the big time of year over there." He told me that the only times it slows down are after midnight and then early in the morning. He says he will be over there all weekend, too, and I ask him if he needs money that bad, and he says, "no, I got nothing better to do, and I got a few ladies over there, know what I mean?"

Another time I went there and just missed being a witness to a car jacking. A young man had walked into the car wash with a gun and told everyone to get down. He took the first car in the line and drove off, leaving the vehicle's owner and his girlfriend stranded. The police were called and they arrived while I sat there and waited for my car, which was the next one in line. Freddie Valentine's brother Bob sat next to me and told me how these kids these days have no discipline and no respect; they aren't afraid of nothing and don't know what's in store if they end up in jail. Bob also worked at the car wash on occasion. Freddie himself told me that he had been working there since he was a teenager on the West Side. It was in moments such as these that I clearly saw the car wash as a window into a particular social domain.

Sitting there just a few minutes, waiting for my car, I learned more than I would have in hours of poring over hospital records. This is not to downplay the importance of such an approach. To the contrary, what I would like to emphasize here is the complementarity of differing methods and perspectives. The preceding examples all illustrate the powerful role played by local environments in shaping one's exposure to a disease such as tuberculosis. The Polish homeless men, the gossiping neighbors on Curtis's block, and the car wash workers all inhabited social and physical realms that were severely circumscribed by local economic conditions.

BBQ AT THE CARLTON ARMS

Another site that was often associated with tuberculosis in many large cities was the single room occupancy hotel, or SRO. Along with jails, hospitals, and homeless shelters, SROs were one of the "usual suspects" as far as TB transmission was concerned. In New York, outreach to all these institutional settings, including SROs, became a major focus of TB control efforts which continues to this day. In Chicago, SROs were not as plentiful, and more of them closed down every year throughout the 1990s. In general, they were not themselves a major focus of TB control efforts, but a few of them turned up more often than others as addresses in the TB case reports, and these did receive some special attention. One legendary institution was the Carlton Arms, located in the Loop and boasting one of the cheapest weekly rates among the downtown men's hotels. This place was wonderfully suited for the transmission of airborne infection. The rooms, in addition to being very small and close together, had wire fencing over the tops of them. As a result, the same air was shared by all the men who slept, drank, coughed, laughed, sang, smoked, or shot dope on a single floor. During my years working TB in Chicago we had many patients who lived there, and after awhile I got to know some of the regular residents, and would sometimes stop by just to see what was happening.

A continuing drama at the Carlton was the owner's struggle against the city, which was attempting to gentrify the Loop, and had by 1999 forced most of the other downtown SROs to close their doors. One long-term resident was a guy they called Willie, who had formerly been a security guard, but had been reduced to a sliver of his former self by years of heroin addiction, HIV, AIDS, and finally tuberculosis. I first met him while working with the Health Department on a mass screening of the Carlton Arms, where we paid each resident a modest sum to get a skin test, submit to a chest X-ray, and cough up a sample of sputum. I was in charge of the latter activity. We had the men march down the stairs, line up on the sidewalk, and instructed them to hack up as much lung-butter as they could into plastic cups. These were then sealed, inserted into cardboard cylinders, and sent to the lab for bacteriological testing. (The sight of this process occurring on Main Street could not have pleased the real-estate developers in that area.)

The following notes describe my first encounters with Willie, recorded after I went back to the Carlton to read the results of all the PPD skin tests.

7/16/98

The place almost seems fun after a while. The guys there seem to enjoy it, or maybe that's just the effect of the weather; everyone feeling better in the summer months. I go there alone today to read the PPD's that were placed on Tuesday during the mass screening. We had a team of ten or so there then; now it's just me and the Carlton faithful. I pull up outside the front door and have them come down and show me their arms. Over half of them are positive, most 20 mm or more. "You're not surprised, are you?" asks Booker, the genial deskworker who acts as gatekeeper every time we do this stuff over there. I'm starting to feel like he and I are friends.

One of the tattooed white guys who work downstairs is telling me how the whole place is going to go condo once the restaurant which they are remodeling opens and starts to make some money. "What's going to happen to all these guys?" I ask. "Who cares?" he says. I just shrug. He says he caught TB just working there. "I been working here for eight years already, I may be working here the rest of my life." I look up at the fire escapes with the doors open to the hive-like mazes of rooms upstairs. Condos seem unlikely future occupants of that space, but in this city it wouldn't surprise me. Booker doesn't believe it; he says they've been saying that for years, and it hasn't happened yet. "We're still here," he says. Although he acknowledges the possibility that they may one day make a parking lot out of it; then he will look at the space where the Carlton stood and say, "Ah, the memories." "When the restaurant is open, they will have this door sealed off and make us go through the alley," he says. "It looks like an alley but it's really a street. Every time someone new moves into the neighborhood, they tell them, "Oh, they're going to tear that place down soon. But we're still here." Booker jokes about the HIV virus being a conspiracy passed through free food or something. The skinny old dude with the toothless mouth tells me matter-of-factly that he has been shooting dope for forty years. That much of my life, gone, he says, tells me he makes three hundred dollars a week and spends most of it on drugs, but he is still sharp in his position as building security, "You wouldn't believe how many thieves I caught and sent down to the 12th Street station," he says.

Not long after the screening, Willie (the skinny old dude) came down with TB himself, and I was assigned as his caseworker. It turned out that Willie had been in the building for so long that the growing burden of his presence was tolerated, even though it was obvious that his health was slipping away from him and he needed medical help. "I'm afraid he's gonna die in there," said Booker. I would go see him every day, carrying his pill bottles with me so I wouldn't have to dig them out of the piles of dirty old clothes and other assorted junk that filled his dark, cramped closet of a room. One day Jasper, the owner of the hotel, asked me to come in his office and said pretty much the same thing. He told me that Willie had worked for his partner for years and years, and so he always let him keep a room and make a few bucks around there, but it wasn't a nursing home, and he wanted to know if I could take him out of there. I said that they could call an ambulance, but he would have to go voluntarily. But they had tried this, and Willie refused to leave, not wanting to surrender his autonomy, even for the sake of his health.

Eventually, however, he did need to go to the hospital, and was sent from there to a nursing home on the South Side. I visited him there once, and he was as feisty as ever, saying he liked it because he had his own room, with a window, a television, and a private bathroom—all things he had lacked at the Carlton. I sat there and listened to him as he told me stories about the women in his life. Because they gave him all his TB medicines every day, I no longer had to see him on DOT, and so I lost touch with him for awhile. Then, in May 2000, I stopped by the same nursing home to check on another patient. While I was there I thought I'd check on Willie, also. I hadn't seen him in a few months and I figured he might be looking better; maybe he might even be ready to walk out.

I found, instead, a mere shadow of a man, sitting in a chair, being fed with a spoon by a nurse. The skin on his forehead was shiny and about to peel away, like a plastic film, and he squirmed in pain between swallows. The nurse told him he had company and he opened his eyes enough to see me, but I don't know if the sight registered. "Open your eyes," she said, "Don't you want to see your company?" I still thought maybe some communication would be possible. I half-expected him to launch into a tirade, or at least to ask for money. He did neither. After she left, I sat there with him for a little while. He was perpetually wincing in pain and he looked like a shrunken puppet. This was AIDS, the old-fashioned way, I thought. An ugly, painful slipping away. "Willie, can you hear me?" I said nice and loud. "Yeah," he said, his eyes open for a moment.

"How are things going?" I asked. And he made one very coherent response: "Slow motion," he said, "slow motion."

I wondered how it must look to him, if there was any past, any memory, anything besides a drifting set of stimuli, some coming from inside, some coming from outside, no difference between them. I may well be a ghost, and he practically is. A guy like this deserves some heroin, I thought. Slow motion, indeed.

"Well," I said, eventually, "I'm going to go now, let you get some rest," as though time for rest was in short supply.

"Okay," he said. I got the feeling that he was beyond the pale, and wouldn't even notice I was gone, or remember who I was, or that I was even there.

As depressing as his situation at the Carlton Arms had been, I couldn't help wondering if this fate were somehow worse, the end more drawn out, dying in slow motion, as he said. I wondered if he missed the Carlton Arms, the daily camaraderie and confrontation. I also wondered if shifting his location really did anything about the underlying problems of poverty and addiction, which had in fact opened the door for his disease. Like the rest of the men at the Carlton Arms, he was part of a largely invisible world of daily hardship and subsistence that the prosperous city of the 1990s had no time for. In a sense, their plight epitomized many of the issues entangled with TB itself. I found the place fascinating because, as the above field note states, it seemed to have a real appeal for people in spite of its squalor. Some of the men had been there for thirty or forty years. So, in July 2000, as I was getting ready to move out of Chicago, I decided to go to the Carlton Arms to do some in-depth interviews with the men who lived there. A couple weeks earlier I was looking at the Carlton Arms for a former patient who had recently been released from prison. At that time I was a little surprised that it hadn't yet been closed down. Booker said, "We got the wagons circled and we're just waiting for the last showdown." This inspired me to chronicle the place, in some way, shape, or form, before the final day of judgment arrived. So I went there one afternoon, and sat in the lobby reading the paper while the TV blared and the fan blew the stale air around. Nobody seemed to notice much, or care. I had my tape recorder with me but hadn't planned anything yet, though I had a skeleton of what I wanted. But as I left, Booker said, "What do you want to do? Let me know. When are you going to come back? What do you want to ask?"

I said, "I want to ask them how long they've been here, what brought them here, what they like about the place, what they don't like, and so on."

"So when do you want to come back?" he asked. Booker had studied sociology at some point, back in the 1960s, and he had a good grasp of the idea of social research. I stood there a second, sweating in the close flophouse air, then made up my mind. "Tomorrow, 11 o'clock."

"I'll be here," he said, "you know everybody, that's Blue, Jasper, this is Richie. We'll all be here." I had seen Jasper the previous week at a rally held in protest of the gentrification process taking place in another nearby neighborhood. Booker said, "He goes to all those meetings now. He's becoming a militant."

I came up with a page of questions, ranging from age and occupation to a little life history and opinions about changes happening in Chicago.

Booker had told me, "Come back tomorrow, and bring some money." So I got fifty bucks in fives, prepared to spread it around. "You ready?" asked Booker when I came in. "Yeah," I said. "You bring money?" he asked. "Yeah," I said, "let's go."

He walked in the lobby, cut off the TV and announced what I wanted to do. Needless to say, I soon had volunteers. Within two hours I had cranked through all my cash and had nothing but some audiotape to show for it. I didn't feel like I got as much out of them as I could have, but there was some good stuff. One guy was a trumpet player, who made money appearing around town, on the street, and at events, including the Blues Fest. Three reasons seemed to stand out, from of all those they gave me for being there: Price, Convenience, and Safety. I interviewed ten out of one hundred residents, which might not be a bad sample size, but probably wasn't representative either. After all, these were the guys sitting in the lobby at noon. Nonetheless, I think I got a good range of short- and long-timers, from different age groups. All were black, although there are some white guys staying there.

Booker fell asleep in a chair while I was doing the interviews and afterward he asked, "What about mine? For organizing this?"

I was a little low on cash, but agreed to take him over to the grocery store to get some meat to throw on the grill for the guys. We walked over to my car, parked west of Main, and we talked a little about the interviews. "Their perspective is not very broad," he said. As we passed the new luxury townhouses on South Main, mere blocks from the Carlton Arms, Booker said, "look, it looks like Mayor's neighborhood thirty years ago." The mayor of the Chicago had moved to the neighborhood adjacent to the hotel several years earlier, and many people felt that he therefore had a personal interest in remaking the entire area to suit his decidedly middle-class tastes. Most of the guys I interviewed at the Carlton, however, seemed to think the city was definitely changing for the better—building nice houses, and so on. A few commented that things were getting more expensive, and that police harassment was getting worse. But most did not articulate this, if they did feel it. "They're so listless," said Booker.

After buying a box full of hamburgers, a bag of buns, and some mustard, we stood on the back fire escape of the Carlton Arms, where the summer's daily barbecues were done, across from the roaring "L" tracks. While lighting the charcoal, Booker said to me, "You're showing interest in them will give them some purpose." A couple young guys who worked there had their custom-outfitted, four-door sedans parked in back, and every time a south-bound train plowed through, one car's alarm would scream for about thirty seconds. An old guy came out and emptied the old water from his cooler over the edge of the black-painted steel, onto the gravel and dirt below. Occasionally there would be a dispute over cooking technique. Like all arguments at the Carlton Arms, these were loud and confrontational, and usually amounted to nothing. Booker told me about the rat looking in his window the night before.

Rats, like TB, are a problem in urban areas that selectively afflicts the poor. In the microcosm of the Carlton Arms, both the changing urban environment and the urban ecology of poverty were manifestly evident. The beleaguered SRO represented the crumbling toehold of affordable urban housing and the downward slide of the working poor in general, and the black poor in particular. The waves of money and political power pushed people before them like flotsam in the surf, to be deposited on some other shore, somewhere out of sight. The fact that they were also prone to disease was just another reason to displace them, while at the same time claiming to help them. In the same way that the men at the hotel wished Willie would leave so they wouldn't have to watch him die, the denizens of downtown Chicago wished that the transient, dirty and downtrodden would be polite enough to abandon the old fleabag flop and find a "decent" place to live, preferably in another part of town.

CONCLUSION

Carrying out the work of TB control involved locating individuals and treating them where they were found, while leaving their surroundings essentially untouched. The limitations of this approach to public health should be apparent from these examples. All of the individuals described above were living within the difficult parameters of poverty. With the exception of Reggie, who had stable housing in an apartment that he shared with his mother, all of them had need of assistance beyond the merely medical. Someone like Reggie, who was well-fed, stably housed, and employed, probably had a lower chance of developing disease in the first place, and even if he did develop symptoms, could have been treated with few complications, assuming he took the prescribed medication and was not exposed to a drug-resistant strain.

The same was not true of the others. Stanley and Josef faced difficult futures with or without TB. For Stanley, a TB diagnosis actually provided access to resources that he would not have otherwise had, and like many homeless patients, he sought to delay his completion of treatment so that these benefits could continue. In spite of his self-confidence concerning his ability to earn money and please the opposite sex, Mr. Valentine accepted an offer to enter a housing program for homeless TB patients. He may have been "working the system" to some extent, but in spite of all his hustling, he was barely scraping by. Looking through his medical records, I saw that one of his previous visits to the emergency room had stemmed from an assault by baseball bat. He was a man who lived within hard circumstances—some of his own creation, to be sure, but many not. These are the people who tend to be exposed to TB and suffer the most with it. A critical epidemiology of tuberculosis tells us this much, clearly: poor tuberculosis patients, by and large, do not pose a significant threat to the health of the affluent, any more than the homeless threaten the housed. On the contrary, they are threatened more by TB than anyone else.

Chapter 6 deals with other "hard cases" such as Willie and Mr. Valentine. In my years working with TB, I encountered many who had similar circumstances and outcomes. Stories such as theirs can give one an entirely different perspective on the problem of tuberculosis, placing it within the frame of a canvas which is both broader in scope and more intimate in detail than those employed by other methods alone. This canvas would also contain the backdrop of the inner city world with all its daily stresses and dangers. The sociological imagination, as defined by Mills, necessitates the ability to shuttle between many levels of analysis while maintaining focus on the central issue: the connection between private troubles and public issues (Mills 8). This chapter has attempted to do just that: to present a tangible picture of tuberculosis in the 1990s: who got it, how they got it, where they lived, and what those environments were like. Tuberculosis is inseparable from these circumstances. If we are going to situate the sociological, cultural, and economic forces that influence health and all its correlates, then we must see them in their proper environment; we must talk about local context and the communities where people live. Ethnography can be an invaluable aid to epidemiology and public health because it provides a means of seeing these contexts as important variables in and of themselves. In Chicago this means talking about the neighborhood, not only as a unit of population, but as an active and powerful presence in peoples' lives.

5   Welcome to the West Side

Hanging Out in TB Alley

Scattered clouds flap like tattered
   flags,
Rips in the sky beyond the horizon
When the masts of the city
Rise from the morning.

In the park every day
Buick, Honda, Chevrolet
Burned up, like buffalo carcass
Slaughtered beasts picked bare by
   buzzards
Bones by the side of the road.

The towers downtown stand solemn
   as queens
The last big pieces on the scattered
   board
While all about them scared and
   blind
Trapped squares of black and white.

Out here the land lies randomly
   arranged
Like the junk in an aquarium;
Crumbling castles, busted buildings,
Rusty tunnels and bridges to swim
   through
And light drifts down like rain from
   the blue.

Bottom dwellers breed—
Catfish-rat-dog-pigeon
Hooker-bum-preacher-suit-sucker
Hang apart but stuck together
Fight for the right to feed.

Saved every day by the words we say:
Pass the bottle, lend me a dime,
We all one blood, we all do time.

Fistful of dollars on every corner
Dirty Harry cruising his mean
   submarine.

A single voice pulls a song like
   an oar:
You all don't know, you all don't
   know,
You all don't know me like the Lord
   do know.

A soft voice says between sips
   of wine:
I don't know why, I don't know why
I would never live nowhere but
   the West Side.

       —Chicago 1994, by the author

ONE DAY I was eating at a soul food kitchen located beneath the "L" tracks on the West Side. It looked like a shack that had been swept up by a tornado in Mississippi and plopped down in between two brick tenements. There were a couple small windows facing the street, and in the winter these were always steamed over and only dimly translucent. Inside, the peeling walls were adorned with paper plates on which menu items had been scrawled in black ink. A single black man, in his sixties and wearing a chef's hat, prepared everything from pancakes and eggs to fried catfish and slid the plates across the small counter without taking a step. A beat-up old boom box with the cassette door missing played an old tape of Booker T and the MGs. In addition to myself and a friend from graduate school, there was a young woman wearing a gas company uniform and another guy from the neighborhood there. The place was so small that we nearly filled it between the four of us. While we ate, we talked about different things: the weather, where to get a good haircut, what the neighborhood was like in the sixties. When I said I worked at County General Hospital, the gas lady posed an interesting rhetorical question: "What, you kill people?"

The neighborhood guy then chimed in, "They tried to kill me." He showed all of us the cast on his arm and he said he had been run over by a car. "This is a different cast from the one they messed up at County," he said. "Some doctor put it on all funny, and wouldn't do it over." Instead the doctor simply told him, "Go on home."

"Man," I said, "it seems like everybody on the West Side has been run over by a car." When I said this, the other folks in the restaurant laughed. I made the comment based on the experiences of TB patients I had known: at least half of them, it seemed, had been struck by an automobile at one time or another, and some suffered permanent damage. One woman had pins in both her knees, another had a huge ugly scar disfiguring her leg as a result of a hit-and-run. The guy responded, "That's because these kids drive so crazy. They shouldn't even give them no license."

"In the early morning if you go through Cleveland Park," I said, "there's always cars smashed up by the side of the road."

"That's where I got hit, Cleveland Park," the guy said. "I was just trying to get across the road." The broad, sweeping boulevards which cut through the park invited cruising, and were often used as alternate routes by people seeking to dodge highway traffic. The foot-bound poor suffered the consequences. Like so many other problems which might be considered catastrophic were they to occur somewhere else, hit-and-runs had become a fact of life here. Between the recklessness of youth and the carelessness of intoxication, life was tenuous indeed. This was the reality of the West Side.

Though quite easily accessible, the American inner city remains in many ways a foreign environment to those who don't live there. Many people pass through the inner city of Chicago every day on their way to and from work. Rarely, however, do these people stop their cars, much less get out. This is especially true in "burned out" areas like the West Side. When I began working at County General Hospital in late 1993, the West Side was new to me. As a college student in Chicago from 1987 to 1990, I had resided in a densely populated lakeside neighborhood with a very diverse and relatively transient population. The West Side, in contrast, was predominately black, and many residents had lived their entire lives there. The West Side was also a place that was generally not frequented by people who *didn't* live there. Many people in Chicago were frankly afraid of it. But as a field-worker for the public hospital, I was obligated to return there many, many times over a span of several years. Simply put, there was a lot of sickness concentrated in the area. For most of the 1990s it had the highest morbidity rates for TB of any neighborhood in the city. In the course of doing my work I came to see that TB was only one of many nested issues. This will be apparent in the pages that follow. For now, I would simply like to describe the neighborhood as I came to know it.

For the casual passer-by, the West Side in the 1990s appeared rather empty. Many of the buildings, both commercial and residential, had been razed since the riots of 1968. As of the late 1990s, there had been some new construction in areas, but it was sparse and uneven. Some patches of land seemed to be going back to prairie. Indeed, the city seemed to be practicing a form of scorched-earth policy, clearing the ground in order to start all over again. When I first entered the area and began making connections within it, however, I began to see a fascinating social reality existing below the surface devastation. It resembled, to me, the remains of a close-knit village, decimated by a war, then stranded on the moon.

In their out-of-print classic *Street Signs Chicago,* Lew Kreinberg and Charles Bowden argue that the idea of the neighborhood as a genuine folk society is a delusion, given the capitalist imperatives that actually drive urban settlement patterns. "Neighborhoods," they write, "have never been the point of Chicago, or of any large city. The city has been about the lake, the canal, the river, the railroads, the airport, mills, factories, banks. Neighborhoods have always been afterthoughts" (Bowden and Kreinberg 18). In another passage, however, they express what seems to be a contradictory argument: "Forget the charts of the sociologists or the ZIP code bureaucrats or the politicians, and find neighborhood in a private geography of flat, store, saloon, job, maybe church, usually school. A place understood with one's own eyes, hands and feet, ground measured and experienced at the level of daily life" (Bowden and Kreinberg 72).

It was exactly this "private geography" which I sought to document through the methods of ethnography. At the same time, I remain mindful of the structural forces that shape these social worlds. As patterns of disease distribution prove, neighborhood boundaries do constitute salient social divisions, and the *idea* of the neighborhood continues to resonate deeply in the minds of both sociologists and urban dwellers. Though forces of gentrification may reduce many "improving" neighborhoods to marketing concepts, in poor parts of the city the neighborhood is still seen as a living, if ailing, entity. In my own research the neighborhood surfaced again and again, both as an actual geographical location where I physically *went,* and as a reference point in the minds of my interview subjects.[1] As Chapter 4 revealed, in doing tuberculosis fieldwork I ventured into many idiosyncratic social spaces. The situations and stories of the ill people that I encountered provided windows into their local worlds, as well as illustrating the external factors that contributed to disease transmission.

This chapter focuses on one neighborhood in Chicago, and on particular people within that neighborhood. It is an area where some of the most dramatic patterns and problems of the postindustrial city are made manifest, where one may see illness in its habitat, as it intertwines on a day-to-day level with complex issues of race, class, gender, and poverty. The circumstances and events I recount here represent only a sliver of life on the West Side. They are not meant to accurately portray the community as a whole. Some of the lifestyles of the very poor—the addicted, the alcoholic, the homeless, the hustler—gain disproportionate attention due to their relative prominence within an area characterized by declining population and economic stagnation. TB is a disease which preys primarily on the poor, and its path cuts across many different dimensions of poverty. Because of this, it can serve to remind us of the interconnectedness of many issues. As Paul Farmer has stated, it is necessary to show "both individual experience and the larger social matrix in which it is embedded in order to see how various large-scale social forces come to be translated into personal distress and disease" (Farmer 1996, 261). To do so, we must consider the social environment of the ghetto as an important factor in the health and well-being of those who live there.

But first, some historical perspective is needed. *Ghetto* is a word originally associated with the Jewish populations of Europe, who were segregated within specific sectors of cities (Zorbaugh 140, Clark 11). In today's American vernacular it usually refers to predominately black neighborhoods located inside cities of all sizes. In both cases it is the fact of segregation (de jure or de facto) for reasons of race, religion, economics, or behavior that is the key to the ghetto. Since the 1960s and the Black Power movement, the term has also been used in a manner that indicates pride in a place that one can call one's own.

The word *slum*, though often associated with the ghetto, has a different set of meanings associated with it. It might be useful to briefly contrast these meanings here. In *The Gold Coast and the Slum*, Zorbaugh wrote that "The slum comes to be characterized . . . not only by mean streets and ramshackle buildings, but by well-defined types of submerged humanity" (Zorbaugh 129). "Human derelicts" of all types were drawn to slum areas because of low rents and lax standards of conduct. But in Zorbaugh's time, the slum was not necessarily an area of racial or religious segregation. The slum was, in fact, by its very nature not homogenous, but cosmopolitan: "The cosmopolitanism of the slum means more than a polyglot culture. It involves a breaking down of prejudices, until in an area like 'Bughouse Square' social distances are reduced to a minimum" (Zorbaugh 150). The slum did contain segregated areas within it, however. These segregated "ghettos" constituted "little worlds" of social relations where immigrants of like backgrounds—Italians, Irish, Poles, Persians—could feel as though they had a place (Zorbaugh 141). In Zorbaugh's time, it is worth noting, the ghetto was quite different from the slum in the sense that it was ethnically segregated but economically diverse. Such a neighborhood, inhabited by African Americans who had migrated from the South, is described in depth by Drake and Cayton in *Black Metropolis*. Sometime between the writing of Zorbaugh's book and the writing of Clark's, the term "ghetto" had come to be associated primarily, if not exclusively, with black Americans.

The situation of poor black people in northern cities, while not without parallels to other poor groups, has some legitimate claims to exceptionalism. In 1968, Suttles wrote: "Oddly enough, it is the lowly status of the Negroes that makes them such a portentous enemy. Because of the universal fear of stigma in being associated with them, it is assumed that no group in the area can halt their invasion" (Suttles 119). It is an irony of history that the segregation of blacks in urban areas coincided in many ways with the integration of other groups into the broader society. Prior to 1900, as Massey and Denton documented in *American Apartheid*, black people were less likely to be confined to ghettos than they are now. According to the authors, "The era of integrated living and widespread interracial contact was rapidly effaced after 1900 because of two developments: the industrialization of America and the concomitant movement of blacks from farms to cities" (Massey and Denton 26). In the period from 1900 to 1940, black people became ghettoized, and ghettos were blackened. A double irony is contained in the fact that the continuing, and sometimes increasing, residential segregation of black people has coincided with expanded opportunity for black people in American mainstream society. In 1993, Massey and Denton concluded that ". . . one-third of all African Americans in the United States live under conditions of intense racial segregation. They are unambiguously among the nation's most spatially isolated and geographically secluded people, suffering extreme segregation across multiple dimensions simultaneously" (Massey and Denton 77). Of all American cities, Chicago was the most racially segregated as recently as 1980 (Massey and Denton 64).

The decades of the 1960s and early 1970s are important historical reference points for the ghetto. The passage of the Civil Rights Acts, changes in federal welfare policy brought on by the War on Poverty, and the social strife that occurred in that era are all benchmarks in the lives of these communities. It is an era which many of my own interview subjects also hearkened back to. Clark's and Rainwater's books on ghetto life are instructive for the very reason that they illustrate how little some things have changed since the 1960s. Clark wrote, in 1965, at the height of the Civil Rights Movement: "The symptoms of lower-class society afflict the dark ghettos of America—low aspiration, poor education, family instability, illegitimacy, unemployment, crime, drug addiction and alcoholism, frequent illness and early death . . . The most concrete fact of the ghetto is its physical ugliness—the dirt, the filth, the neglect. . . . The only constant characteristic is a sense of inadequacy. People seem to have given up on the little things that are so often the symbol of larger things" (Clark 27). The term "tangle of pathology," which Clark coined in his book, was later adopted by Daniel Patrick Moynihan, and became common currency in the poverty discussions of later years. In the late 1960s, there was also a spirit of nationalistic pride that arose in the ghetto, epitomized by vigorous individual voices such as that of Malcolm X, Stokely Carmichael, and Huey Newton and the Black Panther Party. Many of these leaders saw the ghetto as a sort of homeland, and the city as a major site of contestation—even of war—with white authority (Allen 193; Van Deburg 113; Castells 117–118).

This war had many casualties. Malcolm X was killed in Harlem in 1965. The 1968 riots following the assassination of Martin Luther King, Jr. reduced much of Chicago's West and South Sides to flaming ruin. They marked both the apotheosis of this rebellion and the beginning of the end of Black Power. In Chicago, the young Black Panther leader Fred Hampton, who had articulated a radical Marxist perspective on the ghetto, was assassinated in 1969 by the Chicago Police Department, working in cooperation with the FBI. The West Side neighborhood where the killing took place had to be roped off during the funeral to control thousands of outraged onlookers (Goldfield 292). George Jackson, an influential revolutionary voice who originally hailed from Chicago's West Side, was gunned down by guards in California's Soledad prison in the early seventies. These are now considered minor figures in American mainstream history, but they are still remembered by older members of the black community, especially on the West Side.

In 1992, author George Bailey wrote these lines about the West Side of Chicago: "I have walked down main arteries and neighborhood streets where an inordinate number of people, especially black and Latino men, sit the days away, eyes averted, waiting for something to happen. They appear on stoops and on street corners, and in warmer weather, under trees, sitting on cast-off furniture . . . They constitute the faceless, rapidly spreading urban underclass, left behind, caught up in a system which has rendered them null and void" (Bailey xi). This description was typical of those written about the ghetto in the 1990s. In between the writing of this passage and the turbulent decade of the 1960s lay decades of disappointment and despair. The hopes raised by the Civil Rights and Black Power movements had been largely unfulfilled, and this fact was keenly felt on the West Side. The "promised land" glimpsed by Martin Luther King seemed to recede in the distance during the Reagan eighties. For many black men and women, the years between the sixties and the nineties became lost years—lost to imprisonment, addiction, injury, illness, unemployment, or a combination of these. The ghetto of the 1990s, unlike the ghettos of the past, was segregated on more than one level: racially, economically, and culturally.

Many black neighborhoods are still dense with social relations carried to northern cities from life in the rural South. As James Edgar Wideman has written about his mother's place in her neighborhood in Pittsburgh: "Her relations with people in that close-knit, homogenous community were based on trust, mutual respect, common spiritual and material concerns. Face-to-face contact, shared language and values, a large fund of communal experience rendered individual lives extremely visible in Homewood. Both a person's self-identity ('You know who you are') and accountability ('Other people know who you are') were firmly established" (Wideman 73). For better or for worse, long-term, extended relations remain a crucial and incontrovertible fact of life in poor urban neighborhoods such as these. Social networks, however, can be both a blessing and a curse in the best of conditions. As discussed in Chapter 4, the social network—both of house and of street—plays an important role in the community-based treatment of tuberculosis, as well as the transmission of the disease.

The economic and physical deterioration of the ghetto community, the adaptation of social networks to those conditions, the positive and negative impact of these networks on individuals, and the internalized feelings of inferiority and anger that accompany this process are all closely linked phenomena. The ghetto as deviant subculture and the ghetto as oppressed colony are both powerful ideas which surfaced repeatedly in my daily work with TB patients in poor neighborhoods. Often these two images of the ghetto, which might seem to contradict each other, existed side by side in people's minds. Both are, in this sense, real. This chapter deals with my entry into the world of the West Side ghetto and some of the people who I encountered there. In addition to my own observations, it will focus on residents' views of their troubled community: its history, its present condition, and its unclear future.

DOWN ON THE CORNER

One individual, whom I will refer to as "Billy," used to hang around a neighborhood liquor store, situated along a major thoroughfare about five miles away from Chicago's downtown business district. This liquor store was a much-frequented establishment, and Billy, who had lived in the neighborhood since the 1950s, was a fixture there. Nearly everybody in the neighborhood knew him (though not necessarily by his given name) and he knew almost everyone who came there. This was especially true of the other drinkers, most of whom had shared bottles with him at one time or another. My first intersection with this West Side neighborhood came through Billy and "his corner." I first met him at County General because he had active pulmonary tuberculosis. I saw him nearly every day for the better part of a year due to his illness, and I often stopped to see him for purely social reasons. It was while hanging around the corner with Billy that I was introduced to some of the local people, and through him I learned something of the neighborhood's history.

Billy could be clinically described as a forty-four-year-old African American male, a chronic alcohol abuser with a past history of tuberculosis and homelessness. Because of his health history, he was very familiar to other members of the tuberculosis team at the hospital. The first things that

I noticed about him when I went to see him in his hospital room were his goatee-style beard—he later corrected me and called it a "Van Dyke"—and the tattoo on his arm which read "A Love Supreme."

The tattoo was the first thing I asked him about. Referring to the John Coltrane record of the same name, I asked him if he played jazz. His response was, "I like to listen to jazz music and I used to play a little piano. I can play piano by ear. I come from a very musically inclined family." As I was to find out later, Billy had many lines that he used over and over again, and this was one of them. Whenever music came up as a subject of conversation he was bound to say, "I come from a very musical family." He usually stated this as a precursor to a song rendered in low, rumbling monotone. Sometimes he would spin around on the sidewalk, showing off his dance moves as he sang. "I know a lot of dusties," he would always say.

I did not find out a great deal about Billy's family and life history during our first meeting. In the following months, as I got to know him, certain reference points came up again and again. As an objective set of facts, Billy's life would not seem much different than that of many other African-American men of his generation living in this city. Born in a rural county of North Carolina in 1950, in a "log cabin hospital," Billy moved to Chicago's West Side with his family in 1959. His father worked at a cement plant in Indiana for thirteen years and was able to purchase the two-story home that the family occupied on one of the old boulevards. The home was still in the family when I met him, as ownership had passed from Billy's parents to his older sister and then, after her death, to her daughter. The web of names and relations that Billy could reel off in answer to a simple question was remarkable, but it was not necessarily unusual. The majority of patients that I encountered at County General had similar kinship ties, extending back to the South, throughout the city, and often to other cities as well.

Billy was close to his family in many ways. The statement "he's got people," which was commonly uttered about Billy by his street acquaintances, implied that he had kin, and kin were seen as a valuable resource. Again, this might not seem unusual, but this statement was always made in a certain context—namely, in reference to Billy's "condition." The fact that Billy was both a kind, respectful, and intelligent man and a hardcore and apparently hopeless alcoholic was a source of concern to all those around him, not only to his kin but also to others who were also in his "condition." I found this out later, when my relationship with Billy moved from the hospital to the street.

Soon after he left the hospital, I discovered that the address listed on his medical chart was the house of a neighborhood acquaintance. Billy did not actually stay there—though occasionally he slept under the porch. One of my coworkers, who had worked with Billy in the past, informed me of this before I went to look for him, so it was no surprise to me when I found him not at the house but at the liquor store on the corner. This liquor store was a hub of the local community, or at least a certain portion of the local community, and Billy had been a regular on that corner almost from the time that his family moved to Chicago in 1959. He told me that the store had been there "as long as I can remember" and when I asked why people gathered there he simply said "that's where things be happening." Billy's life history was complexly intertwined with this social environment. He was almost as much a part of the local scene as the liquor store itself, and as a sort of public figure the facts of his existence belonged not only to him but to all the others who had knowledge of him and his problems. A good example is that of Billy's "condition," his addiction: how he got there and how he might be helped. The fact that he was an alcoholic was known to all the regulars on the corner, as was the fact that he had "people," who had tried many times in the past to help him "get himself together." One person on the corner told me that Billy used to rollerskate all over the neighborhood and was once known for his grace on skates. When I asked Billy about this he laughed and said "Yeah, that was back in the sixties" and then went on to explain where the roller rink was and demonstrated some of his fancy dancing moves. For Billy, the sixties served as a reference point, almost a time of innocence. Once, when I asked him how the neighborhood had changed, he said that it had gotten worse, "things are more confused." The period he was comparing it to was the sixties, when Jefferson Avenue was a booming strip of shopping and nightlife and there was more of a friendly, trusting feeling among people in the community. This idealized image of an orderly community was often conveyed to me by older residents of the neighborhood, usually as a point of contrast to the present state of things. "Nowadays," Billy said, "you can't hardly even trust your best friend." He attributed this change to the widespread use of hard drugs.

Billy could speak of hard drugs from experience. He started mainlining heroin in 1968, when he was eighteen years old, and he twice went to the penitentiary for armed robberies, which he had committed to support his habit. His first trip to prison was in 1974 and he was there for four years. He was out of prison for about six months before he went back, this time serving half of a six-year sentence. Billy earned maximum time off his sentence for good behavior and after his third sentence in prison (for residential burglary) he "closed the safe and forgot the combination," giving up the life of crime. He did go to the pen one more time for violating parole, but his parole officer gave him a glowing recommendation and his sentence was brief.

When I asked him about this, Billy recounted these events slowly, as though he was journeying back into his memory, as though he had tried to forget them. Indeed, I didn't even know about his prison history until a friend of his mentioned it to me. In the first six months of our acquaintance he had never talked about it, although other aspects of his life were familiar to me from repeated telling. For instance, he often volunteered information about jobs that he had in the sixties, (working as a secretary's aide at a brokerage firm on State Street, flipping hamburgers, loading beer at the Chicago Stadium, picking sweet potatoes in North Carolina), or about other individuals in the neighborhood and his relationships to them. From this I gathered that his criminal past was something of which he was not proud.

Billy's biography placed him within the community in a particular way. He occupied a particular position, or role, though this was not necessarily stable. From the time of his last release from prison in the mid-eighties until the time I met him, Billy had been in and around the same neighborhood that he first entered as a boy in 1959. Elijah Anderson's study of a street corner on Chicago's South Side, *A Place on the Corner,* divided the street corner into three distinguishable status groups—"regulars," "hoods," and "wineheads." I might apply the same categories to Billy's corner, but I will avoid this approach, because the major figure in my street-corner story seemed to defy those kinds of categories. Billy was a winehead, and he was a regular, and he was once a hood, but none of those labels described what he actually *was.*

By the same token, Billy's corner had its own character, its own life, which distinguished it from other places in other nations, other neighborhoods, or even other corners in the same neighborhood. This was the human, the individual, the personal level of the place. In *Street Corner Society,* William Foote Whyte stated that he was trying "To build a sociology based upon observed interpersonal events" (Whyte 358). At some level, he could not separate the social structures of "Cornerville" from the people and activities that made them up. He started with the place and the people, and found that they expressed themselves better than any theory could. My own discussion of the West Side, therefore, must start with the corner where I met Billy. This was my doorway to the world of the West Side. This neighborhood had a remarkable quantity of face-to-face relationships that had endured over time. For better or for worse, Billy's personal history and that of the neighborhood were inseparable. His identity was linked in a basic way to its corners, its buildings, its parks and its people. His public life, in which nearly every waking hour his behavior was on display to others, gave much of his experience the external quality of an artifact, which could be described and analyzed from multiple perspectives other than his own.

This became apparent on the day that I met Kenny, another longtime resident of the neighborhood. Kenny approached me on the corner and asked if I had twenty-five cents. I said "Yes, but what if I need it?" and he replied, "If you needed it, I would give it to you." I gave him the quarter and he went and bought a bottle of wine and returned and we started to talk. Billy was there too, and the two of them, within a matter of minutes, managed to flood me with information not only about the corner, and the neighborhood, but about each other as well. Kenny told me how Billy used to be. He affirmed the fact that Billy used to rollerskate around the neighborhood, and said "You know what? He was good, too. He used to have a lot of talents. He used to draw too. He used to do some crazy shit, too, but you know what my sister says about Billy—you clean him up and he's a fine-looking man." And then he added, for emphasis, ". . . and he can be helped."

I told Kenny how, earlier in the year, Billy had been sent to the hospital with a concussion and spent three days on tubes with a needle in his brain—then was discharged back to the street and promptly got drunk again. "We almost lost him," I said.

Kenny looked at me hard and said, "You serious?" Then he turned to Billy and demanded, "You ain't still drinking, is you?" Then he turned to me again and said, " I'm glad you told me that shit, 'cuz he ain't going to drink no more if I can help it." The attitude conveyed by Kenny in this exchange was one of stern but heartfelt concern, one brother setting another straight. "Today you asked me for a drink, and I gave you one . . . but I ain't never going to give you a fucking drink again," he declared to Billy. Kenny looked over at me several times and said, "I'm glad you told me that." He told me about how Billy had made himself a lot of enemies over the years with his big mouth and his behavior while drunk.

Then Kenny walked away to speak with someone else, and Billy was able to talk to me alone. Normally Billy was the one on the corner making most of the noise, but Kenny was a talker who put even Billy's big mouth to shame. Throughout the preceding conversation Billy had done little more than smile and nod. When Kenny stepped away, though, he said to me, "Some of the things he says about me are true." Then went on to add, "He's a . . . you know . . . a 'special kid' . . . he got problems in the head . . . his momma is worried about him gettin' in trouble, bein' in a bad environment . . . he just got out of the pen and he might end up back in . . . you see how he is . . . he got, like, too much energy . . ." As he told me this Kenny was whipping his wine bottle against a brick wall, lending unintended credibility to the statement. Billy then said in a low voice: "He's probably lucky to still be alive."

This situation could be interpreted in different ways. One could focus on the fact that each one was "talking the other down," while both obviously had severe problems of their own that they sought to deny. One could discredit both accounts, simply because of their flawed sources. Or one could consider the fact that I was there, a white man and representative of the medical establishment (Billy always introduced me as his "nurse") and conclude that each one was trying to impress me in some way with his judgments of the other. Or you could simply see each one's concern for the other as genuine, albeit tangled in a context of shared struggles, failures, and self-knowledge that only gave it more meaning.

Morality in this environment is always relative, and enmeshed in human relationships. Death is a very real presence, and Kenny and Billy both lead lives that could end quickly. Each of them was aware of his own situation, even when judging the people around him. Billy usually added "not like I'm no better" when he criticized others on the corner, and Kenny was the first one to say to me, "I'm a winehead," while at the same time stating that he loved the neighborhood, but detested all "the two legged creatures that's in it."

"I could give up drinking" he said, after asking me if I could help him get a job. "You know what I need? You know what I need to give up drinking?"

"No," I replied.

"A reason." I looked at Kenny and he looked me in the eye and repeated, "All I need is a reason."

I ran into Kenny again about a month later, outside a Salvation Army soup line in a neighborhood several miles away from the corner. I gave him some bus tokens and I said "You owe me a conversation," and he simply said, "Let's talk." I asked him about the neighborhood, what had changed, what had stayed the same. He said, "The neighborhood has not changed, it's the people. Used to be *unity,* a lot of it." Again, this seemed to convey a sense of a more ideal community existing in the past. I was interested in this idea, and so I followed up on it.

"How do you define 'unity'?" I asked. He thought about this and responded, referring to the gangs which were always fighting in the area, "Unity means a Spirit can get along with a Warlord. They can be friends . . ." He described how gangs had lost a certain quality, and now they didn't care about anything anymore. I asked him about Lord Tiny, the late founder of the Spirits, whose name was spray painted on the side of Richardson's liquor store, below the slogan "Spirit City." He said "I used

to see him around. Tiny didn't smoke or do drugs. He wore this motor-
cycle jacket . . . he was a loner . . . he weren't no gang-banger . . . but he
was a leader . . ." Kenny thought a minute, nodded to himself, and smiled.
"Tiny was cool . . . not like those that carry on after him . . ."

"Are you saying that gangs have lost their manners?" I asked.

At this he became excited. "Yeah man, that's it, that's exactly it . . .
they've lost their manners . . . man, tell me, were you in a gang? . . . Gangs
have lost their manners . . . manners, morals, principles . . ."

I mentioned that Billy also talked a lot about "respect," and Kenny
agreed, nodding and saying, "Billy places a lot of value on respect . . . Billy
is cool . . . Man, I remember I used to see him around and I tell you, Billy
was the prettiest thing on the block . . . he always had women coming
after him . . . yeah, he knows how to respect a motherfucker . . . but you
know what? He don't respect himself."

"What about that corner where you and Billy hang out?" I asked. "Tell
me about that."

"You used to be able to meet your friends down there all the time
. . . it was a get-together corner. People used to barbecue over there. But
it's changed. People come up there to buy drugs now, not to meet their
friends . . ."

I asked him about the conflict between the younger and older generations, and he said, ". . . the older generation won't move . . . you know
some of them got sons who sell drugs around there." We then got into a
discussion of why the older generation, which placed value on respect,
was not able to instill respect in the younger. Kenny attributed this to role
models—how drug dealers are the most attractive ones around the neighborhood, and how there's a shortage of strong fathers—an argument
often used in the media. Before I let him out of the car, though, he made
an interesting statement: "We're a beautiful breed of people on the West
Side. We got a lot of knowledge and you know what? We got a lot of
unity."

"Oh yeah?" I asked. "You were just telling me there is no more unity.
Where is it hiding?"

"I don't know. You're the psychiatrist. You figure it out."

It is ironic that he would dump the responsibility for capturing the
spirit of his community right back in my lap, when I was trying to get the
answer from him. But this conversation highlights Kenny and Billy's oft-
conflicting attitudes toward the place in which they lived, as well as the
lives they led there. This ambivalence was profound and deep. One of the
things Billy often said to me was "I got to laugh to keep from crying."
Although this is a cliché, his use of it revealed an acute awareness of his
own condition—both bodily and spiritual. The seeming contradiction of

Kenny's statements—that the West Side community which is both with and without unity—characterized the torn quality of peoples' lives there.

TWO-LEGGED CREATURES

In the book *Slim's Table*, Mitchell Duneier depicts a group of working-class black men living in the ghetto. His empathetic portrayal of their lives and worldviews offered an alternative to the negative stereotypes so often perpetuated by the popular media, and by much sociology as well. Through their behavior and their language they show their values of respectability and personal responsibility, values not commonly attributed to black men in the ghetto. They did this in the face of quite powerful socioeconomic forces, a fact which affirmed their dignity and autonomy, and repudiated simplistic ideas about the effect of the environment upon the individual. These men, wrote Duneier, ". . . live with an acute sense of moral isolation" (Duneier 83).

Duneier's work was rightly applauded. But because of its focus on the positive and negative portrayals of black men and their values, it neglected the role of those very forces—historical, economic, and political—which made the ghetto such a difficult place in which to maintain one's values. The men in the book discuss this problem, but they do so largely in reference to the "negativity" of the other individuals in the ghetto—criminals, crack heads, drunks, prostitutes, and so on. The people that I talked to—Billy, Kenny, and others—also seemed to focus on the "two-legged creatures" that surrounded them. Occasionally they mentioned that Jefferson Avenue, where the street corner was situated, used to be a thriving commercial thoroughfare that was mostly destroyed by the riots of 1968. It was never rebuilt, and still resembled something of a war zone.

They didn't often mention that they lived in a community whose potential leaders have been killed or jailed; a community which was patrolled by police who can arrest men and women at will. Even less often did they mention the systematic disinvestment which left many such neighborhoods without local jobs or any markets other than drug markets, or the decay of the school system throughout the seventies and eighties. These are all factors which were real and could be documented, and which contributed to the physical and mental and moral isolation of everyone who lived there. But it was easier to focus on those people whom they saw—gangs, police, homeless people, prostitutes, addicts, and other "two-legged creatures." Thus, the idea of the ghetto as a "deviant subculture" took root even in the minds of those who live there.

Billy himself might in fact be seen as one of those very "negative" individuals fueling a stereotype that in turn incriminated the whole community. His behavior, as an ex-convict, an ex-drug-abuser, unemployed, absentee father, and public drunk qualified him for that distinction. But Billy expressed values of respect which were very similar in content to those values about which the men at Slim's table talked. Kenny admired this about Billy, and Billy admired it in others. For instance, when talking about Lord Tiny, the late founder of the Spirits, Billy said, "He was kind of rational . . . he got respect by giving respect . . . not like these kids today, who just want to act tough, but couldn't fight their way out of a paper bag." When seen in another light, Billy emerged as quite a different figure—a considerate, friendly, and intelligent man for whom life had not yet worked out as he might have hoped. Though he still planned to "get it together, on the inside."

I once asked Billy what made him keep coming back to the neighborhood and to life on the street, when he knew his family would let him live with them. He said that he missed it when he was gone, and that he wanted to know what had been going on, but he also stated that there are few people that he really missed. I asked him what his family said to him about his life in the neighborhood, and he replied: "They tell me what I already know, things in the 'hood have changed, and hangin' with certain individuals who don't mean me no good is wearin' me down and tearin' me down." It was this crucial self-awareness which made him so human, and so fascinating. Studies which show people as simplistic sociological products rather than complicated creatures of will can miss this dimension.

Billy finished his TB treatment, and for a while his drinking seemed to slow down markedly—though he still drank every day. More and more often I found him fairly sober, and when he was sober he was a very likeable man. After getting a much-needed haircut, the staff at the clinic remarked on how much better he looked, and watching him joke and flirt with the women there, it was possible to see why he might have been popular back in his prime. At times like these it was possible to think he might be following his father's advice: "Have more sense than a white-faced mule, boy—know when to come in out of the rain."

But these encouraging facts did not alter certain others. A couple weeks after coming to the clinic he cracked his hip bone in some incident on the corner, probably while drunk, (I couldn't get a clear story about what happened) and could only get around with the aid of an aluminum walker. A week after that, I went to find him at an apartment where he'd been sleeping on a cot in the living room. No one was there. I found him down on the street, clinging to a metal gate and shaking like a scarecrow as he flagged me down. He had spent the night sleeping outside in mid-December. Two days later he was back to his old self, and was even walking unaided. I marveled again and again at his resilience. Yet it only made me wonder what the next trauma would be, and if he would survive it. There were two men on the street when I found him that day, and as I helped him in the car they said to him, "Billy, what the hell are you doin' with yourself?" and to me they said, "You're a good doctor, man." Their compassion was real, but it seemed to be tempered by the knowledge that even if he didn't die this time he would have many more opportunities.

SPYING ON AN EYESORE

Billy was very helpful to me whenever I needed to locate anyone else in the neighborhood, as he was able to "put the word out" on the street, and would report back to me whether or not he had seen so-and-so. My first meeting with Isaiah came about in this way. I was looking for him because he had left the hospital AMA (Against Medical Advice) with a somewhat urgent case of TB. I knew his name, age, and so on, and I suspected that he resided in the same area, but had no idea what he actually looked like. Isaiah, like Billy, was officially homeless. But Billy knew him, and knew that he hung out on another corner a few blocks down from the liquor store.

Though familiar with the social hub of the liquor store I did not know much else about the specifics of street life in this neighborhood. I knew that there were unwritten rules and patterns of association, but I did not know what these rules and patterns were. There was a submerged web of "loose ties" and "close ties" which connected many people, and TB also seemed to spread through these associations. Often these connections would not be apparent until long afterward, if they ever were.

Through Isaiah, I became familiar with another specific space within this zone of overlapping associations. Like Billy's street corner, it had both physical and social dimensions. To the untrained eye, it was nothing but an empty lot, strewn with rubble and debris, containing one tall old tree and little else. It was located behind a small functioning convenience store, across the street from a large church on one side, with a couple different storefront churches, small businesses, and apartment buildings across the street on the other side.

I describe Isaiah's spot as empty, but it is exactly this "emptiness" which I hope to contest. The text that follows has several sources: my daily journals, some photographs taken by Isaiah himself, and recorded discussions in which we discussed the pictures that he took. Together they provide a vicarious immersion in the world of the West Side, as Isaiah and his friends knew it.

9/01/98

I dropped off a camera for Isaiah yesterday; he snapped a picture of me while I was standing there, and today I went back and saw him, and he said he's been taking a lot of pictures already; pictures of the neighborhood. He says he almost got one of a guy getting arrested for drugs, but the cops threw the guy in the car so fast he missed it.

While he and I are standing by my car, Rock and Cisco pull up in Rock's black car. They get out and Rock is drinking Diet Pepsi; he sees me and says, "Hey, it's Killer Paul," and I say to Isaiah, he thinks I killed Stormy, and Isaiah says no, he's just joking. In a couple minutes after saying hello to everyone else Rock comes over and shakes my hand, calls me "Killer Paul" again, and I say "me?"

I say, "You're paying the undertaker already by smoking those cancer sticks," and he says, "I know, I'm trying to quit, they say every one is a nail in the coffin." I tell him I'll come by his house sometime, but I won't try to stick him with any needles, and he says, "They got me sticking myself with needles now," and I ask why, and he says they told him he's got diabetes, or "sugar." He knew that he had it already, he says, because he had all the symptoms, which he read off of a poster somewhere, but it was worse than he thought.

While we are talking an unmarked police car cruises by, and Rock says, jokingly, "They're looking over here, saying, "What's that white boy doing here? I hope they try something so they can be embarrassed."

Before I leave, RJ asks me to help him "get himself together" so he can get on SSI. He figures by me being a doctor (I tell him I am not) I can do something. I tell him he has to have a medically verifiable condition, and that he needs to go to the hospital and get that done there. Then RJ's wife tells me again about her back problems, from getting hit by a car and falling down the stairs, and how she has pain, and I tell her for the second time, how she should go to the ER and get a referral for orthopedics, otherwise without a medical card she will never be seen.

This account illustrates the concentration of medical need, the unavoidable presence of illegal drugs, the racially charged surveillance of the police and the role of the medical system as gatekeeper to ever more restricted public welfare. Rock's joking with me about Stormy's death was also indicative of a deeply held suspicion. Rock refused to have anyone "stick him" with any needles, and he had refused to be tested by me for TB for this very reason. As a young man he had endured some painful medical procedures, and he believed that black people were foolish to trust doctors or any other medical personnel. I didn't blame him for his suspicion of me, given the history of Tuskegee which he often cited. Nevertheless, he saw the potential advantage of having me around if the police pulled up. "I hope they try something, so they can be embarrassed," he said, relishing the idea of playing one authoritative institution off against another.

Isaiah's life, like Billy's, was wrapped up with that of the neighborhood, and his observations reflected those connections. The following excerpt reveals some of his empathy for the people around him, and the effect of their fortunes on his own identity:

9/14/98

I pick up Isaiah's photographs and drive over to the West Side so we can look at them together . . . The first thing he tells me, before I can mention the photos, is that some guy named Big John died today, or rather, died a couple days ago but was only discovered and removed from his apartment on Warner Blvd. today. Isaiah watched in sorrow as the firemen and paramedics went in to remove the body with masks on because the smell was so bad. He said he was really hurt and angry because, as he said, "the so-called friends" who were supposed to look in on Big John didn't do so, and he ended up suffocating from the heat. "Can you imagine, sitting there, unable to do anything, having your life flash before your eyes, unable to breathe because of the heat, dying like that?" He kept talking about it. I asked him if Big John hung out on the corner, and he said, "Once in a while," but he hadn't seen him in a couple of weeks.

It was clear that Isaiah was quite upset with this incident. For me it revealed, once again, the presence of death on the West Side, a daily companion. Isaiah himself said as much: "I've seen so many go, I'm afraid that pretty soon I'll be the last dinosaur."

As we flipped through the photos, I asked Isaiah to tell me what each one was a picture of. Though many of them seemed like almost random snapshots of the area in which we were standing, to Isaiah each one had content and meaning. There was one that seemed to be merely a picture of a sidewalk, but Isaiah said that the picture showed that the grass on one side of the street was better tended than the grass on the other side. When I asked him about the grass on the near side, he said, "that's the neighborhood grass. Miserable." I asked him about the expression, "the grass is always greener on the other side of the fence." "Well," he said, "it's true."

Another picture seemed to contain nothing but a bright glaring sun and some clouds, but in the corner of the photo was a small winged shape, and I pointed to it, and he said, "That's a helicopter; they got the neighborhood under surveillance." He laughed about the situation of himself pointing that little camera up at the agent of surveillance: spying on the spies. "They been surveillin' us; I figure it's time we start surveillin' them," he said.

The humorous vision of this role reversal reveals the steep power differential that exists between residents of the neighborhood and the world outside: you have a helicopter, I have a disposable camera. Compared to that of the police, or the news media, or the medical establishment, Isaiah's power was quite minor, and most of it was devoted to his daily struggle to survive and maintain himself. In this area, however, he had earned the respect of his peers. Isaiah's ability to escape from medical institutions, including psychiatric wards, was the stuff of local legend. The following excerpts discuss Isaiah's peculiar propensity for freedom, which always leads him back to the neighborhood, and the sense of isolation he feels when he gets there:

12/21/98

I ask about Isaiah and Hank says he hasn't seen him yet today, he hasn't seen him since the funeral. "What funeral?" I ask.

"Lincoln," he says.

"Lincoln passed?" I ask. (I had tested Lincoln for TB back when Isaiah was first diagnosed.)

"Yeah. He was sleeping in that truck. He got the pneumonia. Four guys died last week," says Hank, and ticks off the names; Bishop, Shepherd, Lincoln, and one other.

"Did they die of natural causes?" I ask.

Hank doesn't know. One of them was a woman only thirty-two years old. Another one had cancer.

The guy in the pick-up truck, who feeds the pigeons two bags of rice every day, pulls up, shows me some admission papers, and tells me he just brought Isaiah to Bethlehem Hospital last night. Isaiah was shaking, about to have a seizure, so he brought him over there. He told him he needs to dry out, completely, and said he'll sign him into the psycho ward if he wants, just like last year.

If he's in there he can't sign himself out, says Hank. Last time they had him in three strait jackets, and he still got out.

Hank and the pigeon guy both went to visit Isaiah last year when he was in there for a month, they say. The pigeon guy is going to go see him today, says he will bring Isaiah some change to make phone calls with, and he will sign him into the psycho ward if he wants, keep him there for thirty days to dry him out good.

I leave my card with the guy, ask him to give it to Isaiah. He puts it in the envelope with the rest of the papers. I tell them goodbye and leave the red pickup truck and the maroon Chevy there on the lot, at the start of a cold grey day.

12/23/98

I saw Isaiah this morning; he made it out of the hospital today, though he says they kicked him out, not once, but twice. He left in the daytime and had to go back in the evening because there was a needle still in his arm. He showed me the mark. He said he had called an ambulance to bring him back to Bethlehem to have the needle taken out, but the driver refused to do it; so he got to the hospital on his own.

He told me the story about the three strait jackets; how he left Bethlehem Hospital while still wrapped up in one, and managed to steal two more and sell them in the neighborhood. I asked Isaiah how he got the other two out when he was tied up in the third, and he said with a grin, "Where there's a will, there's a way." He says he got out of the straitjacket by rubbing against the brick wall behind the barber shop until it came off, because, he said, he had to be free.

At Bethlehem they don't even like to take him in anymore because he always leaves. One time they cut his coat off—a coat that I gave him—and he walked home in his hospital gown in the dead of winter. . . . He started talking about how he would like to see some of his kids on Christmas, but they live about fifty miles away and he has to get out there to see them. He doesn't know the address or phone number but he knows where the house is, he says. He says he doesn't like to be alone on Christmas, but if it comes to that he will go to the church where he doesn't know the people, but at least he knows that they believe in God and want to get along with their fellow human beings. He will walk along the streets and look at the lights and think about the way things used to be.

"Sometimes," he said, "it's like it's not the same Chicago."

This last statement by Isaiah is indicative of the ongoing transformation of the city and the mingled feelings it brings. Isaiah's comment about the "miserable" grass on his side of the street, and the green grass on the other side, as shown in one of his photos, reflects an attitude prevalent in poor neighborhoods and often mistaken for fatalism. This, I would argue, it is not. Rather, it reveals a certain wisdom engendered through survival in the face of persistent and worsening poverty. The paradoxical crisis expressed by Isaiah is also captured by the words of Bowden and Kreinberg: "This is the catch-22 of city life and everyone knows it. If your neighborhood is bad enough to need fixing, it cannot be fixed because it is too bad to risk money on. Unless it is so bad that a better class of people are attracted by the dirt cheap housing or it gets so bad that it can be bulldozed. Then the ruins will bring forth the bankers" (Bowden and Kreinberg 38). The paradox for many of the inner-city poor, simply stated, is this: no one wants "better neighborhoods" more than they do, but "better neighborhoods," under current definitions, probably means getting rid of them. The culmination of thirty years of urban decay, for those stubborn enough to persist until the tide turns, will probably be eviction. Fighting poverty in Chicago often means relocating poor people, and poor people know this.

DAILY SOAP OPERA

Poverty is as much a part of Isaiah's world as are the buildings and the streets themselves. Evidence of it is unavoidable: the frequent deaths, hospitalizations, and everyday dangers are so commonplace as to be mundane. Isaiah is more sensitive than most when it comes to these things. The others, like Hank and Rock, acknowledge the death toll with graveyard humor or apparent nonchalance. Rock refers to me as "Killer Paul," due to his stated belief that I was the one who killed his brother Stormy by bringing him to the hospital for his tuberculosis. When Hank tells me that Lincoln passed away, it is as part of an informal record-keeping: "three dead in one week." Lincoln was old, but his death was brought on by the unfortunate fact that he had to sleep in a car in the middle of December.

The dependence on subsistence labors such as collecting cans and doing odd jobs around the neighborhood is indicative of the prevalent privation. So is the widespread reliance on different forms of state subsidy. The common experience of poverty is also revealed in the constant sharing of scant resources, from wine to warmth, a practice extending even to the pigeons. Such sharing, as these accounts illustrate, also includes personal information. The intimate knowledge Isaiah has of other people's health and income circumstances reveals relations of sometimes uncomfortable familiarity. Poverty can wear civility thin, and the constant threat of violence in this neighborhood is another fact which lurks around the edges of Isaiah's narrative. In the remainder of our interview time, Isaiah described some of the episodes which brought him to the hospital so many times. Aside from recurrent seizures, which stemmed from a gunshot wound to the head incurred in the 1970s, Isaiah had also been sent to the hospital for injuries administered by local muggers. Billy once clobbered him on the head with a rock after an intoxicated altercation in front of the liquor store. The following excerpt from my field notes describes another such incident, in which Billy was on the receiving end of a blow from another "friend."

6/01/96

I saw Billy on the corner yesterday; he showed me the split in the top of his head, sewn up sloppy as an old baseball, sent out to the field one more time. He's been bashed around the bases unbelievably much, it seems. I gave him a dollar and encouraged him to go in to the hospital to receive the injections that he needs. His eyes seemed a little unsteady, though it was the first thing in the morning and he hadn't yet had a drink, I thought I detected an absence of his usual flair. Finally he managed a rhyme, and I was a little relieved that Billy was still Billy.

It was his old friend Shaky who did that number on him with the Louisville Slugger. He said that Shaky has been sick, his belly all bloated like he's about to give birth, and his brain half gone. Some friendship, when you can let a brutal beating slide; just another day on the street.

Dramatic events like these are nearly everyday fare in parts of the West Side, and places such as the parking lot provide a forum for discussing them. Isaiah's concern with the condition of his neighbors is revealed in his expressed sorrow over the fate of Big John and the health of Cisco and Johnny and with the struggles of the local churches and businesses. Not to be minimized, either, are the alternating bouts of boredom, which the violence and gossip helps to fill. In Chapter 4 I referred to Granovetter's ideas of "strong ties" and "loose ties," especially as they relate to transmission of disease. In these testaments and vignettes of neighborhood life, we can see how "dense networks," formed over many years, coexist with a sort of casual detachment or hardness to the sufferings of others, even close friends, so that their fates and failures may be witnessed and commented on as though they were a daily soap opera.

Aside from the relations which populate this space and make it the contradictory social crossroads that it is, Isaiah's account also tells us much about the greater forces which shape the lives that intersect here. As Isaiah says, this space is at the very center of an eyesore, and the forces of progress are closing in. What this will mean for Isaiah and the others is apparent but unstated. The engines which drive this seemingly inevitable process are also unnamed. The ominous photo of the helicopter shows an overarching awareness of an encroaching power. In sociology we give socioeconomic forces abstract names such as gentrification, deindustrialisation, or privatization, but for Isaiah and his friends they are simply the workings of the world, a world which is controlled by people who are elsewhere. Occasionally a powerful agent might be identified, such as the City, the Mayor, the Police, or the White Man. Sometimes these agents have human faces: specific police officers, social workers, construction workers, health workers, and other street-level bureaucrats.

Sometimes the onus for the neighborhood's decay was placed primarily on the residents themselves. "The people that live here burned it up theyselves," Cisco stated with contempt, a sentiment reminiscent of those maintained by many people living outside the neighborhood. As stated above, the idea of the ghetto culture as deviant and deficient is hard to shake, and many who live there appear to share it. More often, perhaps, destructive elements within the community itself are identified, as when Isaiah states that "people have stopped caring," referring to his street corner associates as "misfits" and "biological mistakes" or when Billy bemoans the "younger generation," or when Kenny attributes the neighborhood's decline to the "two-legged creatures" that live there.

This internalized stigma, however, exists side-by-side with another perspective, less often expressed in front of me, but nonetheless real. In its most basic form, it consist of an instinctive awareness—verified by everyday experience—that the ghetto is the victim of gross neglect or outright oppression. People on the West Side are quite aware of how their neighborhoods are perceived, not only by whites, but by other blacks as well. They, in turn, often perceive themselves as social pariahs in white society.

I interviewed some people on the West Side in the summer of 1996, around the time when President Clinton signed the Welfare Reform Bill (officially titled the "Personal Responsibility Act") into law. We were standing in an alley, where some men were sharing a hot dog, and a couple other men made some interesting remarks to me. The first man, whom I will call Mack, stated that any blacks who were found walking around on the wrong side of Warner Avenue would be picked up by the police and arrested for loitering. Whether or not such practices were a matter of police policy, people on the West Side definitely sensed that they were being actively patrolled.

Further comments by Omar made this point even more explicitly. In language reminiscent of Frantz Fanon, Omar declared:

> The only thing they're not doin', is they're not puttin' black people in chains anymore, like they used to do in slavery times. Other than that, we in chains anyway cause we are confined in a square area. If you go down to 11th and State and look at how the police know where you are at—don't know me at all, but can come find me whenever they get ready, cause they know where the black community—the map down at 11th and State right now is blocked off in red, that let you know where all black people are at. And they got a circle around it, where how far black people can go, and if you pass that limit, you goin' to jail . . . if I go out there right now, walk around right now, the police officers out there, they will even go get the neighborhood gang, the white gang that's in the neighborhood, say some black studs right here, and they'll come over and let them jump on me, and turn they back and say they didn't see this happening, and take me to jail, after they come and jumped on me, and the police officers done that.[2]

Here the idea of the ghetto as an oppressed colony can be clearly seen. Earlier in the conversation, Omar had expounded on the differing standards that apply to whites and blacks in American society. In doing so, he employed a "bottom-up" analysis of the economic and medical systems:

> There's two different laws for whites and blacks. White laws are easier, black laws are harder, and anything a black do, that a white guy would get away with, it cost a black guy money to get out of jail on it. And they know we don't have the money to get out of jail on that, because they won't let us have any money in this community no way, cause we don't have any jobs here, they don't put jobs here, they move all factories out of the black community, they put 'em in white communities, or make you travel to a distance where you can't get to work, and then you still under the minimum

wage. Bill Clinton raised the wages, the other day, to $4.75, and $4.75—
and then it don't come into effect until October—$4.75, you spend that
much on bus fare getting to work for a whole week. So when you get your
check, how can you raise a family, with kids? How could you buy 'em food?
How could you buy enough clothes? How could you pay, if you're not on
welfare, how you gonna take 'em to the doctor? If a black person go to the
doctor, he has to sit in the hospital twelve hours before he even get waited
on. You be dead. White people get waited on automatically at hospital.
Period. So we lose either way it go. You can't work, you can't eat, only thing
they put in black communities is liquor stores. Liquor stores and drugs.
Black people don't produce no drugs. Black people don't produce no guns.
So where did it come from? How in the hell can you come across the ocean,
with pistols, poppy—what they call them things?—heroin plants. Opium.
How in the hell can they get here if white people don't bring 'em here? Black
people don't own ships, they do not own factories for them to produce
weapons. You know, so they dump 'em. I seen a movie a long time ago, and
it said, heroin was only for black people and Puerto Ricans, man. You
know, I don't understand. When white kids started using heroin, and mar-
ijuana, they made drug abuse programs for it. After then, they started opening up clinics. Then when white kids started getting addicted on drugs, they
open up drug clinics.

Here Omar addresses another factor often blamed for the plight of the
ghetto: drugs. Beyond their purely physical effects, drugs can play different symbolic roles. Drugs may be simply equated with those who use
them: "These crackheads, these junkies." On other occasions, as above,
drugs may be seen as a malevolent force or a dark conspiracy originating
in the power structure, or the white world. A guy named Arthur, who
makes money fixing lawnmowers, snowblowers, and automobiles in an
empty lot, told me that he wanted to escape the community because
nobody there cared about anybody. "I'm sick of every bit of it," he said,
"Nobody cares. They don't care about themselves. How can they care
about anybody else if they don't care about themselves?" When asked
what made the neighborhood turn bad, he told me simply, "Drugs."
Regardless of their sources, drugs as a whole are seen as the major con-
tributor to the ghetto's slow rot.

Bringing the neighborhood "back," then, becomes synonymous with
ridding the community of drugs and drug dealers. On this point, some
people in the neighborhood held views that seemed quite conservative.
The following interviews, conducted in 1996 in a soul food restaurant on
West Jefferson Street where many old-timers and street people used to go,
gives a quick snapshot of the neighborhood as it stood in the mid-1990s.
Each reflects a different perspective on the changes in the ghetto. First I
spoke to the owner of the restaurant, a woman whom I will call Justine:

Paul: Why don't you tell me a little about the restaurant, and how it started, how long ago it started?

Justine: Well, I been here thirty years, so, it has changed, dramatic, it has really changed, because a lot of the places burnt down, tore down, a lot of peoples moved out, lot of businesses, gone out, so I'm just one of the lucky ones still here. So, uh, but since its building back up, I believe its gonna be better. It gotta be better.

Paul: How is it building back up?

Justine: By tearing down and building more, more homes, just like over on Washington Street; they're building, they're just building these little townhouses, making it better, so people will have better places to live, and getting these old buildings tore down, that's helping the neighborhood, because it's just rat dens, prostitutes and whores, dope houses, and they done a good job by tearing them down . . . that's our main, that's our main problem, to get all these buildings down and get these dope dealers off of the street, prostitutes off the street, and it'll be a better community for all of us.

Paul: Now, why don't you talk about the way this neighborhood was back in the sixties, back around the time of the last [Democratic] convention.

Justine: Well, it really wasn't as much dope on the street as it is now. That's one thing it wasn't; it was more, it wasn't, well the streets was more safer to walk, so, but like it is now, most of the old dope dealers is in behind bars, so just these young, this younger generation, so, it was lots better, cause it was safer for you, but now, it's, it's terrible . . . It used to be, we didn't have to go way West, South, North to shop, you could shop right here in the area, but now you got to go out of the area to buy anything, it's not like it used to be, but I hope and pray that we will get back into it where we can shop in our own area.

After speaking to Justine I made the acquaintance of a man in his forties, whom I will call Darrell. Darrell told me that I looked just like his little brother. He expressed a more positive viewpoint of the street life on the West Side than that held by Justine:

I was born in 1956, born around this area, and uh, it's a wonderful area. We don't get off on anything, we just do our own thing, because we have our own rights in this area . . . Everything always click together, and we all love another, and this is a neighborhood that everybody get together. We hook up on our nickels, pennies and dimes, and try to buy ourselves a little wine, because we all have our personal problems, and we all have to deal with our own thing. . . . This is the ghetto.

Justine and Darrell represent different positions within the neighborhood. She is a longtime business owner and hopes to see things get better. She sees good developments on the horizon for the neighborhood, as buildings are demolished and gang members and drug dealers and prostitutes are arrested. Darrell, on the other hand, is probably one of those people whom Justine is just as glad to see go. He refers to the common practice of "getting together" to buy some wine as an example of local solidarity. But the fact is, if the neighborhood goes upscale, both of them may be forced to move out. Justine's breakfasts of eggs and coffee for $1.99, her menu written in magic marker on cardboard, featuring items such as grits, ham hocks and pig ears, may not be welcome in the "New Chicago" either. Both of their reminiscences concerned some of the pivotal events of the 1960s in the West Side; the riots of 1968, following the assassination of Martin Luther King, Jr., and the death of Fred Hampton at the hands of the Chicago Police Department in 1969. They also reveal some of the issues of power and agency discussed in the pages above. Further comments by Darrell make this clear: "We're just chess pieces. They move us. You understand? Other than that, we have no power. We have no political power." The realization bluntly expressed by Darrell might also be deemed either fatalistic or realistic, depending on one's point of view. Again it reveals the ambiguous experience of living inside an "eyesore." By the year 2000, Justine's restaurant had closed its doors, but the ghetto remained.

The ghetto neighborhood, like the ill individual, lives a sort of shadow existence. Living on the West Side is both a psychic and a physical trial, and one wonders why people would return there if they had a choice. This conversation with Jeremiah—another acquaintance of Billy and Isaiah—took place while he was in the hospital, on one of numerous occasions. I asked him what he thought about the city where he lived, and why he always returned to the West Side. He simply replied: "I been to other places, but I just don't like it like Chicago . . . I just know places, I just know people here. It's hard to make any kind of change, you know." Here again is revealed the same pattern: familiarity creates its own social reality. You go there because you know people there; you don't go anywhere else because you don't know anybody anywhere else. This is true not only for a certain set of people but also for a certain style of life. Ghetto life is both boring and exciting; there is nothing to do, and any day you might face death. Within the ghetto, there exists a different set of standards than that which prevails outside, and they appear to be mutually exclusive. In other words, those who succeed in the day-to-day subsistence and survival of the ghetto are, almost by definition, incapable of succeeding in the "straight" world.

One day Jeremiah was sitting inside my car in an alley on the West Side. This alley was another social crossroads, similar in some respects to Billy's corner, Isaiah's vacant lot and Hank's car. This was the place to which Jeremiah always returned when he left the hospital, no matter what the state of his health. He and I were casually talking while I administered his medicines. In this conversation, Jeremiah referred to different people passing back and forth. His comments illustrate feelings of familiarity and trust, but also anger and distrust with local networks. This conversation shows how the social relationships which give a place meaning can also be linked to all sorts of negative feelings. Jeremiah had just referred to me as being a doctor, and I quickly corrected him.

Paul: I ain't a doctor.

Jeremiah: You as close to being a doctor as anyone out here . . . Ain't nobody shit . . . These niggers dope fiends . . . Half these, most of these niggers dope fiends. Period.

When I asked him what people did to support themselves in their drug habits, he responded in this way:

Jeremiah: That man hustle good as a motherfucker . . . (laughs) That fucker be hustlin', boy. He got money. That nigger have money, man. I'm talking about hundreds. He a lucky motherfucker. That fat nigger there, too. Fat motherfucker. I can't stand that nigger either, man. He don't want to put me in charge of the rent and shit. He won't take no money from me, ain't that a bitch? . . . It's a few people over there that trust me . . . But they ain't got shit theyself. . . .

Paul: So how many other people out here that don't do nothin'?

Jeremiah: Man, everybody out here do somethin'.

Even though Jeremiah emphatically stated that "ain't nobody shit," still he claims that "everybody do somethin'." No one is legitimate, in straight world terms—as he presumes that I am—but everyone has a hustle. People in the ghetto, as these comments show, tend to view each other instrumentally, as means to a particular end.

Jeremiah's characterizations of different people are determined in large part by the ways in which they make their money and the things that they do with their money. He sees other people in terms of what they have done and will do for him, money-wise, and in terms of what he owes to whom, and who owes what to him. But precisely because this is a ghetto, such social instrumentality coexists with a long-term familiarity with the people around you. So at times it seems that even though you know everybody, but you trust nobody. This is the paradox of intimacy and paranoia that both Isaiah and Jeremiah illustrate in their statements and in their actions. It is not something which is unique to the ghetto, not by any means. But it is made more intense by the bareness of everyday life there. As another man stated about his street corner acquaintances: "Now, right now, the reason I stopped hanging on the corner, with the guys, is cause I don't know what they got. Okay? I don't drink behind 'em no more, nothing like that, and I don't mess around with that old stuff no more. See what I'm saying?"

To offer a point of contrast, a Latino man, who lived in a different poor neighborhood, expressed some similar insights about the role that money plays in the street. This man, whom I will call José, was a chronic alcoholic who had been hospitalized with a case of inadequately treated pulmonary tuberculosis. I was curious about what drew him back to the street, aside from his obvious lack of money.

> I like the challenge . . . I like the challenge. The way it is, you know. Everybody's like struggling, their way. Everybody's dirty and stuff, but, we're all, we're human beings, and you find out that sometimes a wino is a better person than that guy walkin' down the street that's all dressed up. Cause sometimes a wino will help you out, you know. Like, I'm the type of guy, if I see a lady struggling with two bags of laundry, she can't make it, I go, "Senora, here I'll help you with a bag. You don't have to give me nothing." "Gracias, senor, gracias." Lay it down, hey—we be doin' that on the street. That's the type of guy I am, I don't like to see, you know, people strugglin'. If I'm there, if I can help 'em. I always been like that . . . And I got a lot of friends on this Street, all I got to do is walk down the street, and people give me cigarettes, a dollar, you know, cause they all know me as a good guy. And I am. Well, I think I am, except for my, everybody's got their faults, and I got drinkin', and I smoke cigarettes. I'm not into drugs. I got enough problems with drinking and smoking. That's enough, you know, that's five dollars, almost, a day, just doin' that.

In this case, the exchange of money was seen as something which confirmeds one's place: people gave him money because they knew him, and they knew that he was struggling. The neighborhood where this man lived was very different than the West Side. It is a predominately Mexican neighborhood, and though it is also quite poor relative to other areas in the city (both these neighborhoods were selected as federal "Empowerment Zones" by the Clinton administration), it contains a lot more "above ground" economic activity. There are hundreds of legal businesses lining each side of the main street which this man frequents, and the flow of patrons to and from these businesses financially benefits those who exist on the margins of the community.

THE LONELIEST BULL

Isaiah referred to the empty lot as "the last spot" to be emptied and cleared, so a new Chicago could be developed. One day, while passing through the neighborhood, I stopped by the lot and heard another opinion on the subject.

3/25/98

I went over by Hank's car . . . Geronimo was in there, smoking and drinking and wearing a black beret pulled over at an angle, like an artist or a revolutionary, and he and Mick both shook my hand and he got out of the car and came over and talked to me. He turned up the radio and he said, "You remember that? That's The Loneliest Bull." He told me the story of how Quincy Jones went to Spain and saw a bullfight; and there was a bull with eight swords in him who fought for 4½ hours and everyone cheered this bull because he was such a brave warrior, and so he wrote this piece of music, "The Loneliest Bull." He told me how he used to have a band, back in the sixties, before he got married, and he told me how great a guy I was and how I had balls for going wherever I needed to go to help somebody. Some people would say that I was in danger just by being over here and being white, he said. He was gripping my hand tight as he said this, and again I had the uncertainty as to whether or not it was a threat.

I asked him about the neighborhood, how they're clearing out all the buildings, and every time I come through it seems another building has gone down, and he said they're clearing all this out, moving everybody out to the suburbs because this is soon to be the prime real estate in all of Chicago. "We are not stupid," he sad. "We may drink a little wine, but we know what's going on. Those people in the suburbs are sick of driving four or five hours to work and all the floods and so on, and now they want to live over here, but they don't want drugs and prostitution and gangs and all of that going on right next door, so they're slowly clearing the land." Geronimo works in construction and says he has the blueprint at home; they've been wanting to do this for thirty years, he says. Then he goes into his thing about Vietnam, how he came back in 1972 and he was spat upon and couldn't get a job because he was a vet and he was black, and how they don't allow intelligent, talented black people to have a chance.

I stood there listening to Geronimo and looking across the vacant lots at the stragglers drifting through, trying to sell something or bum a smoke or a drink, and I considered how the ghetto, for all its problems, has long been at the same time a so-called "site of resistance," where the indoctrinations of the dominant culture were seen clearly as ruling-class propaganda. The ghetto, in this sense, was like "The Loneliest Bull." It had always had courage and spirit in spite of its oppression, and its most effective outlet had always been its rage. The black urban rebellions of the 1960s had spurred important political and economic concessions from the white establishment in major cities (Hill 49). Paradoxically, however, the success of a certain sector of the black middle class in business and politics had left the ghetto itself weaker and more isolated, as prosperous individuals left the ghettos for the other areas now open to them. The loss of manufacturing jobs also had a very real effect on these streets. By the 1990s, those who stayed in the neighborhood but did not participate in the illegal drug market had a hard time earning cash. People like Isaiah and Cisco and Johnny, who hustled for the little money they could get on top of whatever assistance they might receive, depended on the disposable income of their neighbors: the owners, patrons, and guests of the barber shops, liquor stores, pool halls, and churches in the local neighborhood. These are people who knew them, and who they knew would at the very least feed them.

But as the population of the elderly and the working classes is thinned by death, illness, and market-driven relocation, the situation of those left behind becomes more and more stark. As Jamie Peck has argued, "Capital is engaged in a restless search for more profitable sites of accumulation while labor continues to require the stability and support of community life" (Peck 15). Unfortunately, one cannot necessarily exist without the other, and poor communities have few bulwarks to defend them against the ravages of job market fluctuation. We are often reminded of the perpetual crisis endured by children in the inner city. But what of men and women like Isaiah, stretched between a past that was also materially poor, but which was relatively rich in social relations, and a future that is uncertain in either category? For them, the poverty of the postindustrial neighborhood is bleak indeed. With eight swords in its hide, there is only so long a bull can last.

Isaiah's comments concerning his photographs contain a wisdom born of experience: there is them that have, and them that don't, and rarely the two shall meet. Implicit in his observation, I believe, is the knowledge that his own fate is somehow tied up with this piece of turf where he has spent a good part of the last forty years. At one point, when looking at a photograph of neighborhood men talking, or "bull-jiving" under the tree in the empty lot, Isaiah says, "All this ain't nothing but nostalgia. All this is gonna be gone, and these guys won't know what hit 'em." But when I ask him about his own nostalgia, he simply says, "You call it nostalgia, I call it memory." Again, we see the apparent contradiction, of which he is a living example. Memory, in fact, may be the most significant value which the neighborhood now possesses. The "eyesore" that is perceived by outsiders forms a good chunk of Isaiah's own world, and it is doubtful that its social meaning will be recognized when the bulldozers finally arrive.

CONCLUSION

Billy was my initial informant in the neighborhood, and his presence there remained a touchstone for me. His physical deterioration was also a tragicomic barometer of the withering effects of unchecked alcoholism. Five years after my first encounters with Billy on the street corner, he was no longer a daily fixture. His seizures and his injuries, both of which stemmed from his drinking, had landed him in a nursing home a hundred miles from the neighborhood. I kept in contact with him, and agreed to pick him up and bring him to his sister's house for the Memorial Day weekend. However, I refused to drive him to the neighborhood, as he tried to convince me to do. Inevitably, however, he ended up there. The following narrative concerns the events that occurred when his acquaintances in the neighborhood sought my assistance in removing him from an environment which they themselves deemed destructive.

6/3/99

I saw him there yesterday and it was all I heard wherever I stopped in the neighborhood. "Have you seen Billy? He's been sitting under that tree since Saturday."

The beginning of summer had washed West Jefferson Street's most poetic drunk onto the shore of Richardson's liquor store. He sat on a lip of concrete with a scab black as a birthmark staining the side of his face. I stopped and asked what had happened. "My head met this cement over the weekend," he said. He said that he was still living in Joliet, at the nursing home. So apparently he was not hell-bent on escaping from there. Just a little vacation.

But today when I went back around the way, I ran into Ruth, with whom Billy used to stay. She got up from one of the crates under the tree in the parking lot on First Avenue and walked up to me, pleading, "Paul, you got to get him back. These people out here don't mean him no good."

. . . I said, "he's a grown man, I can't make him do anything he doesn't want to do." But I also said I'd stop by and check on him.

There he sat still, though he had by now managed to track down a milk crate to sit on, and he had some company under the tree; an older guy with a sharp black hat, like a blues man's hat, and glasses, and a tall thin younger guy. Henderson was there, too, and Mitch Sutton.

I stopped the car and got out. Henderson approached me and told me that Lester had said that he was going to give Billy money to get back home. "There goes Lester now, in that yellow car," he said, pointing to a faded paint job rumbling away through the alley. Soon enough Ruth showed up, too, and I also saw Jessica crossing the street. It seemed like the whole neighborhood was gathering round. Mitch and Henderson greeted me by name, but the old guy in the black hat asked if I was a cop.

Ruth was crying, begging Billy to get up and go with me. Billy was there with a plate of food on his lap, wrapped in plastic, dropped off by one of his neighborhood benefactors. All of a sudden there was a small crowd gathered there below the tree, a whole dramatic scene centered on Billy. Everybody wanted to know what I was going to do; I told them I didn't know: What could I do?

But it couldn't be resolved between me and Billy because there were too many voices, and then Billy said that he was ready to go, after all, so I said "Come on," and they practically picked him up and dragged him over to my car. I opened the passenger door and they almost shoved him in . . . all the while he protested, "I can get in the car my god-damned self!"

With the door closed I pulled away, waving goodbye to the crowd. Then we had to decide what to do. But first I had a question: "What just happened back there?"

It was a sort of community event, subject to interpretation: a West Side *Rashomon*. They thought they were doing one thing, and he saw another. As Billy says, "every eye closed ain't asleep." He was watching them the same as they watched him.

Billy said, "The first law of nature is self-preservation. They act like they is so concerned. They wanted to keep me there. Misery loves company. They didn't mean me no good. That's what pissed me off. I said let me go, let me go, let me go, but they kept grabbing me."

What struck me most about this street corner drama were the seeming contradictions it contained. On the one hand there was a demonstrable concern, a desire to help a fellow human being by delivering him from the depths of the neighborhood to a distant safe haven. I served as a sort of deus ex machina in this scenario: upon me they projected the power to remove him, to protect him, to save him. On the other hand, what this concern implied is that his associates, the people in his network, wanted him to be taken away from that which was destroying him—the neighborhood in general, but also themselves. "He don't need to be out here," they said, "he's going to end up killed." He didn't believe that they really cared; he talked about how his "so-called friends" wanted to "keep him there" because, as he said, "Misery loves company." Yet he apparently wanted to stay—and in fact, even though I gave him ten dollars and dropped him at the train station, he returned to the corner later that day.

How does one explain this sociologically? How does one go outside the peculiarities of Billy's personality and see the social forces at work in this situation? The best answer that I can come up with is deceptively simple: to take Billy seriously, and to consider both his behavior and his words as valid pieces of the puzzle. Where one ends up, then, is face to face with a paradox: Billy is drawn back to a particular place (which is as much social as geographic) while at the same time he recognizes its perils. He is drawn there, again, for a deceptively simple reason: it is all he knows. It is a part of who he is, and a part of him is frozen there. He has put in time, and human beings tend to invest themselves in those places that they inhabit, no matter how empty or decrepit they may seem from the outside. The decay of physical space and the destruction of human bodies, by causes both external and internal, can be linked through this ever so human attachment.

These examples convey a sense of the social world inhabited by many of Chicago's TB patients. It is important to understand the pathos and intensity of this type of neighborhood life for two very important reasons related to tuberculosis. One pertains to the causes of tuberculosis: the physical and social environment depicted here powerfully affects the health outcomes of those who dwell within it. In the 1990s, many TB patients in American cities inhabited harsh social landscapes such as these. They did not create these landscapes themselves, but they had to live within them and adapt to them. In the hospital they found temporary physical respite, but when they left the hospital they returned to unaltered circumstances. The same world that "wears them down and tears them down" remains there to greet them when they get out.

One might conclude people would pursue any opportunity to escape these destructive environments, and those who chose not to do so were either deficient or self-destructive. This becomes a circular argument, a catch-22: if you cared about yourself, you would leave the ghetto, but you can't leave the ghetto until you care about yourself. Men and women who are accustomed to living on the street are often drawn back to it when they get out of the hospital or prison, even when offered housing alternatives in other areas. In the eyes of the "straight" world, this makes them irresponsible, criminal, or crazy. But such a dismissal does not do justice to the situation's complexity, or its social content. Though battered by forces of social and economic change, the ghetto space retains its pull upon the people who have lived inside its "private geography." Men such as Billy, Kenny, Isaiah, and Geronimo exist on the very edge of an abyss. In political and economic terms, they are practically meaningless; their world is stigmatized, devalued, and slated for destruction. They know this, and yet they persist, playing out the old patterns.

This is where the other, more elusive aspect of the neighborhood comes into play, and this is the other reason why it is important to understand the social context of tuberculosis. In the hospital, patients often find their physical needs met and their social needs starved. What draws them back to the neighborhood, apart from the power of an addiction, a defect of character, or an appetite for destruction, is the simple fact that they have a place there, and a role to play, no matter how insignificant it may seem to an outsider. As Bowden and Kreinberg eloquently wrote, "People belong to neighborhoods, because they can't find much else to belong to. Neighborhoods are occasions, places where people hang their hats until they get the chance to move on. They lack the persistence, the organization and the strategy of the groups that exercise power. That's why they lose" (Bowden and Kreinberg 40). Fractured and torn as it may be—and as much as they might claim to hate it—the neighborhood remains, outside of the family, the most significant repository of memory and meaning that these men and women possess.

6   Hard Case Histories

Narratives of Tuberculosis, Homelessness, and Addiction

TUBERCULOSIS AND TIME

A FAMILIAR phrase among black Chicagoans is: "I'm going through changes." Its implications are nearly always negative. When we heard this statement from a patient in the clinic, we knew that a litany of woes was coming. If things were changing, it usually meant they were getting worse. Martha, my supervisor, would laugh and recite the line from the old blues song, "Born under a Bad Sign": "If it wasn't for bad luck, I wouldn't have no luck at all."

Time in the ghetto tends to be cyclical. For many people, the only markers of importance are the beginning and the end of each day, and the monthly dictates of various checks, bills, and appointments. In between these points, one seeks not to advance, but to simply survive, maintain, and when possible, enjoy. Echoing Lewis (1959) and Anderson (1994), scholars and pundits often claim that the culture of the ghetto poor is "oppositional" to that of most Americans. The poor, they say, have a chronic case of "present-day orientation," which simply means that they fail to think about tomorrow. As a result, they are unlikely to "defer gratification," a quality deemed essential to success in mainstream economic society. For deferred gratification to make any sense, however, one must have a reasonable expectation that there will be some positive change or reward in the future. Even though some people in the ghetto may seem to lack a sense of history—as do many Americans—they are nonetheless people with a past, with memory and with experience. Unfortunately, for many poor people the present looks a lot like the past: same shit, different day. This can make the task of history difficult.

Different communities follow different clocks and calendars. In Native American communities, when events start late someone will inevitably state that they are running on "Indian time." The phrases "Puerto Rican time" and "black time" have a similar meaning, and just about every ethnic group probably has their own version. Each of these only has significance in relation to the unstated: official time, or what one of my patients might have called "peckerwood time." Peckerwood time is rationalized time, the white man's time: the clock as an abstract entity, elevated to higher importance than that of human use or meaning. Built into this time concept is the assumption of universality, that we all experience time in the same way, and the expectation that we need to get somewhere, to progress or ascend, for our lives to be meaningful or important. At job interviews we are often asked, "Where do you see yourself in the next five years?" This is a perfectly reasonable question from the perspective of rationalized time. "Right here," or "Alive, I hope" are not considered sufficient answers.

Illness, like poverty or cultural difference, disrupts the sense of time that society imposes on its members. Anyone who has been acutely ill, even for a short period, has experienced the warping of time that occurs when the body's functioning is impaired: the seemingly endless minutes awaiting the next cathartic heave of the stomach, the hours sliding away in fevered sleep. Like the poor, those who are shut out of society by virtue of their illness or disability develop "timetables" of their own, ways of breaking chunks of undifferentiated time into manageable units (Roth 21). The effects of illness interact with the bitter pill of poverty to create a double dislocation for those unlucky enough to be afflicted with both. Unfortunately, this makes it even harder for others to relate to such individuals, especially if they are encountered only for short periods, in the grip of a strangling condition. Narrative accounts of illness, which attempt to place the seismic convulsions of the body within the context of a person's experience over time, can help to communicate the pain of this dislocation, thereby increasing understanding and aiding in the process of healing (Brody 1987; Kleinman 1988, 1992; Frank 1995, 1997, 1998.)

Tuberculosis treatment lends itself to a narrative approach, because it takes at least six months, often longer, to complete a standard course of TB therapy, and relationships between individual workers and individual patients often grow and persist beyond the usual boundaries of patient-provider interactions. It thus becomes possible to view individuals longitudinally. This "long view" of people can also serve as a counterweight to snapshot sociological judgments—quantitative or qualitative—which may fallaciously link behavior to some set of deficient values: a deficient character or a deficient culture. As Georg Simmel has written, "We cannot know completely the individuality of another" (Simmel 10). No person is ever absolutely knowable, and some people may present very different faces to different people at different times. This is especially true when people face the grinding trials of acute illness and persistent poverty.

By presenting case histories based on relations with people that evolved over relatively long periods, I hope to disarm many of the prejudicial tendencies which are embedded in medical institutions and their methods of documentation and categorization, especially when it comes to the homeless and indigent. As Chapter 3 showed, even those hospitals that regularly deal with the poor are capable of such prejudice. Homelessness is often seen as a sort of existential or behavioral category, centered within the individual, rather than as a temporal material condition, a result of definable social circumstances. Narrative allows us to see homeless persons as part of a larger whole, both socially and historically: people, who come from someplace and go somewhere, and who accumulate experiences and make decisions within understandable parameters. These are not "illness narratives," in the sense that they chronicle a person's subjective health experience; rather they are stories about particular individuals as they interacted with me, and the medical institution I worked for, over a period of time. Like episodes of illness, however, patient-provider encounters and relationships are saturated with social meaning. These accounts will necessarily be incomplete, as I am far from omniscient, and I knew these men and women for only a fraction of their lives. They will, for the most part, tell my side of the story—though excerpts from recorded interviews will present some of their words unaltered. However, these "tales of treatment" serve a valuable function as an expression of the human side of both medical statistics and sociological theories.

It is against the uneven, intersubjective ground of actual experience that any theory, method, or philosophy must be tested, just as political theories always find their true test in the street. The street, in these three cases, is located on the West Side of Chicago, Illinois. The patients to be discussed, Isaiah, Stormy, and Jeremiah, were all African American males in their mid- to late forties. At the time of this writing, two of them were deceased, and the other was still hanging on in the neighborhood. They were all mentioned in the previous chapter in relation to their lives within the neighborhood community. In this chapter they will be considered in relation to their bouts with TB and medical treatment. This is, after all, why I knew them.

All had histories of alcoholism or drug abuse, some had seizure disorders, and all suffered from sporadic homelessness. As such they were somewhat typical of the tuberculosis patients encountered at County General, where I was employed, though not necessarily representative of TB patients in general. County General dealt with some of the most "hardcore" cases of TB in the city of Chicago, and these men would all have been placed in that category. Because of their demographics—or "risk factors"—they were all considered to be potential "problem patients," likely "noncompliant" or "delinquent" takers of pills. Such presumptions might have been practically supported by the reported past behavior of these men. Nevertheless, as the following narratives will show, they differed significantly, in their personalities, behaviors, beliefs, and relations with the medical system. In short, they had different stories, and the details are significant in each case.

Case 1: The Trail of Isaiah

My first knowledge of Isaiah came when I was notified that he had "eloped," or "absconded," which meant he had walked out of the hospital against medical advice. He had done so despite the fact that his sputum samples were swarming with mycobacteria. Now he was loose in the community with active, untreated TB, presumably without any medication, and potentially spreading disease. Such a patient would normally be hospitalized, in isolation, until it was deemed safe for him to return the community. The most important task for public health purposes, in a case like Isaiah's, was to find the patient as quickly as possible and medicate him sufficiently to eliminate risk of contagion, thus "breaking the cycle" of infection. Ideally he would be returned to the hospital and treated with full confidentiality. However, if the patient refused to return to the hospital, the same ends could also be accomplished in the field—although it got a little muddier out there. Achieving that end is what this story is about, at least from the point of view of my own duty. For Isaiah, the meaning of our first encounter was somewhat different.

7/07/97

How to describe West Jefferson Street in early July? Sidewalks jumping like a field of grass with jitterbugs, drunks, junkies, and hustlers. Not to mention the folks who just like the street life. I go out there to ask about Isaiah, who absconded from County General today, leaving his IV stand in the hallway outside ward 61. From reading his hospital chart I learned that he was a hardcore alcoholic prone to seizures and fistfights, with a history of TB in the past and all the symptoms of a blossoming recurrence, including a positive sputum smear, indicating that he is currently infectious. All of this, as well as the West Side address, matched almost exactly the profile of my old buddy (former TB patient) Billy, and so it occurred to me that Isaiah might be found in the vicinity of West Jefferson, perhaps in front of the popular community center formally known as Richardson's cut-rate liquors.

In the pulmonary office at the hospital I found a copy of Isaiah's old TB clinic chart, and sure enough the address listed was identical to that often used by Billy. That was it: I was on the trail. It's times like that when a little history in the "hood" helps out. While looking for Isaiah I found several other people that I knew, three of them old or current TB patients themselves. One was Billy, of course. The others were Denise, holding her new-born baby, Denise's sister Lisa, pregnant and drinking a beer, and a guy who lives in Aurora and gets his TB treatment (DOT) out there . . .

We traded small talk for a minute while I waited for Billy to return from the liquor store with the bottle of Thunderbird which I enabled him to buy by lending him a dollar. In all this time there is no sign of Isaiah. He is still a phantom to me—I have no clue what he looks like. I half expect to see him come strolling down the street in his hospital gown. No such luck. Billy will surely see him and tell him I am looking for him, if he doesn't know already. This process may take a little time, but I am confident I will find him.

7/11/97

I actually found Isaiah today in front of Richardson's cut-rate liquors, though at first he denied it, and said he was someone else. "That guy walking down the street with a black coat and a cane is Isaiah Washington," he said. "You can't miss him." I was skeptical because someone else had just told me that this was him, but I said "Okay," turned around, and caught up with the man in black. He was standing at the bus stop when I walked up and asked him if he was Isaiah. "No," he said angrily, "I was just cussing him out about not taking his pills. He yelled at me and threw the pills on the floor."

The pills he was referring to were the pills I had left with Isaiah's cousin Hank the afternoon before, sealed in a small, plain paper envelope.

"Was he wearing a blue jacket?" I asked.

"Yeah, that's him."

"Well, that guy just told me that you were Isaiah Washington."

He then pulled out his wallet and showed me his state I.D., even though I didn't ask him to. "Do that look like Isaiah Washington?" he asked.

"No, it sure don't," I said.

"You see," he continued, "We got like a little club over there. And I been getting on him about taking his pills because we don't want it to be catching."

When I returned to Richardson's the other guys didn't try to cover for him. "He just went round the corner," they said. I caught up with him in the alley, talking to two other men who were sitting down on a curb. He had three plastic bags slung over his shoulder and a black fisherman's cap on his head. "Man, why you want to pull that shit?" I said. "I just want to talk to you for a minute."

He walked around the corner away from the other men and then stopped and stared at me. Two times in a row he asked, "Why you be wondering who I am?"

I said, "I need to talk to you because you got a sickness inside, and you can run but you can't hide."

"I don't spend much time in one place. I be moving around," Isaiah said. With his bags slung over his shoulder, and his fisherman's cap, he looked like a hobo, outlaw or frontiersman. He was wearing a long sleeve jacket zipped up in spite of the summer sun. I could see the scar on his lower lip just healing up from the fight that sent him to County General in the first place.

7/14/97

I found Isaiah, or rather he found me, around the corner from Richardson's ... He was carrying the big plastic bags again, and wearing a patterned vest and the denim fishing cap. I picked him up in my car and he bought a 7-Up at a small corner store and swallowed the pills in the passenger seat beside me. He didn't ask for any money. He showed me the empty packets from the pills I gave him since Thursday—including those he had supposedly thrown on the ground.

After Isaiah let me speak that first time, I was able to convince him to give our Directly Observed Therapy (DOT) program a chance. Each day I would meet up with him, at his convenience, and he would take his prescribed pills in my presence. Then, at the end of the week, I would give him ten dollars in cash. This money, and the occasional bus token, was the only material incentive that the program offered. Even so, this ten bucks could be very persuasive—revealing, perhaps, how poor most of our patients were.

The preceding episodes illustrate several issues in tuberculosis treatment. One is a straightforward issue of power. The similarities between medical field-workers, such as myself, and the police, both in terms of what we actually do and the distrust that we encounter, ought to be apparent enough. Like police officers, field-workers cultivate relationships within an area and then use them to accomplish their own ends. The social networks of the street can be either a hindrance or an aid in locating a particular person.

When I entered housing projects or other areas where illegal activities were common, I was often asked if I was a cop. This was partially due, no doubt, to the color of my skin. The segregated inner city allows for quick detection and categorization of racially designated outsiders. Stereotypes are employed by both sides—residents and tourists—and when entering these zones one has the feeling of being inspected. At the same time, one has the initial feeling of being a spy. In some instances I was referred to by people who knew me as being "practically black," or "having some black" in me. This was not meant literally, but as a sign of my relative trustworthiness. It also implied that no one but another black person would be genuinely interested in helping black people.

In fact, both police and social workers in the ghetto are commonly (and accurately) perceived as agents of powerful institutions, patrolling a population that is seen by much of the public as potentially dangerous and in need of pacification and control. This awareness cuts both ways. Think about it: a poor man, afflicted with a deadly disease, is tracked down, in the streets, because he has no address, no telephone, no next of kin. The very language employed by the health institution—"absconded," "delinquent," "noncompliant"—resemble those terms employed by the criminal justice system, and highlight his culpability. It does not take much imagination to realize how a patient in such a position might feel. What if someone from the hospital where you were treated for a stigmatizing condition showed up at your place of work, asking where you were, telling people—directly or indirectly—what illness you had? A middle-class person might sue for less, yet this is common practice. Alert sociologists will note the conflicting agendas evident here. Field-workers serve to extend medical control outward from the hospital into the heart of the community. Day by day, the field-worker attempts to build a relationship which will facilitate the proper ingestion of medicines. In this way, the social becomes instrumental: it is a means, rather than an end in itself. For the patient, of course, the relationship may be instrumental also. Sometimes the relationship takes on a life of its own.

Unlike a cop, a fieldworker carries no gun and no badge, and has virtually no authority of any kind other than that granted by the hospital or the health department: in other words, very little. They are not doctors themselves, so the opinions of field-workers concerning medical matters are easily disregarded. Some do act like cops, taking the hard-line stance that people with infectious diseases who don't take their medicine are indeed analogous to criminals, because their behavior threatens the health of the community. Others see the failure of some patients to take their pills as "their own problem," choosing to focus their energies instead on patients who, they feel, deserve it. In spite of their personal feelings, however, the fact remains that field-workers must deal with patients in their own terms, in social scenarios where the patients maintain a degree of personal control that they do not possess in the institutional setting of the hospital or jail, where they are first encountered. Interactions between health workers and patients in the field, therefore, are intensely negotiated relationships. This negotiation takes place on a daily basis, as the following examples will illustrate:

7/24/97

Isaiah was quite drunk early in the morning yesterday and the day before, but today he seemed fairly straight and sober. Two mornings ago he rambled on and on about pathology, microbiology, and artificial humans. Then he began reciting the Gettysburg address and said that people around the neighborhood hate him because of his education and call him the white man's child. He also said that he has shrapnel in his back and that the Internal Revenue Service will not let him die. Then he looked at me and said "You kind of understand me, don't you?" and I answered "I'm trying to hang with you, Isaiah."

7/25/97

Isaiah announced today that I had earned his trust because of the letter I wrote for him yesterday, stating that I was watching him take his TB meds every day. I did not say anything in the note about his infectiousness, but apparently what I wrote was sufficient. I also asked him about the artificial humans, and he stated that the technology exists to make machines like people and pretty soon they won't need a man and a woman any longer. The year 2000 is the year that humans will begin to destroy themselves, he said, and by 2501 they will be gone.

7/30/97

Isaiah was again appearing dejected and stated that he might not want to keep taking his medicine. "What is they interest in me?" he wanted to know. "Who?" I asked. "The hospital" he said. I then told him that the lab results had revealed that he did indeed have TB. "How bad is it?" he wanted to know. I tried to explain that there was no cause for alarm, that TB was totally treatable and actually not that dramatic. But he seemed to want the drama. "Bring me another cup" he said, "And then I can know for sure. I don't want no man, woman or child to be infected by me." I told him that wasn't very likely as long as he stayed out-of-doors most of the time and didn't live with any women or children. But our communication didn't seem so good today . . . We sat there for a long time as I tried to get him to help me out with the testing of his contacts . . . "Things are going to get tough for me when we do that" he said, referring to the testing. I said "It won't even be that big a deal, it'll be over and then they will forget about it." He looked at me long and hard and I had no idea what he was thinking . . . I treat our relationship carefully, afraid I might shatter it and make him cross that thin line of refusal into the land of noncompliance.

He said something today about how all the guys around there thought of him as a foreigner because of the way he talks. He says it's because he grew up in a mixed neighborhood in the sixties, and so he will occasionally say something in Spanish, and the other men will doubt his blackness. . . . He also mentioned some guy who lives in the neighborhood who has bleeding sores all over him and how he tries to avoid that guy.

7/31/97

This morning Isaiah wouldn't take his pills at all. He looked depressed, said, "I'm not on the program today." He said this a couple times. I said, "Come on, Isaiah, I'm not out here for myself, I'm out here for you." He looked at me silently with sad eyes, like he tends to do, and replied, "I know." I sat there in the car and he stood there shuffling his feet for a second, then wandered back over to the group sitting under the tree without saying anything else.

This was about 7:30 in the morning, and the air was still cool though the sun was bright and the sky was deep blue and clear of clouds. I sat in the car for awhile thinking he might wander back and change his mind, and trying to think through what I might do to help him change it. I am not someone to want to force pills on anyone, but in this case I don't want to be lax, at least not yet. He might still be contagious, after all. I looked over at him sitting in the easy chair under the tree, apparently singing to himself and playing imaginary guitar and drums too, and it occurred to me that brother Isaiah might be defined by some people as mentally ill.

Finally I wrapped a dose of meds in a piece of paper and drove up alongside where he was and waved him over to the car. I wasn't sure if he would come over, but he did. I handed him the packet of pills and said, "Look, take these later on if you feel like it then. I'll be back tomorrow to see you again." He took the pills and said that maybe later he'd be more inclined to take them. I said, "You need to take them, man" sincerely, and he nodded and said "I'll be out here tomorrow between 7 and 8." I said "Okay, see you tomorrow," and went on my way.

8/04/97

Isaiah was still underground as of this morning. After making the rest of my stops I circle back to the 'hood and there he is, sucking on a bottle of Night Train in a paper bag and talking about how he "doesn't hang around with infectious people." I am afraid that the alcohol will make him ornery like last week but he comes over and takes the pills without a problem. He even reminds me to give him the two red ones.

He makes some comment about how all the names I keep in my "orange book" belong to infectious people. "Some of them are, some of them aren't" I say. The orange book he refers to is simply a plastic folder where I keep the daily monitoring sheets for all of my clients. But Isaiah still apparently thinks I have some secret governmental information of those carrying contagion. . . . He kept talking about how people around there have all sorts of diseases and that's why he tries to keep his distance. The distrust and enmity he expresses toward his own friends is a little distressing.

8/06/97

I made it out to West Jefferson Street by 7:30 A.M. or so, and Isaiah was not there. Neither was anybody else. The field of wildflowers had been mowed down and the block was desolate as a ghost town. It was a cool morning and the wide open sky reflected the emptiness of the earth. I circled around Richardson's but didn't see Isaiah or Billy there. I decided to try again an hour or so later. There was a cop car flashing on the north side of Jefferson as I headed east. I wondered if the whole neighborhood had been raided and jailed.

8/07/97

Again this morning Isaiah was nowhere to be found. I got out of the car and walked over to where the men sat beneath the rolling clouds, like villagers waiting for the rain that never comes. The men looked up, waved in indifferent recognition. They said they had not seen Isaiah, as far as they knew he was still in the hospital. I said he wasn't there. One of them said, "I bet he walked out; I bet he pops up today."

8/09/97

I headed over to Jefferson Street to look for Isaiah again. At this point I am starting to worry. Patients will sometimes disappear for days, weeks, or even months. But sometimes they turn up dead.

When I got to the corner, though, Isaiah was there. He was in a pretty good mood, having walked out of County General the night before. "I even got a pair of blue pants" he said, and laughed out loud. . . .

Indigent patients arrive at the hospital in varying states of mental competence and awareness. Each time they are admitted, if their old records are not located, they are assigned a new unit number, and a new record is started. As a result, they frequently possess multiple identifiers. This is what had happened with Isaiah: I had been looking for him under his full legal name, but he had been admitted under a nickname. Because his last name was so common, and the unit number was different, his admission went undetected by our TB team. Such inconsistencies in institutional (as well as individual) memory may contribute to the "poor historian" tag, since physicians are unlikely to trust testimony that cannot be independently verified. In this case, Isaiah might have been re-diagnosed as a new case of TB, or might have been presumed "noncompliant" if his diagnosis and treatment were recorded under separate unit numbers. Piecing together histories on such patients can require considerable detective work, especially when these wrinkles multiply over time.

8/26/97

Isaiah had a birthday on Friday. He took the day off from DOT, just as though it were a job. He wanted to try to see his kids. I gave him his ten dollars a day early. Yesterday he was back on the corner. I asked if he had seen his kids; he said he saw two of them, and that made him feel a little better, as they were happy to see him. He took his pills again without any problems. Our routine has become regular and non-problematic. The men on the corner know my name and wave at me when I come and go. Isaiah told me that the guys who hang out under the tree are mostly old-timers, mostly drinkers, not dope-fiends like those who hang out by Richardson's where Billy is.

8/27/97

Isaiah's clinic day came at last. He said that he would be ready to go when I got there but he wasn't. He was already stinking of wine and was wearing the same green pants he's had on all week. He said that he would like to change his clothes so I told him I'd come back in an hour, after seeing my other patients.

When I came back Isaiah still had not returned, so I pulled around to Jefferson Street and asked after him. This block, like so many others on this stretch of West Jefferson, has never been fully rebuilt since the riots of 1968. Half the street consists of vacant lots and boarded-up storefronts, but people still live in the apartments above some of them, often renting or staying informally. Isaiah's cousin directed me to a black painted wooden door. I pushed it open and called upstairs. Isaiah answered, said he'd be right down. When he emerged almost ten minutes later he was wearing different clothes, but they looked just as dirty. He had a white plastic bag full of stuff with him as well.

On the way to the clinic we talked some about health practices in the area, because one of his tree-buddies came up to me and asked me if I was a doctor and could I do anything about his asthma. I answered no on both counts before I pulled away and then Isaiah told me that he brags about me, says I'm a good "medical field technician" and that's why that guy thought I might be able to help with his asthma.

Isaiah says that there are not enough clinics around the West Side. He said it's like the Old West; if you want something you'd best get on your pony and ride to the next town. I said there's plenty of doctors over there (at County General Hospital), it's just a question of getting in to see them. He said, "Yeah and even then they're swamped, so that's why a lot of people around here still use home remedies, fish oil, and stuff like that."

I ask him if this is really true and he says, "Yes, it's mostly home remedies around here." . . . Later on, after Isaiah has been in clinic, I see Dr. Taylor, the medical director of our program who handles a lot of our indigent patients. I say, "So I guess you met my buddy Isaiah." He responds, "Yes, and he reeked of alcohol." My supervisor [a public health nurse] tells me that Isaiah needs to wash his face. I say, "you know, it's too bad because I think he could make a good impression."

With Isaiah's first clinic visit an important hurdle had been cleared. His dosage was reduced and DOT continued on a twice-weekly basis. His illness had been effectively managed and any chance of his infecting anyone else had been greatly reduced. Medically speaking, then, DOT had been a success. In addition, Isaiah had spoken very highly of Dr. Taylor. From this point forward, the symbiotic social basis for the DOT was established. Two months later, Isaiah's treatment was over halfway completed, and he was helping me locate another lost TB patient on Jefferson Street.

Now Isaiah would sit in my car and talk to me at length. He said that no one in the neighborhood was interested in the things that he was: chess, backgammon, physics, biology. He said that if they knew he wasn't black, they would kill him in a second. He said he was Irish, Indian, Mexican, and he only looks black on the outside. Months went by this way: I pulled up on Jefferson Street two mornings a week, and waited. Often I did not see where he came from, but he was there just the same, rain, snow, or sun. He sat in the car and told me the latest thing on his mind, be it his cousin's knee operation, the amorous encounter he had the night before, or the recent outbreak of herpes he heard about. Isaiah, the walking risk factor, had somehow become the model TB patient. He told me that, as of the first of the year, he wanted to quit his drinking for good.

I asked Isaiah, as the end of his treatment drew near, what he thought I wanted that first time I came looking for him. "I thought you'd come to put me back," he said. "When you wake up with a needle in your throat, four IV's in your arms, and a tube stuck up your penis, it makes you feel like a guinea pig." He said that he was a person who was used to having his health, to doing what he wanted to do. His episode of illness had interfered with that, and so he sought escape as soon as he was able. I then asked him how he felt when he first got sick with tuberculosis. His statements reveal his perspective of both the hospital and the community, and the important roles that each of them played in his life:

> Isaiah: Well, when I first thought I had it, it was kind of frightening . . . because to me it seemed like a common cold or something, but I noticed that the cough was kinda rough and dry at times, and the mucus was sometimes thick and green or thick and white, and once in a while it was more harder for you to hold water down, and you sweat even when you, you know, it's cold outside, you're sweatin.' And, at times, you not able to rationalize that having sort of a sickness that you're not used to, so you go to the hospital, you get it checked out, and then someone tells you that you have TB.
>
> Then you have to realize that something's wrong here. You know, you might get frightened, but you got to face it. I faced it, and it was not that easy at first, because, as I know from a fact, I ran off from the County because I was frightened. I don't care if you have proper time to sit down and have somebody explain it to you, fear is the thing that you have to deal with personally as well as socially. Medical fears, you can put aside only with the help of friends, people, your doctors, and your community. People that surrounds you supports you to get this checked out, and I for instance am glad I had that.

Paul: When you talk about fear, was it the illness itself that had you scared, or was it the, something that the doctors or the County was doing to you, or a combination of these?

Isaiah: Well, it's the combination, really, because disease, see, when you say the word disease, the first thing you get is what the media and a lot of other places paint up in your mind. Some of these people do not have actual knowledge; what they do, they overdramatize. Then, you winds up fearful. As far as the hospital. . . . They give you the impression that if you got it, you probably come in contact with somebody that had it, then you, just now finding out, but no telling how many people you have encountered, in contact with. And then you faced with the fact that, if I did this to somebody, what is my option, what is my responsibility? And it's a fear, itself, a mental and emotional fear that drives you to start thinking irrationally, you start to get scared, run, run, run, run, run. But there's no hiding. There's no hiding. And like I said, emotionally, physically, it's draining, cause you wants to sit down and talk to somebody but from the moment you mention TB to some peoples out here, they look at you like you just said plague, or leprosy. They, they got to back off from you, peoples start walking away from you.

Paul: So you think there's a lot of negative images surrounding TB still?

Isaiah: Yeah, but it's, it's, some people that they just see the word TB and they got a funny look on 'em. They start lookin' at you. You'll be sittin' at the desk talkin' to someone and they'll get up and walk away from you like they got to do something very urgent, and they, when they come back, they keep their distance about two or three feet from you. And you wondering what's wrong. You wondering what's wrong, and then, when you're into the hospital, or something, you got doctors that tells you the good things that you can deal with about this, and some of the bad things too. You get confused, and you constantly wants to know, what gonna happen to me, how will it hurt me, what is this gonna do, is it gonna be swift, fast, or, you know, slow: bit by bit.
. . . The hospitals can help you, clinics can help you. But you got to put yourself in the position to think: when you go to these people, be honest with them, let them know what you goin' through. You know, psychologically you're nervous, psychologically and morally you're, you're thinking you're a threat to society when you're not. And it's gettin' to be sort of like you're outside the place and lookin' in, lookin' in at the crowd, but you want to go in, but you're afraid to, cause they say you got something. And then the moment that you tell somebody you got TB, some people shun you, peoples you know for ten or twenty or thirty years. They look at you, they back away from you. They act as though that you done something or you got something lot worser than a knife or a gun, or a bomb. You know, it's sort of, it's like bein' placed in a jar as a specimen. And everybody lookin' at you. But they don't want to touch you.

Billy once said to me: "Never judge a book by looking at its cover, because the element of surprise is a monster." In this case, the surprise was not a monster at all, but rather the reverse: beneath Isaiah's demographics and diagnosis lived an intelligent, independent, and somewhat troubled man, existing within a dense set of enduring social networks which he loved but also deeply distrusted. These ambivalent feelings are not unique to relationships in the inner city. All of us sometimes feel angered, confined and misunderstood by those who are closest to us. Familiarity may indeed breed contempt. Daily involvement may foster intimacy, but it can also sharpen one's sense of resentment. What was very different about Isaiah's West Side, as opposed to many other communities, was the powerful social stigma attached to it, and the predominately negative images of it that were internalized and projected onto others. "These people out here," said Isaiah, "are misfits. Biological mistakes. I study 'em like National Geographic would study 'em." Nevertheless, he was one of them, and if they were endangered species, then so was he.

Another episode involving Isaiah illustrates again the contradictory nature of relationships within the neighborhood. In October 1999, long after his tuberculosis therapy was completed, Isaiah was at the usual spot when I stopped by, and he was walking with a noticeable limp. Cisco and some of the other guys were there. I asked Isaiah what had happened to him. He said that he had fallen down and cut his leg, and that it was still oozing blood and pus. He said he had cleaned it up at the shelter, in the shower, but he didn't tell anyone in the shelter about it because he was afraid they would send him to the hospital.

I told him that he probably should go to the emergency room, and so did all the other guys. They started yelling at him, saying that they didn't want "to lose another buddy." They said that he shouldn't worry about getting his wine, but should take care of himself first: "What you got to do?" they demanded. "What's more important than your health?"

Isaiah didn't budge, though he did become agitated. "I'm not worrying about no wine," he protested. He said that he would go to the hospital later, but he had something to do first. I told him that if his leg was infected—and it didn't look good, judging from the stains on his pants— he could possibly lose it, and even die. Finally, I said, "All right, guys, Isaiah knows what we think, he knows what he should do, now whether or not he does it is up to him." My experience with Isaiah had made me believe that he would not do anything if he thought he was being pressured into it, and if it seemed to impinge on his autonomy. So I left him there like that. Eventually, he did make it to the hospital and the knee was tended to. But the street corner debate concerning the injury reflected the social nature of illness and injury in this environment.

CASE 2: THE STORY OF STORMY

For those who live there, the West Side has a personality all its own. Stormy, one of Isaiah's associates from Jefferson Street—and the subject of the next narrative—once told me that everyone who has lived in the neighborhood comes back eventually. "Why is that?" I asked. "There's always something goin' on," he said. We were standing on a street corner while a group of women—one of them another former tuberculosis patient—yelled and screamed at each other. "You could make a soap opera on this corner," he continued, "and it would beat out anything they got on the tube now."

Stormy's story was more puzzling to me than Isaiah's. I first met him while looking for Isaiah, and Stormy later helped me with another patient, a woman who also had a diagnosis of TB and who frequented a neighborhood pool hall, which was actually more of a private club. This pool hall was located behind a locked door and a boarded-up window on the corner of Franklin and Jefferson. There was a big kitchen, because the place used to be a restaurant. Stormy lived in a room which looked like a broom closet, which he shared with the water softener. As it turned out, Stormy and Isaiah had been friends for years. Several cases of TB—including Isaiah, Stormy, and this woman—were in fact associated with this private club, even though it was never officially identified as a locus of TB transmission. It was another one of the nodes where social networks overlapped in this West Side community, similar to the car wash, the street corner, and the parking lot described in previous chapters.

When I first met Stormy, I had no knowledge of his TB diagnosis. He did not look very healthy—he was extremely thin and walked with a cane—but he was also an active intravenenous drug user, so it was hard to tell if his emaciated state was the result of illness or addiction. In all likelihood, it was both. But the story of how I managed to "discover" Stormy's TB diagnosis is interesting in and of itself:

1/24/98

I was entering data in the computer on Friday, getting ready to go home, when I came upon the name of "Allen Jackson." Now, "Allen Jackson" was a non-entity to me, just another name to be placed on the list of the lost. My supervisor had simply told me that he was unable to be found. But there was a phone number in the computer, so I decided I would try it, just in case.

I punched in the numbers and let the phone ring. A woman answered and I asked if she knew Allen, and said that I was calling from County General. She said "I know where you're calling from, and Allen's not here. He's living on Jefferson." The way she said "Jefferson" made me think she must mean my part of Jefferson Street, the part with its own magnetic personality. "Where on Jefferson?" I asked. She said, "I don't know, I'd have to have someone go look for him and call you back. Somewhere around the 3700 block."

She called me back and told me the exact address, 3717 West Jefferson. Then it hit me: "I know right where that is. Does he go by any name other than Allen Jackson?"

She replied, "No, not really. They call him Stormy."

"Stormy?" I said. "I know Stormy." I thanked her and headed back out to the street as soon as I could. I pulled up to the pool hall and hopped out of the car. I was feeling the burden of responsibility for not knowing about Stormy's TB earlier, and I hoped that he hadn't gotten too sick, so that there would be permanent damage and more people infected.

Stormy came out and said "Hi Paul," and I motioned him over by the door and quietly explained the situation so it couldn't be heard over the blues music and clicking of cue balls in the background. He was not angry but appreciative; I told him he should go to the emergency room and he said he would, and he thanked me over and over again. He asked if I would be working with him later, coming to see him take his medicine, the way I did with Isaiah, and I said "yes," and he said, "I would like that."

Stormy went to the emergency room shortly, and he was admitted with a diagnosis of tuberculosis and AIDS. I went to see him there in the hopes of interviewing him for this study:

2/01/98

I attempted another interview on Friday, with Allen Jackson, aka Stormy, but he had just received an injection which made him drowsy and he seemed pretty wrapped up in *The Jerry Springer Show*. I sat there with him and got caught up in it too. He said people around the neighborhood watch the show regularly and some days life on the street corner resembles the show. He says he would watch it every day if he could . . .

Stormy is quite straightforward about his drug use. I ask him if he is still shooting heroin and he says yes; I ask him how often and he says "every chance I get." I ask him where he gets the money and he says he borrows a little bit here, a little bit there. Because of the multitude of loan sharks in the vicinity he is able to borrow money, dollar on the dollar, so that his monthly check is normally gone as soon as he gets it.

After several weeks at County General, Stormy was transferred to Maple Grove Hospital, a long-term care facility which was also run by the County. I did not know this at the time, but Maple Grove had an unfortunate reputation amongst some Chicago communities. Some even referred to as a "death camp." For a man in Stormy's position, being very ill and malnourished and borderline homeless, it seemed like a sensible place to go, where he could get all his meals, a warm bed, and the medical care that he needed. In fact, the first time I visited him at Maple Grove, he did show improvement. But each succeeding time I saw him there, he seemed to get progressively worse.

The following field notes detail some of these visits with Stormy at Maple Grove, as well as my visits with his family and friends. Several of his brothers and sisters stayed in the same building on the West Side, and I had tested all of them for TB shortly after I found out about his diagnosis. Or, I should say, I tested all of them except for his brother Rock, who refused to let me "stick" him with any needles. A conversation with Rock and Stormy's other brother, Cisco, is recounted below as well:

2/27/98

Stormy looked good, with his hair freshly cut, close to the skull on the side. He is still very thin, of course, but he looked healthier than he did at County General. I had intended to tape our conversation today, but after getting there I changed my mind, even though I had the recorder in my pocket. I felt like it was better just to sit, listen, and learn some more first. We talked about his family, people on the street, cops, gangs, drugs, the younger generation, all these things. I told him I'd like to hang around that pool hall some time and he said, "I was thinking about that, if you might want to sit there some night and watch everybody come and go." I told him how those young guys were looking at me that one time, and he said, "They wouldn't bother you, not if I told Rufus to look out for you." Rufus, it turns out, has family in the Spirits (a local gang), and the pool hall is in Spirits' territory.

Stormy told me I should get his brother Johnny into the clinic, and that I should also make sure I test his other brother Lewis, who they call "The Rock." He's stubborn, "just like a rock," says Stormy. Then there's a guy they call "Baby," because he always uses that line from Kojak, "who loves ya baby?" He's part of the pool hall crew.

I told Stormy about Jeremiah, how he shot dope til the day he died, because Stormy says he is now serious about kicking it. He says he thinks that he and Jeremiah got out of prison around the same time. I told him I saw pictures of Jeremiah when he was stocky and muscular, and how the street and the drugs wore him. "That's how it does us," says Stormy. "I wish I'd never laid eyes on the shit." He eats his Maple Grove-style beef taco while we talk. When the meal arrived, he asked me if I wanted some, and I was about to eat one of the tacos until I realized that I still had the mask on.

Every so often the phone rings; it's a woman Stormy met in the hospital, wondering what he's up to, if he's going to be able to go and get his check. It is, of course, check day, and Stormy is supposed to meet with a social worker to arrange a pass so he can go cash it and get a little money. He seems set on staying in Maple Grove at least ninety days. The place appears to be treating him decently so far, although for excitement it can't compare to West Jefferson Street.

While I was at Maple Grove, I told Stormy about the book entitled *The Corner*,[1] written about a street corner in West Baltimore. I said to him, "you could probably write twenty books about West Jefferson," and he said, "Shit, you could write forty."

What was it about the West Side? I discussed this question with Stormy, since he was a long-term veteran of the street life in that part of town. He said that even South Siders were afraid of the West Side, although to him it all seemed the same. I told him I had heard that a lot of the folks on the West Side came straight from the South, in the fifties and sixties, and that South Siders looked down on it, and saw it as being wild and uncivilized. "That's true," he says, "the ones that comes straight from down South want to prove themselves, to get in the gangs, show how tough they are." I asked him about the conflicts over there between the older and younger generations and he said it's not as bad as it was a couple years ago, when there were fights almost every day. "What happened?" I asked. "I don't know" he said. "Maybe half of them got sent to jail," I suggest, and he laughs and says, "Yeah, a LOT of 'em is in there. And it's going to get worse now that this new guy is in charge of the police."

As far as the police went, Stormy said, "There ain't nothing going on around there that they don't know about, and half of it they got their hands in. Once in a while they will make a bust, and if they don't like you, if you're a loud-mouth asshole, they will take drugs off someone else and put it on you so they can lock you up longer." At this time, Stormy seemed like he was progressing, and I looked forward to him getting out, even though it was not clear where he would go. The next time I saw him there was over month later.

4/10/98

. . . at Maple Grove today. . . . Stormy seemed tired and somewhat sad. When I showed up he asked me if I was going back to the West Side; I said that I could, and then we asked the nurse if he could get his weekend pass. He got his stuff together while I went and picked up his meds from the pharmacy. . . . Stormy said he is sick of the food there (at Maple Grove), and that's one of the reasons he wanted to spend Easter with his "peoples." He also said he didn't want anyone from the street to know he was home, and he wanted to avoid drinking. We got his stuff together and I got Stormy over to his sister's house by 2:30 P.M.

I feared that he would go straight back to the corner. But after the Easter holiday, Stormy did return to Maple Grove, and I went to see him there one more time in May.

5/8/98

. . . I went down to the third floor where Stormy was. Almost immediately I realized that he was not getting better since the last time I saw him. In fact he seemed to be worse. His health has visibly declined since leaving the street. He seemed to slip in and out of recognition of who I was and where we were, and would start talking about things as though we were continuing a discussion which I could not remember initiating. Then he told me he had been seeing angels peeking in his window at night, for the last three weeks.

I put on some rubber gloves and pulled some socks over his swollen, scaly feet. We couldn't even get them in his shoes. He wanted to take a walk out to the cafeteria, but after about a half an hour I realized that he wasn't going anywhere fast and I would need to move along if I was going to see the other people on my list. I helped him get up and waited til he got out of the bathroom before I left. "Have you ever had a problem standing on your own two feet?" he asked me.

"No," I said, "I've been lucky."

"It's a hell of a feeling," he said. "You want something so bad, but you can't get it." I could see that he was dying, dying for a cigarette, dying for a fix maybe, dying for a little bit of freedom, but trapped in a hospital bed and a sick body.

Maple Grove was a long ride from the central city, and since Stormy was receiving all his meds there, I was not required to go visit him, and I didn't have a chance to do it again. However, while making my rounds on the West Side, I did stop by to see his family, whom I had met while conducting the contact investigation. This encounter was also quite illuminating.

6/12/98

Last stop before heading back to County General is by Stormy's family's house, where his brothers Rock, Johnny, and Cisco (first time I met him) are sitting on the porch. "Go on, keep going," yells Rock. As I walk up to the steps I say, "You're making me feel rejected," and he calls me the "Grim Reaper." "Don't try to stick me with nothing," he says, "or I may have to fight you, see if I can kill the Reaper."

Rock thinks that the white man sees the black man as a guinea pig. He asks me about the Tuskegee Experiment; he asks me to tell Cisco all about it. I tell him what I know about it, but Cisco says, "They couldn't have done that to those men if they didn't sign no papers agreeing to it," and Rock yells at him about how ignorant he is, saying that those doctors that worked for the government gave those men syphilis.

I said it was my understanding that the men already had syphilis, that the doctors told them that they would be treated for it, but then deliberately withheld treatment to see what would happen if the disease ran its course. Rock won't let anyone stick him with needles or anything; he says that's why Stormy is lying there on his deathbed at Maple Grove, because he let himself get stuck by the white man, and that AIDS is another experiment aimed at the black man. Cisco and Rock argue back and forth like this, Rock yelling, "You don't believe me 'cause you think I'm a stupid, ignorant nigger!"

Cisco simply says, "What harm a white man ever done to you?"

Cisco has arthritis that makes his fingers look like bunches of grapes. "Can they do anything about this here rheumatoid arthritis?" he asks. During the yelling, Johnny sits silent and his wife comes out with an embarrassed half-smile on her face. I ask if anyone has been out to see Stormy. Rock says he's going to go as soon as he gets a license plate on his car.

Again, one sees illustrated here the dialectic between dependency on institutions and distrust of them; a conspiratorial world view, expressed by Rock, balanced against raw medical need, evidenced by Cisco's questions concerning his arthritis. Ironically, Rock would later tell me that the doctors had him "sticking" himself, due to his newly discovered case of "sugar," or diabetes. He had read an informational poster or pamphlet on diabetes and recognized many of the symptoms in himself, but resisted seeking medical care at first. When he was a young man in the sixties, Rock had been the object of some questionable surgical procedures, and he never forgave the medical profession for the pain it caused him. Nevertheless, he needed their help.

At the time of this encounter, we all knew that Stormy was getting worse. So it was not a big surprise to me when the news came, via Stormy's sister-in-law, that Stormy had died at Maple Grove.

7/20/98

Trail of swallowed pills broken today only by the news of Stormy's funeral, and even that only threw me off by about a half an hour. I picked up Geronimo and he accompanied me to the funeral home on West Jefferson to pay respects, greet the family, and then get going because, as he said, "I got other things to do." I said, "I liked Stormy," and he said, "I liked Stormy too. He wasn't a bad guy. He had his problems, but he wasn't a bad guy." Stormy, as far as he knew, had never robbed, killed, or hurt anybody. Apparently they shared an apartment for a time while Geronimo was having some "domestic misunderstandings," as he says it.

I had found Geronimo on the corner of First Street and Franklin Avenue, where Isaiah and his crew of drinkers hung out. I asked if he knew about Stormy, and he said yes he did, and I asked if he would like to go to the service, and he said, yes he would. "Anybody else?" I asked. "What about Isaiah?"

"I don't think that's a good idea," he said. Isaiah was standing off by himself, on the other side of Melvin's car. "He's been walking around in circles for two days, won't talk to nobody. Just in one of them moods."

We parked at the laundromat next to the Praise Temple Church where Stormy's brother was the pastor. We saw Cisco standing outside greeting people with a black tie and coat on. He thanked me for coming and said he was looking for Rock. Geronimo and I went inside the church where Stormy's body was lying in state and we sat down in a pew. He talked to the woman sitting behind us casually. He had tucked in his shirt but was still wearing his round mirrored sunglasses. A pack of cigarettes was visible within his shirt pocket. We sat there for awhile, then I went outside to answer a page and saw Rock out there. I went back in and soon the family entered and was seated, while the woman minister recited the words to the Psalm about green pastures.

After they were seated, Geronimo and I greeted them: Cisco, Rock, Cornelia, Johnny, and Rosetta. I thanked them for telling me about the funeral and they thanked me for coming. Cornelia and Rosetta were crying, while the brothers were stoic and silent. Geronimo and I left after paying our respects, though we did pick up an obituary on the way out. Then we were back on the hot street. I drove Geronimo to the corner. I thanked him for accompanying me and he thanked me for bringing him. I told him how I felt bad about bringing Stormy to the hospital in the first place, since it seemed like he just went downhill once he got in there. On the street he was sick, but at least he was functional. That's what made me wonder.

Geronimo then told me about a relative of his, who convinced her husband to go to the hospital upon the advice of a doctor. He was a sick man, but he functioned okay. Within a couple weeks of entering the hospital, he was dead. He said that she then thought that maybe it was her fault for convincing him to go, but there was no way of knowing for sure.

I had just read some sections of Laurie Abraham's *Mama Might Be Better Off Dead*,[2] which described circumstances eerily similar to those surrounding Stormy's demise. A patient in Abraham's book was sent to a long-term care hospital, on the advice of physicians, and she ended up dying there. (Meanwhile, the money spent by Medicare and Medicaid was astronomical.) While Stormy had obviously been ill, I had a hard time believing that a man who was perfectly coherent mentally could so quickly dissolve into a near-vegetable while under medical care. Some city residents, as I stated above, consider certain hospitals to be death camps. They think that the medical professionals send people there to die. Rock's view of the conspiratorial professions played about the perimeter of my mind. I began to wonder if, beneath the clean surface of Maple Grove, was concealed a dangerous mediocrity, if not a malevolent intent. In this sense, I was perhaps internalizing some of Rock's paranoid perspective.

As a sociologist, I also wondered about the various social factors that might have contributed to Stormy's decline. County General sent many TB patients to Maple Grove, and usually they improved there, if only because of the regular meals and the rest that they received. I had heard many complaints about the place from patients themselves, but usually these related to the inattentiveness of the staff and the tastelessness of the food. I relate the story of Stormy here because he seemed, on the surface, to be someone who did everything right. He went to the hospital as soon as he found out he had TB, then he agreed to go to Maple Grove for the extended care that he needed. He obediently submitted himself to the ·guidance of medical expertise. According to the logic of his brother Rock, this was a deadly mistake. Within a few short months he dissipated mentally, and then he died. What, besides the illness itself, might have sped his decline in the hospital, rather than slowing it?

I had genuinely liked Stormy. He helped me out when he was in the street, and had told me a lot about the things that went on there. After his death I started to wonder if, in a strange way, the life of the street, while wearing away his body, had also somehow sustained him. When he gave it up, he had nothing to occupy his mind—the daily soap opera of the street corner was over, and the TV versions could not compensate for its absence. In the same way that he missed his "peoples," he missed the street food, the juicy Polish sausages and french fries full of unhealthy fat, and the street drugs, which had led to his contracting the virus. These things were destructive, and this much he knew. But they had filled a gap that he perhaps could not address in any other way. When he removed himself from the street, he also cut off the daily infusion of energy provided by the perpetual struggle for survival. The hospital, with its bed pans, daily pills to swallow, and four walls to stare at, could not provide what the street did. The hospital was an absence, rather than a presence; it provided removal, but offered no replacement. He may have been headed toward premature death in any case, but the hospital, with its blank, sterile boredom, had sped up his sentence rather than suspended it.

According to Simon and Burns, "The corner is rooted in human desire—crude and certain and immediate" (Simon and Burns 74). People are drawn back to it the same way that they seek out the addictive substance itself—because it provides a fix, however temporary: "As it is for every other watering animal, the watering hole is the only truth you can afford. It owns you, uses you, kicks your ass, robs your mind, and grinds your body down. But day after lonesome day, it gives you life" (Simon and Burns 74). The corner and its addictive fix of dangers are not "natural" or inevitable phenomena, but they may be comprehensible responses to a life of chaos. If we seek to remove them without addressing the human needs with which they are intertwined, and the social conditions from which they spring, then we may simply be committing a sort of social amputation. In doing so, we risk losing the life along with the sacrificed limb.

Medicine, in a Foucauldian view, not only defines people in a certain way, but also actively surveys and polices them. It does this, in part, by regulating and constraining desire, be it desire for sex, for food, for drugs, for excitement, or for justice. Desire, in fact, is patently unhealthy. In the case of the so-called "underclass," the unemployed urban poor, desire often takes a shape which is officially defined as pathology. Never mind that laws and other social factors themselves may drive and constrain the process by which drugs, sex, and violence erupt in poor communities, guaranteeing that a certain percentage of poor black youth, for example, will be either addicted, imprisoned, or dead before they reach the age of fifty. Those that survive within such a harsh system often do so through adaptations which normative systems—educational, legal, medical, religious—define as deviant, criminal, immoral, or insane.

The medical system, which ostensibly intends to heal, can do so only through a radical denial of the very forces that wound, decay, and disable people on a daily basis, but which also provide the meat of their daily mental lives: the very substance of their desires. Death of a physical kind follows the psychic and social death which the system has already imposed. As Judith Butler has argued, it is exactly those who are "socially dead"—gay people, prostitutes, drug users—who are marked by public discourse as threats to the normal (Butler 27).

Months after Stormy's death, I was talking with Cisco, and he expressed some of his feelings for his deceased brother, in a typically plainspoken manner:

11/23/98

Later on, after leaving the office, I stopped by Jefferson Street because I saw Cisco there, sitting outside the new pool hall with James and Rufus. Rufus re-opened it with a minimum age of twenty-eight required to enter. He did that as a way to keep out the young gang-bangers dealing their shit. Isaiah was inside, crashed dead asleep on a couch. Rufus asked if I wanted to sit down and he went inside and got me a milk crate to sit on. Cisco and I talked about Thanksgiving; he told James how I liked soul food. I asked him if Stormy had been with them last year. He said, "You know, I was just thinking about Stormy today. I miss the old guy."

I looked over at the corner, remembered Stormy standing there with his cane, when he was living inside the old pool hall, before he went to the hospital. "Stormy was a good guy," I said.

"Everybody liked Stormy," said Cisco, "except the ones that he tried to get over on, because they had got over on him." He paused, then repeated that phrase he used when I was over at his place a couple weeks ago: "We're living in a hell of a cycle."

Death and disorder are greeted with a sort of nonchalance and grave-yard humor in the ghetto. They are everyday stuff. Funerals of community members, young and old, are a common social event, advertised on flyers in local fast food shops and routinely attended by the whole range of local residents. Geronimo's informal behavior at Stormy's funeral revealed his adaptation to this reality as much as it did his callousness. "These things go on for hours," he said as we left. He spoke from experience.

Occasionally, I have heard individuals within such communities express the true sadness of their situation, both personal and historical, in quite profound and concise terms. Cisco's statement about "a hell of a cycle" captures this sense of tragedy, loss, and entrapment. Faulkner once wrote, "the past isn't dead, it isn't even past." In dealing with men and women on the West Side, one often gets a sense that they are entangled in associations and conditions—historic in origin, yet brutally immediate—that simultaneously strangle and sustain them.

The next narrative offers an example of a patient who, unlike Stormy, did nearly nothing right. He was not a "good patient." Aside from his relationship with me, which entailed a regular ingestion of pills for his TB, he was a medical nightmare. Having resigned himself to death, he would not relinquish the pursuit of any desires, no matter how destructive. Yet he managed to linger on for a surprisingly long time, in spite of being homeless, hungry, and addicted in the street.

CASE 3: THE PROPHET JEREMIAH

Jeremiah's tale, like Stormy's, is a tragic one. I actually knew him before I met Isaiah and Stormy. He was also an acquaintance of Billy's, well-known to the corner where Richardson's is located. His narrative further illustrates the apparent futility of the therapeutic task pursued within a neighborhood context of poverty, homelessness, violence, and addiction. The story unfolds over a period of almost a year, from the time I first met Jeremiah until his suffering ended. He had been diagnosed with TB in the previous year, but had repeatedly failed to follow-up with his treatment. It was in this context that I made his acquaintance.

1/2/96

I go in the isolation room to confront this guy Jeremiah about his delin-quency. He responds readily; he is as friendly as one might hope he would be. Without apology he tells me, "I've been shooting dope. So now I've got pneumonia again." Yet he insists that he's been taking his meds all along.

I press him for a legitimate address but no pressure is necessary. He gives me his current residence and his brother's phone number.

"I've built a wall around myself," he says. "I've been using heroin for thirty years."

The hospital discharged him, but I was unable to find him at the address he had given me. I trekked up and down across the arctic waste of Chicago in winter, looking for Jeremiah, the icy downtown towers unfurling flags of pale pink and purple in the flat blue sky above the frozen city. Standing in front of West Side slum houses that may as well have been in Siberia, I could hardly feel my toes. I was on his trail, but the weather made it hard to track anyone without access to the shelters. I spoke to his sister and she explained that "he used to be real intelligent until he got mixed up with that dope." When I saw him in the hospital, though, he had told me that he wanted to quit drugs. I held out hope of finding him.

As fate had it, it was not long before Jeremiah returned again to County General. Oftentimes the illness itself places a limit on how long a TB patient may avoid the medical system. In Jeremiah's case, it may have been any number of things that sent him back to us: the illness, the weather, an accident, or an injury. I went to see him, to try once again. I started trying to develop a relationship with him. He told me how he felt about his health, his life, and his hospitalization:

2/9/96

"I'm tired, Paul," says the voice from beneath the sheets. "I'm wore out. I keep getting sick. I don't think that I'll ever get well. I just want to die. They gave me ten milligrams of methadone—me, a thirty-year vet. I just shot $40 worth of dope. I thought it would make me feel better, and it did for awhile. But then I couldn't hardly walk. If I could walk I'd go down the hall and tell them how I feel; I would cuss them out. Nothing but skin and bones, that's all I am. Skin and bones. I used to be big. 175 pounds. Solid."

"I thought you said you had a good life."

"I have. But it ain't good no more. I just want it to be over. I'm tired. I hurt all over. I ain't never hurt like this before."

He told me that the only time he ever quit dope for more than a short period was when he spent eighteen months in the penitentiary. He said that he found religion for awhile, but after he got out of prison, he went back to the dope. He moved to his sister's house because the dope dealer was right down the block. In these first conversations we never mentioned AIDS, and hardly talked about TB either. "I'm taking my medicine, too," he said. Remembering that heroin addicts liked sweets, I brought him an ice cream bar and he said, "Paul, you're always welcome." After I gave him two dollars in cash, Jeremiah said I was his best friend. No one else had been to see him in the hospital, not even his family. He said that they were all sick to death of his failure. His wasted torso was a totem of self-abuse.

About the doctors, he said, "I'm just blood to them. All they want is my blood." This view of the doctors' intentions was not atypical. Like many other patients, he acknowledged his own "attitude," but felt that this was his only means of expressing his suffering and his dissatisfaction with the inadequate methadone dosage and overall neglect that he experienced inside the institution. The doctors had managed to depersonalize their relations with him, to the point where he felt that he was "just blood" to them. He therefore welcomed a chance to share his complaints with me, even though there was very little I could do about his addiction. While he was still in the hospital, he expressed to me his questions concerning his recent TB diagnosis:

Jeremiah: You know, Paul? I want to find that out. How I can start being positive? When I been negative all the time? For TB, I'm talking about. I know I got a trace of it. But uh, I don't understand . . . it ain't been that long since I left here. What was it, about three weeks ago? Could it be getting worser?

Paul: Yeah, if you're not taking the medicine.

Jeremiah: I'm taking it.

I didn't really believe him, but I didn't want to threaten the stability of our relationship by pushing the issue too much. We got along very well from the very beginning. In spite this rapport, however, I was again unable to find Jeremiah after his next discharge from the hospital. I drove slowly through the garbage-strewn alleys, like village lanes lined with makeshift shacks, old buses, fires burning in cans, old men sitting on stools. He wasn't there. But once again, his failing health brought him back to the hospital, and I returned to his room to see what I could do:

3/26/96

Jeremiah swears that next time he will allow me to find him; he says he had a dream about us hanging out on the corner. I think I will keep his case for myself, rather than assigning it to another worker. I say "maybe I'll get you a job if you straighten out." He says, "I got a lot of experience," and I reply, "Yeah, the bad kind." He laughs at that and I give him a dollar and get on my way.

3/28/96

Jeremiah gets out of the hospital today. He told me that I am the only one he trusts. He says we will hang out and I will be known in the hood. He says, "I am a prophet, I live off the fat of the land."

According to Jeremiah, the leaders of the street gangs, once radical, had long ago sold out to the police, the Mayor, the Man. The temptation of riches overcame the love of the people. He says that it was some of the gangs who led the rebellion on Jefferson Avenue in '68. Now the gangs is all about money, he says. Jail and drugs got the rest.

I would often ask patients about their lives in the neighborhoods, and the changes that they had seen. Jeremiah's response here is reflective of the neighborhood's history, not unlike other accounts I had heard. By asking these questions I was able learn a little about him and his background, as well as that of the neighborhood itself. His memories depicted an entirely different life from that which he was currently living. He had gone to college for a spell, before going to prison. His failure to support either himself or his family—he had a couple of grown daughters living in the Chicago area—he attributed to his own mistakes, and to dope. His sisters were tired of him, he says, and his close-knit family was pulling apart, or already had. He saw himself as the black sheep, the one who couldn't stay straight. He said he wanted to get it together, to return to a "normal life." Even though he said this, it did not appear that he had any intention of giving up dope. His addiction was the dominant fact of his existence, and it made confronting his TB disease (or his AIDS) that much more difficult.

After many such conversations with Jeremiah in the hospital, he was discharged again. This time I got in touch with one of his sisters. With her help, I located him in an alley about a block away from the corner where Richardson's liquor store was located. There, for the first time, I watched him wash down his pills with a pint of wine. Medically this was not recommended, but he did it anyway. He told me that someone had stolen forty dollars from his pocket while he was on the nod. This was the first time he ever had this happen, he said. "That's my trick," he said. "Nobody supposed to be able to do that to me. Makes me want to hurt somebody." His diminished abilities as a hustler and a thief compromised his position in the street, and he knew it. Yet he wouldn't leave the street, at least not for very long.

Every morning he materialized outside my car or at the end of the alley like a frail phantom. I still wasn't sure where he was sleeping; I thought he was probably spending the nights in a shelter somewhere. One morning after he took his pills I bought him a coffee and a bacon and egg sandwich at Joe's Restaurant, across the expressway from the police station. He wouldn't go into Joe's himself because he had sold some faulty power tools in there some time ago, but he still preferred their food to any other in the neighborhood. I asked him if he found out who stole his forty dollars, and he said, "Yes, but he went to jail." He then made a remark about how bad luck catches up to those who do harm to others. I said,

"What about you? Why haven't you had bad luck after all the people you ripped off?"

He answered, "I do have bad luck. I have AIDS." We both laughed at that, even though it was no joke. Such comments reflected the graveyard humor that I alluded to earlier, but Jeremiah's attitude toward his disease was both fatalistic and brave, because in a sense he actively defied the stigma that it placed on him. He did not try to hide the fact that he had it, and he claimed that he was disliked because of this. In one conversation, he told me how his sickness had affected his social standing in the neighborhood. About one guy, whom he pointed out in the alley, he said: "He won't take no money from me, ain't that a bitch?"

I asked him why, and he said, "Because I got AIDS. That's discrimination." I asked him how long he had known he was infected, and he said twelve years, though people in the neighborhood had only known about it for five or six years. I asked him if they treated him differently when they first find out he had it. He said, "a little different. But they just started that shit lately, real bad. . . . The shit get me mad, man. You hear me, Paul? . . . I'm MAD, man! I can't go no-where. . . . People don't like me, man! They think they gonna get somethin'. . . . They think I'm gonna give 'em something, man." At another point, he told me, "They hate me 'cause I got AIDS. . . . I got AIDS and I'm outspoken about it." Along with his diminishing health, he carried the internalized burden of this stigma with him at all times. AIDS meant death, social as well as physical, and having accepted that end as inevitable, he plunged forward, without slowing down. Because I saw him almost every single day, I observed his downward slide.[3]

Once I was unable to find Jeremiah for a whole week. Later I found out he had landed himself in jail. On another occasion, when I was driving him to the clinic, he asked for two dollars. I gave it to him and he ran into some housing projects and returned less than five minutes later. He had bought some methadone to stall his dope sickness long enough to make it through the morning. Periodically he would be readmitted to the hospital, but he would return to the street immediately upon discharge. At one point, his lips were raw and bloody from the effects of the HIV virus. Then, after a short stint in the hospital, they seemed to be healing. I asked Dr. Taylor about Jeremiah's TB meds, to make sure they were correct. Because he had been on and off of therapy several times, there was some risk of him developing drug resistance. Dr. Taylor looked up the lab result on the County General computer, decided that Jeremiah's TB disease was still sensitive to all meds, and that the standard twice-weekly therapy could continue. Then he looked up Jeremiah's CD 4 count on the hospital computer. This provides the best measure of a patient's actual functioning immunity. A normal T-cell count for healthy individuals is between 500 and 1,000. Jeremiah's CD 4 was listed at 4. I asked how Jeremiah's lips could be healing if his immunity was so low. He replied that it was mainly because of the antibiotics. Jeremiah, the junkie zombie, was kept alive only because of what he ingested or injected. At this time, he was sleeping in the back seat of a station wagon in the alley.

Sometimes he would say, with perfect sincerity, "I'm trying to straighten out and take care of myself, Paul." Yet I had to wonder: How long before the tortured old heart simply fails? He looked twenty years older than he actually was. Early one morning I went with Jeremiah to Justine's soul food restaurant on Jefferson and bought him an egg-and-hot links sandwich. The owner's daughter was there, as usual, and she jived back and forth effortlessly with Jeremiah. As I was sitting there on the stool, Jeremiah said, "You like it here, don't you?" In a small way, I was sharing his world. At one point, Jeremiah said, "Nobody's gonna fuck with your car, peoples likes you around here." Another time he said to me, "Man, you're cool. You got some black in you. You ain't no natural-born honky." As I stated earlier, I did not take these statements literally; rather, it seemed to imply that I was trustworthy, at least to some degree.

At times Jeremiah's world was quite frightening. The following field notes chart some more shows some of the ups and downs he experienced.

8/14/96

Jeremiah was drunk this morning over by Richardson's, bragging about some fight he got in last night. "I knocked him on his ass," he said. "This dude tried to kick me off the corner, he called me a winehead. I said, 'Fuck you, man, I ain't no winehead. I'm a dope fiend.' And I knocked him straight on his ass. I was up here this morning, looking for him again, to finish him off, kick his ass. He gave me this lump on my cheek and bloodied my lip again, though."

He was bouncing back and forth with his plastic cup of pale yellow wine while Billy sat on his crate, sober and sad-looking with a dirty cast on his broken leg. Meanwhile, Jeremiah begged me down for two extra dollars. He started with demanding five, telling me: "I love you, man. I'm serious. You're a good person. When you come visit me in the hospital, I love that shit. My own people don't even come to visit me there."

In spite of his exuberance, this comment reflected Jeremiah's continuing estrangement from his family, and the sense of isolation he felt. My involvement was exceeding the strict requirements of my position, perhaps, but I was still basically a stranger, and I was there because I was paid to be. Nonetheless, I was special to him simply because I seemed to give a damn.

10/15/96

Jeremiah came limping through the rain in the alley off Baltimore Avenue. "I got hit by a car last night," he said. I was supposed to bring him to the clinic today, but for obvious reasons he expressed a desire to go to the Emergency Room instead. Before he would go, however, he insisted on scoring some dope to keep the pain away. He had me drive him past the home of his payee, Big Daddy, who gave him ten dollars, then to West Ford Avenue, where the dealers were nowhere in sight, so then we went to the housing projects and I was sitting there steaming mad while he leaned out the window yelling, "Hey homey, you working? I busted my leg. Bring it over here!" They wouldn't do it, though, probably because of my obvious presence. Finally, we went to his familiar dealers on a street just east of Baltimore. These guys didn't question him, they just carried the stuff to the car.

"What happened to you, man?" the guy asked Jeremiah as he took his ten dollars.

This whole thing tore me up inside and I yelled at him several times but I knew that he would not stay in the waiting room at the hospital without getting some dope first, and he said as much. He said he would walk out, drag himself to that corner for a fix. Even then, the stuff was bad, Jeremiah said, because they let it get wet in the rain. It was nothing but a square of foil with powder inside.

But when I helped him out of the car at the back entrance to the Emergency Room, the severity of his situation overwhelmed all moral judgments. He was simply a suffering man, and the nurse who greeted us there with a wheelchair called him "sweetheart" and "baby" as she waited for him to shift his battered bones onto the stretcher.

I would like to comment on the reaction of this nurse, and how much it impressed me. Health workers are as susceptible to stereotypes as anybody else, and people who routinely work with the indigent poor are not always sympathetic to the plights of people like Jeremiah. Nurses are likely to be somewhat hardened, to say the least. Nevertheless, they are also capable of magnificent displays of compassion—not in exceptional circumstances only, but on a daily and routine basis. After this episode, which made me truly feel as though I had accomplished something by ushering him into the sanctuary of the hospital, and away from the street, I thought maybe a brink had been reached. Even with a busted ankle, however, he could not be pinned down:

10/16/96

Jeremiah was back on the street today, with a new sweater and a pair of crutches. He said they let him go without even considering his admission, and he wouldn't let them stick a needle in his knee, and all he got was Tylenol for the pain. . . . His ankle is swollen up like a tree stump stuffed into an unlaced sneaker. He slowly descended the back stairs with his crutches under his arm, his hair wild but his face calm. He had already had his first bag of dope for the day.

The guy who fetched him for me, Spike, has been babysitting Jeremiah on the third floor, helping him get to the bathroom, and hearing his testament of pain. He said, "Jeremiah's a good guy, in his way."

Jeremiah said, after Spike walked away, "that Spike, he's a good guy. I used to think he was kind of simple, you know?"

In Chapter 5, I discussed some of the sharply contradictory aspects of social life in the West Side ghetto. The knowledge that one's friends can't be trusted coexists with a completely democratic acceptance of one's fellow street dwellers. Relationships are profoundly ambivalent, and that which developed between Spike and Jeremiah was exceptional only in the sense that it seemed to be genuine: both men were surprised by the fact that they actually liked each other.

10/23/96

I dropped in on Jeremiah to see how he was holding up. Spike led me up the stairs to the third floor; it was the first time I had been inside the rooming house where he sometimes stays. Jeremiah and another guy were there, sitting in front of the open stove with their hands held to the warmth. The blue pilot flickered and I saw a cockroach scurry from out of the oven's belly; Jeremiah seemed calm and said his ankle was improving. He asked me for five dollars, which I didn't have with me. I asked if he wanted to go to the clinic and he said no. I couldn't tell if he was high or not. It was raining and chilly and one couldn't be blamed for not wanting to even move.

10/28/96

When I saw Jeremiah yesterday he was freshly drunk and talked about how his ankle was getting better and how the others in the house thought he was crazy for not using crutches. He bragged that on Friday he's getting two checks, not just one, and he intends to sit on his mattress and shoot dope to his heart's content . . .

He limped after me, down the wooden stairs to the back yard and out to my car. I said, I hope you're not going to insult me by asking me for more money. He said "I only need two dollars." I said "Goddammit Jeremiah." I gave him fifty cents.

One day I showed up at the building where he was staying, and I was wearing a blue flannel shirt. He said he liked the shirt, and I saw that his own clothes were dirty and worn, so I gave it to him. To some degree, I was entering into this world of his, and I saw that it was a high-pressure world of complex reciprocal relationships. To accomplish the simple task of seeing medicine ingested, I had to descend daily into this web of trust and deceit, a behavioral tug-of-war.

Many times I questioned what I was doing. For example, by giving him money I was making it possible for him to purchase drugs. However, this money also enabled me to maintain my relations with him, to keep him on his TB meds. He would have found a way to get the drugs regardless—that was my reasoning—and perhaps by getting the money from me some additional stress was saved. In the meantime, I could make sure his TB was cured, and could, perhaps, help him obtain the additional help he needed, with his addiction and his AIDS.

But my days in the field were beginning to resemble forays into the land of the living dead. One morning Jeremiah was sitting by the barrel in the alley when I pulled up in the car. He hobbled to the car like an absurd Charlie Chaplin cartoon; his lips moving but his feet going nowhere.

"I'm tired, Paul. I'm ready to go," he said.

"Go where?" I asked.

"To heaven," he said.

He had gotten jumped and beat up again after he complained about the size of a five-dollar dose of dope. He was really pissed that he could do nothing to defend himself; that seemed to hurt him more than the beating itself. After this incident, he consented to at least try to get into a detox program. I thought maybe he had "hit bottom," as they say, that he could now bring himself to take the hard steps of cleaning up, getting off the drugs, and extending his life. I brought him to the door of the nearest drug detox program. The place was like a military installation. I left him there and parked about two blocks away, then returned to find him being ushered off the premises. Apparently he had a bag of dope in his pocket which he refused to discard.

"I ain't throwing that away! That's ten dollars!" he yelled.

"That ain't ten dollars," I said. "That ten dollars is long gone and all you got is that useless shit."

"Hey, Paul, that hurts."

"You know what they say about the truth."

"The Truth is the Light," he said.

This is an expression I had heard many times on the West Side. Billy, in fact, often used it. It is interesting that Jeremiah offered me this phrase, rather than the one I was looking for, which was "The truth hurts." Perhaps these two phrases are roughly equivalent; each one implies that a recognition of the truth points the way toward change. Recognizing the truth, however, does not necessarily mean that one will respond to it. Seeing the light does not guarantee sound navigation. Jeremiah's vision may have been clouded by addiction, but he saw where he was headed. Yet and still he did not divert from his course.

11/14/96

Jeremiah looks more and more like a dead man.
I hold up a mirror and say
Look at yourself
He glances in the glass, expression unchanged,
at the hollowed-out face, crusted lips, bent frame:
Don't look too good, huh?
I tell him, my pockets are empty, I gave Lucius my last two dollars.
He nods, in need of dope, nearing death,
too weak to even argue.

11/18/96

I found Jeremiah walking down the alley at 9 A.M. with a gray blanket wrapped around his shoulders and his black hat pulled down over his ears. He looked like some sort of nomad or refugee, and his voice was reduced to a snotty gurgle and squeak. He said he spent all night outside in the cold. I sat there beside him in the car, not knowing what to do as he kept trying to talk and kept coughing up phlegm instead of words. It was as though he was trying to talk with his head in a tank of tar.

Suddenly it seemed as though this might be it, that he might be near the end. "I'm dying, Paul. I'm tired, I'm hungry, I'm dying."

"You need to go to the hospital," I said.

"I will go, as soon as I get a bag of dope," he replied.

But I couldn't stand to be a party to that this time. Not with him looking this bad. I took him to get a bacon and egg sandwich at a place on Detroit Street and I brought it to the car and handed the paper bag to him. I went to drop him back at the fire barrel and he said, "Just give me a token and I'll go to the hospital. I'm not coming back (here). I don't want to come back."

But before he got out of the car one of the young studs walked by and they made a quick transaction of cash for contraband and he sat back in his seat.

"Let's go," he said.

I dropped him off at the clinic building with his blanket, his dope, and his paper bag full of food, ready for the inevitable wait to be admitted through ER.

A couple hours later I headed over to the hospital to see Jeremiah. He had been admitted, and he was half-asleep when I entered the isolation room. "Hey buddy," I said. He crossed his hands over his chest like a bed-ridden Jesus and said in a sickening moan: "I'm hurtin'. I'm hurting Paul." I brought a bag of popcorn back to his room later that same afternoon and found the place a mess. A pair of discarded pants and an ugly polyester necktie were draped over the chair by the bed. The covers of the bed were pulled down, there was a Styrofoam cup spilled on the floor and empty juice cups piled on the bedside table. I knocked on the bathroom door, hard, several times, and called his name. There was no answer. I stood there with this stupid hot pouch of popcorn in my hands and the mask on my face and he was gone already. I asked a nurse where he was and she said, "He left."

"What?" I was slightly astounded. "He can barely walk." She shrugged.

So I walked back down the hospital corridor, ripped the bag open and started eating it myself. Apparently the hunger for dope overcame the weakness in his legs and lungs. I could just picture him traipsing through the wet snowy streets, hunting down a pusher so he could return to his hospital bed, a machine of addiction. I was too tired to be disappointed. The only thing I couldn't understand was how he kept going.

Around this time, I sat in the car with Jeremiah and tape recorded several conversations with him. Unfortunately, due to technical difficulties, one of the lengthiest of these tapes was lost. What I remember most from that morning, however, was the pride and anger that Jeremiah expressed. He said that his sisters owed him because he taught them everything they knew about the street: "Do your hear me, Paul?" he nearly screamed. "I taught them everything!" It was as though he wanted some credit for what he had given, what he knew, what he had done, in spite of the degradation of his current circumstances. I was probably the only one willing to listen to this tirade. Certainly his sisters didn't want to hear it, and his street companions didn't need to be reminded how rough it was.

The street has little patience for those who cannot keep up its relentless, grinding pace. At the same time, one immersed in the life of the street has little chance of acceptance anywhere else. This was the ledge on which Jeremiah stood, and its edge seemed to be crumbling. He could no longer keep up, and this was apparent to everyone. He was like the lame elephant left behind by the herd, a sacrifice to the lions. People tolerated him, but just barely; only the truly compassionate, such as Spike, and a man named Curtis, an ex-con who no longer used drugs, took the time to help the sick, lagging man. Others didn't even want him around. He carried the smell of decay and death: the stigma of disease contributed to his marginalization, even within this liminal area he had occupied for so long.

One day I went to find Jeremiah, figuring that he would be out waiting for me by the fire barrel, as he usually was. But the alley was almost empty, as though everyone had been chased out. There were two young guys standing where the barrel had been, and Jeremiah's old buddy Riley, and a woman I didn't know. As I pulled up, a car with a white man inside drove past. The man looked at me as the car rolled by and then out the other side of the alley.

"Who was that?" I asked the young guy in the big black coat with the hood pulled up.

"Po-lice," he said.

"Where's Jeremiah?"

"His sister got him a room at the Hotel Rialto, room 223."

The Hotel Rialto. As many times as I had driven past it, I'd never been inside. It had always seemed like a strange relic from a wartime novel, located on a busy corner on the West Side. I loaded my camera with film and parked across the street from the hotel. I had this idea that I must photograph Jeremiah before he ended up dead. I doubted that would occur anytime soon, because he had fooled me so many times before with his resilience. But I was going out of town for a week, and in that time anything could happen.

It turned out he wasn't at the Rialto, which I found strange. In my experience, information so specific was usually not a lie. I walked down the street to Cassidy's house. A guy named Slick opened the door.

"You seen Jeremiah?" I asked.

"Nope," he said. The day got longer and longer, and I was getting worried. From my office I called up Jeremiah's sister and found out that she had placed him in a house on the South Side and paid the rent. But then she called me back and told me that the rooming house wouldn't keep him, because "he can't control his vitals," and kept "messing himself up." She didn't know what to do and neither did I. Later I drove down to Jeremiah's sister's house on the South Side. There was nobody there. I left his medicine in an envelope in the mailbox. I hoped that he could hold on, perhaps go in the hospital again and regain some strength.

Then, while I was gone on vacation, the streets took their due. Jeremiah died the night I left town and was buried the morning of the day I came back. *It figures,* I thought, *the little bastard cheated me out of a last sight of him.* I kept thinking of all my conversations with Jeremiah. From the day we met he was telling me he was ready to die. A prophet living off the fat of the land, he had said, but his hustling had gotten harder and harder and his legs could no longer bear him up. "I'm ready, Paul," he kept saying. "I'm tired." "It hurts," he moaned to me while wracked with pain in the hospital bed, before he walked out in search of dope to keep him going. He had a lot of heart. That's the biggest compliment I ever heard him give to another, and that was probably the most he could ask for. It was all downhill, it seemed, after he found that he couldn't keep himself from getting whipped by street corner punks.

CONCLUSION

Jeremiah's case was a sort of milestone for me, both in terms of the depth of my involvement and the futility of my efforts. After he died, I went to see his sisters, whom I had previously only spoken to on the phone. "Jeremiah was a trip," said his older sister Jade. I sat down with them at their house on the South Side and we looked at pictures of the family, including Jeremiah. I saw him in his younger, healthier days, and heard stories of what kind of man he had been. Most important, perhaps, was the fact that my own feelings of futility were shared. In fact, my feelings could not compare to those held by his family. Jeremiah's drug use had been a plague upon their house for many years; his sister told me how he used to show up at her place of work on the day she received her paycheck, asking for money. "That," she said, "was a very annoying habit." In the urban black community, women are often called upon to carry the double burden of earning money and raising children. Even sisterly love has its limits, however, and Jeremiah had reached them.

Nevertheless, they would sometimes succumb to his supplications, and always tried to help him in whatever ways they could. It was his sister, for example, who placed him in the rooming house in his last days, and then had to go get him when they kicked him out because of his problems with uncontrollable diarrhea. It was she who brought him to the hospital for the last time. On the way there, she told me, he begged her to drive him past the corner where the dealers were so he could buy some dope to hold him over. She refused. "It's for your own good," she insisted. His reply, in the low rasp that I could hear as though I were there myself, was brutally simple: "Fuck you." That was the last words she heard from her brother. She loved him, but she could only be glad that his suffering was finally over. No doubt she was also glad that he would no longer be a source of suffering for her, either.

The death certificate, which I later saw, stated simply that he had died of "immunodeficiency syndrome." In such manner does the master category of a defining diagnosis collapse all complexities within its own ambiguous space. He died of AIDS, as inevitably as he himself had stated he would. The story of how he initially contracted the disease was buried somewhere in the murky memory that died with him, somewhere between addiction and imprisonment. Poverty was only the backdrop, in this standard view; it made matters worse, but did not spawn the problem. The drugs merely spurred the process along. His sisters, both of whom had managed to avoid any such pitfalls, laid the blame ultimately on Jeremiah himself—and on the drugs.

The same was true of Stormy. His sister had long ago kicked him out of the family's building on the West Side, because he had been unable to regulate his drug use and never paid any rent. Stormy and Jeremiah were both released from prison around the same time in the late 1980s, and both returned to a neighborhood where few possibilities existed that were not related to the world of illegal drugs. Those drugs were perceived both inside and outside the community as a sort of corrosive, invasive demon that sapped men and women of their pride, intelligence, and will. For both of these men, drugs were probably the most powerful factor influencing a painful life and premature death. Disease was as much a result as a cause.

A sociological perspective reveals how a generalized depravation within a limited area may have facilitated the process which these narratives present as inevitable. My life intersected Stormy's and Jeremiah's on a downward trajectory. Though Isaiah completed his TB treatment and hung on in the neighborhood, his alcoholic seizures and frequent trips to the emergency room did not bode well for his chances at old age. Each case is different, but what stands out in all of these stories is the utter lack of material means for combating or ameliorating the destructive power of physical addiction. Combine that with a geographic confinement within the ghetto and social relationships rubbed raw by daily catastrophe, and the result is a lowered tolerance for the constant needs of others, even those of family. This is seen in the exhausted resignation of both Stormy's and Jeremiah's sisters: "I got my own problems," they told me, "I can't be worried about taking care of a grown man."

But why is drug and alcohol addiction necessarily linked to such profound social suffering? Certainly, in middle class communities, addiction often occurs without fatal results. Drug rehabilitation is possible in the ghetto, but given the persistently poor neighborhood conditions, its benefits are notoriously short-lived. The rhetoric of rehab is "once an addict, always an addict," and this itself may be interpreted as an invitation to relapse. Like the criminal record that both Stormy and Jeremiah carried, their drug abuse had become a social identity, permanent as a cattle brand. There are very few other options, in terms of either residence or employment, available for the convicted, addicted felon. One is left with little solace outside the circle of those similarly afflicted. That solace comes in a needle, a pipe, or a bottle.

If they serve no other purpose, perhaps these stories might show, quite concretely, how such conditions collaborate in the degradation and destruction of human lives, and how human beings nevertheless persist: "sustaining," in Agee's memorable words, "for a while, without defense, the enormous assaults of the universe" (Agee and Evans 54). Placing people within both a social and a temporal context and seeing them as active members of families and communities of meaning may help to disarm some of the stigma that adheres to them as individuals and thereby affects the nature of their interaction with medical institutions. Poverty, homelessness, and addiction are serious conditions in and of themselves, and when compounded with disease they can become quite deadly. Compliance with medical therapy, while it may address immediate health issues, does not address these underlying conditions. In the next chapter, I will consider three more case histories, again paying close attention to the issues of stigma, compliance, and social context.

7   Difficult Negotiations

Coercion, Care, and Compliance in TB Therapy

STOCK-IN-TRADE STEREOTYPES

IN THE winter of 2000 I attended a citywide meeting of tuberculosis care providers, in honor of "World TB Day."[1] The Chicago Health Department was celebrating some of its success in controlling tuberculosis, and deservedly so, as disease rates had once again been reduced to record low levels. Most interesting to me, however, was a skit performed by the staff of a public health clinic. It was based on the then-popular game show, *Who Wants to Be a Millionaire?* and as contestants it featured four characters: an alcoholic woman, a homeless mentally ill woman, a Latina woman who claimed that she did not speak English (though it was implied that she actually did), and a woman who lived with her eight grandchildren, all of whom she had exposed to TB. The game, which they called *Who Wants to Cure TB?* was won by the grandmother character, with the help of a health department physician who served as her "life line."

The women performing the skit, who were themselves all people of color, played their roles for laughs. The implicit stereotypes may have been loudly decried if someone else had been responsible, but within the confines of the TB control community, the skit was fairly well received. The reason is simple: such stereotypes, and the more complex realities which lie behind them, are everyday fare in the world of TB treatment. Doctors and nurses employ them on a daily basis, for understandable reasons. A physician who is severely pressed for time may resort to stereotypes as a way of navigating the murky waters of social and cultural difference that surround many patients. Some of the most prevalent social stereotypes pertain to poor black women in particular (Richie 285). The fact that a black woman who is sick and addicted also has several children, for example, may be seen as yet another confirmation of her faulty character. If she is a tuberculosis patient, and she is not taking her medications, this may be interpreted as evidence of her irresponsibility, or even equated with criminality. In the relationship between health providers and poor patients, the differential in terms of both knowledge and power is quite marked. This makes poor patients quite susceptible to snap judgments based on superficial personal characteristics, and they have very few means of legitimately contesting them. The patient may be seen as the problem, rather than the illness, and this can make successful treatment less likely, as patients become aware of how they are being perceived. Ironically, stereotypes that profile certain categories of people as "difficult" or "noncompliant" may themselves help to ensure that they will be.

The desired end of all tuberculosis treatment programs is permanent medical cure of the disease in individual patients, thereby ending the cycle of further infection. Inadequate care or noncompliance can result in recurrence of active disease, further infection of others, and possible multi-drug resistance or death.[2] The highest priority of the DOT program, therefore, was curing patients, and the highest priority of the DOT worker was making sure that patients took their medicines. Though this might seem a very straightforward task, in practice it was complicated by numerous factors, and noncompliance was a persistent and much-discussed problem in our program as well as in TB programs in general. Some have tried to substitute other words, such as "nonadherence," for "noncompliance" or "delinquency" in order to defuse the paternalistic implications that these terms carry (Sumartojo 1311). However, changing the word does not alter the fundamental power relationship that underlies the compliance issue: contained, for example, in the very word "prescribe." I will employ the widely recognized terms "compliance" and "noncompliance," and will discuss them in relationship to tuberculosis treatment.

The proper ingestion of prescribed medication is, of course, a central issue in tuberculosis control, in terms of both curing individual illness and ending the spread of disease within communities (Bayer 1995; Schluger 1995; Booker 1996; Pablos-Mendez 1997; Coker 2000; Naing 2001). Patients who do not properly ingest their medications, for whatever reason, are frequently referred to as "noncompliant" by those who are charged with the task of TB control.[3] Noncompliance itself is a persistent issue among patients with conditions of all kinds. There is no way to accurately predict noncompliance, and for many people it is a logical response to circumstances that they do not understand, and which frankly scare them (Donovan and Blake 509). It is a cardinal rule of medicine that *all* patients are potentially noncompliant (Sbarbaro 325). Many patients question the virtue of the regimens prescribed to them, often for very good reasons. Research on noncompliance suggests that there is no particular demographic or personality type that is *essentially* noncompliant, and that compliance is most likely to occur as the result of a genuine, quality *relationship* between patient and provider, or because of effective social support, and not because of any specific tactic or policy that the provider might employ (Sbarbaro 330; Donovan and Blake 512; Sumartojo 1318). The national tuberculosis control establishment, as exemplified by the CDC, maintains that "barriers" to compliance presented by behaviors, attitudes, and social conditions can usually be overcome through the appropriate application of compassion and sensitivity on the part of the health worker, as well the use of strategic "incentives" or "enablers," such as cash, bus tokens, or fast-food coupons.[4] In those rare cases where patients remain noncompliant despite all good faith efforts, involuntary legal detention is sometimes seen as the unfortunate but necessary solution. Most tuberculosis programs, however, recognize involuntary detention as being both undesirable and expensive, and do not use it as a substitute for other measures (Lerner 1999, 236). Through the mechanism of DOT, these programs place the onus for compliance, and thus treatment completion, on themselves rather than on the patients.[5]

Although public health research demonstrates the danger of presuming any person to be either compliant or noncompliant, a fascination with isolating the psychological essence of the delinquent individual persists. Dr. Taylor was a very pleasant man who treated many of our program's TB cases. He was popular with the patients, and somewhat remarkable in the sense that he approached each one with the same good nature that he evidenced toward everyone else. He enjoyed hearing the stories they had to tell him, and was fascinated with the circumstances of their lives and the ways they managed to survive. At the personal level, he was flexible and nonjudgmental, willing to accommodate the special needs of a population that was often charitably described as "difficult." But on an intellectual level, he was interested in understanding why certain people ended up in certain situations. He concluded that many of our TB patients had never developed into fully rational, self-regulating human beings. He didn't see their failings as crimes, and he didn't hold anything against them, but he felt that they were somehow stunted. He wasn't sure if this was due to family upbringing, social environment, or innate inadequacy, but he believed that there was probably a pattern, and that if we studied them closely, we could learn the reasons.

For this purpose he wrote a research proposal. He wished to employ a psychological instrument to test our patients and obtain some sort of objective measure by which we could analyze, classify, and possibly treat them better. The prejudicial potential of such a project seemed apparent to me, and he might have been more circumspect in this phrasing. But much of social science and public health is engaged in projects of the very same nature, and it's possible that the only thing preventing his proposal from being funded, as he believed, was his lack of the proper theoretical jargon and affiliation with a major research institution.

On another occasion, a psychiatrist contacted our program about the possibility of interviewing some noncompliant TB patients. Dr. Taylor agreed and asked if I could help out, so I brought two people into the clinic specifically to meet this gentleman. One was Jeremiah, who had eluded me for several months before I got him on DOT. The other was Ms. May, an elderly woman who initially refused to believe she had TB, and resisted taking her medicine. I was somewhat proud of my success in getting these individuals to participate in the DOT program, and after the clinic was over I asked Dr. Taylor if the psychiatrist had gotten anything out of the interviews. He replied that the guy said that they were "okay," but he wished that we could have gotten some "truly noncompliant" patients for him to interview.

I said, "Well, they're compliant *now,* but they weren't compliant before. Would a *truly noncompliant* patient come in to this clinic for an interview at all?"

The glaring fact here is that compliance, when it occurs, occurs largely for social reasons. It is only logical to argue that noncompliance is also a social product, rather than a characteristic of individuals. Predictions of noncompliance based on crude demographics often have ideological overtones and reflect prevalent stigmas (Donovan and Blake, 507). Even past episodes of noncompliant behavior might not be a sound basis on which to form such predictions, as these can themselves result from social factors which affected the relationship at the time. According to Goffman, the application of stigma diminishes a person's humanity and rationalizes discrimination against them, regardless of its basis or its intention (Goffman 1963). The following narratives, based on field notes and interviews, deal with women who were initially viewed as inherently noncompliant patients, and who were stigmatized in other ways as well. By drawing on the perspectives of the patients themselves, and relating their behaviors to the larger context of disease, these accounts illustrate the value of the illness experience model (Morse and Johnson 1991) when applied to the complex issue of compliance.

CASE 1: THE ANCIENT MS. MAY

May Johnson had a long history of noncompliance, at least as far as her TB medications were concerned. She lived alone on the top floor of a housing project devoted to the elderly and disabled, located only blocks away from County General Hospital. I had heard the doctors, my supervisor, and my coworkers discussing her case many times in the past. They thought she was crazy, primarily because she steadfastly refused to acknowledge that she had TB, yet would open all the windows in her 20th floor apartment to admit fresh air as a means of self-treatment. The first field-worker assigned to her was a woman who had worked with TB patients at County General for over twenty years. Ms. May refused to let her inside her apartment after only a couple of visits. On the verge of giving up, my supervisor asked if I would be willing to give it a try.

The following notes describe some of my attempts, over a period of several months, to win her cooperation.

6/11/96

They send me to see May Johnson at 1783 West Jefferson, the old folks' housing project near the stadium. No one else has had any luck with her, and they want to know if a white man can maybe get the job done. I play the part of the polite yet persistent professional. She immediately wants to know if I'm a doctor, and I tell her no, and then I am forced to explain exactly what I am. "I work to control the spread of disease in the community. I'm an epidemiologist."

"You know I'm not going to look that up," she says.

Yet that hunched toothless old lady with the black wig clinging tenaciously to her gray head like a cat has some wisdom to offer me. Behind her is a book shelf loaded with dusty encyclopedias. Apparently she used to be a third grade teacher.

She eventually allows for the possibility of me coming to see her once a week. I figure it's a start.

7/24/96

I brought Jeremiah and May Johnson into the hospital today, in my own car, at different times. I had to load Ms. Johnson's wheelchair in the trunk. She was waiting outside at 9 A.M. when I pulled up. "Here I am, Paul," she said from the shadows of the building. To me she was quite civil today, though she did find some people to gripe at in the clinic, including a psychologist who was intent on interviewing noncompliant TB patients.

7/27/96

Thursday afternoon I brought May Johnson her medication. I asked her how she was doing, and she said something like, "I'd be fine if you didn't keep coming out here." After that, though, she invited me in to sit down and started asking me questions—if I was married, and why not.

"That's all right," she said, "You're a young man. You got plenty of time." Then she said that she likes to see young people trying to do good things, and she tries to encourage them. Half the building knows her and respects the intelligence inside the gnarled old body. She is not the locked-away loon so depicted.

8/25/96

This week I accomplished the remarkable feat of getting Ms May Johnson to swallow pills while I watched. She bitched and moaned the whole time, that hunched and ancient soul. One of my coworkers who was previously assigned to her says she gets a little disturbed when that woman suddenly straightens up and looks her square in the eye.

"I never heard of such a thing. In all my years of taking medicine, I never heard of having nobody watch me take my medicine. I ain't no child; I'm a grown person." She sat there and took the pills between complaints such as these.

[During one of my visits] I got a clue about her feelings of anger and alienation [while hospitalized]: "I never felt so neglected as I did when I was at County General," she said. This perception of neglect reinforces the notion that the doctors have no idea what's really wrong with her, and so (she says) they simply keep treating her for something she no longer has (TB), if she ever did. The fact that no symptoms seem evident only adds to this confusion. Meanwhile, she says, the doctors do nothing for her heart, which is her main problem.

10/16/96

I watched a mouse scurry across May Johnson's floor, all the way on the 20th story. Her apartment is pretty clean, too; she says they must come in through the pipe or something. The other day she told me that my coming over made her feel better almost immediately. Now she is suffering not only from loneliness but also has shortness of breath. In and out of the hospital, that is her story.

11/12/96

May Johnson now has it back in her big old wooden puppet head that she does not need any more TB pills because she wasn't treated for it the whole time she was in the hospital. I said, "All right, let me check. I'll be back."

1/27/97

May Johnson passed away on January 20, 1997, Martin Luther King Day. She was sixty-seven. My brother was supposed to do her last will but she had not sent it to him yet, as she was not able to contact her only son in Tennessee.

I saw her on Friday in the hospital and I brought her a *Sun-Times*. She started looking for her purse to give me some money, but I told her not to bother, because I had bought the paper for myself and had read it already. "Well, you still paid for it," she said, but I replied that I was just going to throw it away anyhow. She said that she expected to go home pretty soon, possibly over the weekend.

On Tuesday, following the King holiday, I looked for her on Ward 35.

The staff there told me she had been moved to the cardiac care unit. I walked over there and asked about her. They said she had been discharged.

I called her at home on three consecutive days and there was no answer. I called Medical Records at County General, explained the situation, was passed to the operator, explained the situation again, then to Admitting, explained the situation once more, was put on hold, explained the situation again and was told matter-of-factly that she had "expired" on Monday.

At one level I was not surprised but somewhere else I was quietly saddened, thinking of the ringing phone, the unfinished will, the encyclopedias and pillows wrapped in plastic in the 20th story apartment that I won't have to go to anymore. I thought about her gasping and moaning low in pain and how I wasn't able to do anything, thinking maybe this time her time had come.

It is strange to think that she was only sixty-seven, when she seemed as old as time, a twisted ancient tree.

Another case complete.

The reductionist logic of disease control views the closing of a case as a success, even if it was not the result of effective treatment. Both cure and death (while under therapeutic care) bring an end to the cycle of new infection, and so either one is more acceptable than noncompliance.

In this case, one can clearly see how the character of the patient-provider relationship was closely related to the issue of noncompliance. Ms. May was doubtful, up to the very end, that she ever actually had tuberculosis. Her main problem, she insisted, was with her heart. She suffered from a chronic heart condition, and it was her heart which eventually gave out on her. The whole time that I knew her, she suffered no symptoms of tuberculosis, and there was no medical reason to believe that she was jeopardizing anyone, or even that she was necessarily noncompliant. Her distrust of the doctors was reflected in her attitudes toward them, and she honestly felt that they had neglected her concerns. Emily Martin has compared women's resistance to medical authority to that of laborers who go on strike (Martin 140). Ms. May's questioning of my authority was directly tied to her doubts concerning the medical institution as a whole, and therefore her "noncompliance" served a distinct purpose.

Imagine, for a moment, how you might react if someone whom you had never met came knocking on your door, asking to enter your home and watch you take your medicine. You might very well respond, as Ms. May did, "I never heard of such a ridiculous thing in all my life." She was a proud and intelligent woman, who saw such an approach to her as a sort of insult. Yet I also sensed that perhaps there was a basic need for respect that, once fulfilled, could result in a mutually respectful relationship. I therefore sought to respect her wishes, and her choices, and to explain to her as best I could the facts about tuberculosis, and why it was necessary to continue to take medicine even if one didn't suffer any more symptoms.

Ms. May purposefully tested my patience. But I kept coming over, and for a long time I just sat there and talked to her, or patiently endured her scorn, until she got used to my presence. I sensed that she enjoyed my visits, even if they merely provided the small joy of directing one's frustration at a real human being. Even after she began taking the pills, she claimed to have trouble swallowing them all at once. I started bringing her packs of chocolate pudding that she could eat along with the pills, to help her get them down.

As I became a regular guest in her home, I naturally noticed that she was well known to many people within the building. She had a gentleman bring her food and a newspaper every day, and she paid him for his trouble. She would also offer to pay me when I would do favors and bring her things. When I rode the elevators with her, I noticed how she interacted with many of the other residents, and how they respected her. I saw that she wasn't a crazy person locked away in her room, cut off from the world. Apart from the fact that her age, temperament, and illness imposed a certain degree of solitude upon her, she was a fully functioning social being.

According to Sarah Nettleton, biomedicine has been challenged by sociology on several grounds, including its failure to recognize the socio-environmental context of illness, and its failure to treat "the whole person," especially in the case of women (Nettleton 5). Ms. May's criticisms of the doctors' lack of knowledge of her overall condition, her accusations of neglect within the hospital, and even her eventual death can all be seen as concrete examples of the limitations of institutional medicine. This does not mean that the medical institution was negligent. Quite the contrary: the institution, and the health professionals employed by it, were doing exactly what their jobs demanded. The fact that Ms. May's death occurred (and was, it seems, barely noticed) while the institution was fulfilling its stated functions raises the question of whether or not it is even possible for such an institution to truly address its own shortcomings. Asking a hospital to address the whole person is like asking an auto repair service to improve the habits of drivers. They may try, but how effective can they be once the vehicle has left the shop?

This is important because, as mentioned above, the achievement of medical compliance depends on the establishment of "active, co-operative relationships between patients and doctors" (Donovan and Blake 512). But if the structure of medical institutions actually precludes the development of such bonds—if they are not rationalized economically, for example—then problems such as these will unavoidably remain. Undoubtedly, medical care in this country would greatly improve if all doctors had the time and inclination to hear their patients' stories and understand their points of view. Then, perhaps, it would be possible to realize the true potential of American medical technology and expertise. This is an unlikely scenario, however, because it does not lend itself to economic efficiency, much less profit. It is only when balanced against the high cost of hospitalization that the time and money devoted to DOT makes sense. And this is only because DOT workers are fairly cheap to hire.

On the other hand, the social determinants of health in this case were largely unaddressed by the medical or public health institutions. At the time of her death, I was surprised to realize that she was only in her early sixties. From her physical appearance, one might have concluded that she was a seasoned octogenarian. She was shrunken and hunched, probably due to long term calcium deficiencies, and her heart was also diseased. Given these circumstances, the end may have never been in doubt. Treating her TB disease may have saved her from an even earlier death, but this is impossible to know. Without thorough knowledge of her health history, it is also difficult to assess what else might have been done to prolong and improve the quality of her life.

The saddest thing about her case, from my point of view, was that such a sharp mind was imprisoned in a withered body, living alone in a room on the West Side. Her physical isolation testified to her independence, but her loneliness was also undeniable. In spite of the friends she had in the building, she suffered tangibly from poverty and neglect. There was no grocery within walking distance of her building, only a Kentucky Fried Chicken restaurant down the street. In any event, her condition sharply limited her travel. She was dependent on the Meals-on-Wheels program and the people in her building whom she paid to shop for her and bring her daily papers.. When I was able to personally transport her to the clinic, she was clearly relieved.

Unfortunately, I was never able to interview Ms. May formally about her health and life experiences. As I got to know her better, I grew to respect her opinion, and I was very proud of the progress that I had made with her. I saw how her opinions about the hospital made sense on many levels. The initial estimation of her as "a crazy old lady" was quite far from the truth. In fact, she also saw us as "crazy," for trying so hard to treat an illness that she didn't believe she had. It was only through persistence and respect that this impression could be overcome. Though not necessarily surprised, I was saddened by her death. But her story held an important lesson for me, a lesson I learned many times: sometimes, when attention and care is given with no expectation, it can yield more than one might have expected.

Case 2: The Legendary Linda

Linda was well known to the clinic staff at County General from the time I started working there in late 1993. She was notoriously noncompliant, and if there were an official list of the worst tubercular rogues in the city of Chicago, she would surely have been on it. Over a period of more than five years, she was hospitalized eight times for tuberculosis, and each time she was placed on TB medicines. Starting in late 1993, with the initiation of the Directly Observed Therapy Program at County General, she was offered a program of DOT each time she was hospitalized. On each occasion she agreed, but did not cooperate for very long. Somewhere along the line she had developed serious drug resistance, presumably as a direct result of many failed treatments.

In January 1996, Linda Murdock turned up again at County General. I went to see her, to try to coax some information about where she was living and where she could be found. Sometimes the onslaught of the acute symptoms brought on sudden conciliatory moods in patients. But all I got out of her was that she and her boyfriend Jack lived on the West Side: "We sleep on the street, in the hallways, wherever we can lay our heads." Obviously, this situation did not lend itself to consistent follow-up care. Nonetheless, we tried to work with her. She was referred to another local agency, a program designed specifically for homeless TB patients. There she was provided with housing—paid for by the program—on the sole condition that she cooperate with DOT. She stayed in the program for about a month, then one day she disappeared, and the case worker was not able to find her. Eventually she returned to the hospital, as we knew she would. Her illness placed a sort of iron limit on her escape attempts. I use this phrase deliberately to capture the way her behavior was seen by the TB control community. In the eyes of the hospital and health department, she was a fugitive from therapy. She either didn't know what was good for her, or didn't care, and in either case, the best solution was to lock her up.

Linda fit into a preexisting symbolic language in this respect: she was a breeder of bacteriological weaponry, threatening the population at large. At the time of our encounters with her, however, there were as yet no effective legal mechanisms for detaining tuberculosis patients in Chicago against their will. Many viewed this fact as a serious impediment to effective disease control. Nevertheless, it forced us to work with the other tools at our disposal, which essentially included only the power of persuasion and a limited program of cash incentives. When she did finally return to County General in the fall of 1997, after an absence of over a year, one of her lungs was badly damaged, though not destroyed. But her past record of treatment didn't seem promising in terms of her future recovery. The regimen for MDR patients is much longer and more diffi-cult than the regimen for plain old drug-sensitive TB. The second-line medications are less effective than the standard drugs, and the side effects are also worse. The combination of these two factors makes compliance even more unlikely.

We decided, however, to take another shot at working with her. In fact, we didn't really have a choice. She was technically our responsibility, hav-ing been diagnosed at our facility. In September of 1997, Linda Murdock came back to the hospital, via the jail, and she said that she had found a new man, whose name was Claude. Jack (the old boyfriend) and the street life were behind her, she said. She asked me if I could go by her new man's apartment and tell him where she was. She gave me very precise instruc-tions on how to find him; I followed those, and there he was, in a build-ing that looked like the last thing standing after a nuclear bomb. It was an old hotel, with the window boarded up and litter strewn throughout the halls. A sound of wind or running water rippled through the darkened corridors smelling of human waste. On the second floor I knocked on a gated door and a man asked "Who's there?" I told him I was from County General and he opened the door. A door across the hall opened also, and both men were concerned about Linda. They seemed sincere, and I thought that following her in the field might actually be possible this time.

While I was attempting to contact Linda's social network, she was trans-ferred to Maple Grove Hospital, the long-term care facility. The plan was for her to complete her treatment as an inpatient where she could be closely monitored until she was cured—a process that would take up to eighteen months. She was there less than a month, however, before she signed her-self out and found her way back to the city. I managed to locate her on the West Side, at Claude's new apartment, but she had no medicines with her. Apparently she had left Maple Grove without receiving any.

So we carted her in to the clinic and got her started on meds. The doc-tor decided that we would try, once again, to treat her as an outpatient on DOT. The biggest potential problem was the complexity of her regi-men. "Second line" drugs, used to treat MDR TB patients, must be split into morning and evening doses to reduce adverse side effects. DOT workers didn't normally make regular visits after working hours, which meant that her evening dose would go unobserved. I was to see Linda and Claude every morning, five days a week, until she was cured. I would watch her take her morning pills, and then I would set up her evening dose in a compartmentalized plastic pill box. Claude would encourage her to take the first round of pills while I was there, and he claimed to watch her take the rest of them at night. Often I had to spend significant periods of time sitting there before she would finish. Claude would fix her breakfast first, and she would insist on eating it before ingesting her medication.

Months wore on. The following entries describe some bumps along the road to Linda's eventual cure.

2/4/98

Today . . . Linda Murdock was brought in to the clinic successfully, where she spent ample time with Dr. Taylor, discussing the problem of her weight loss, which has not ceased and is somewhat troubling. I saw her take her pills every day this month, unless she is slipping them under her pillow, which is possible, but she also seems to exhibit no symptoms.

When I arrived, she came down the hall to let me in, and when I asked "Are you ready to go?" she responded, "I ain't goin'," and I said, "You've got to go," and she persisted, in that nonchalant defiance she has, and I was on the verge of getting upset when I realized that she was kidding, and that she fully intended to go. She smiled slyly at me as I realized my leg was being pulled.

Inside the apartment, Claude kidded me about watching the beginning of *Ducktails,* his favorite TV show, and I sat there, half-ready to doze off, while they all got ready. I dropped Claude and Slim on Jefferson Street and then carted her to the clinic. I left her there, told her I'd be back in an hour or so, and went to see about another patient. . . .

2/6/98

Linda has been throwing up all morning, Claude says, and from his look and tone I believe him, even though he has been drinking already (a golden glass of beer sits on the window sill when I arrive—his morning jolt). She wants to take her pills later in the day, and since she took them late yesterday, I agree to that. Besides, I would rather err on the side of caution in her case. At this point I don't think she would go to this length to bullshit me. I give her the packets of pills, morning and evening doses, for today and the rest of the weekend, and instruct her to take them today, and to stop taking them tomorrow if the nausea continues, and then not take them again before Monday, when I return. That way we can better determine if the pills are making her sick, or if it's morning sickness, or something else. Considering her weight and the seriousness of her case of TB, it's best to be careful. We can always bring her back to County General next week, if necessary.

2/22/98

Claude told me Linda was still "smoking that shit" (rock cocaine), every time she got a few extra dollars in her pocket, and that's why she can't put on any weight. He hadn't seen her since the day before, when she walked up to the corner and didn't come back. "Just leave the medicine here with me," he said, "I'll make sure she gets it. She'll be back here later on."

I didn't want to waste my time worrying about Linda, but I was concerned just the same. What steps should I take if I felt she had a drug habit, and that it was interfering with her TB treatment, thereby endangering her life? And what if I admitted that I cared about her? But what if she wouldn't admit it to me that she was even using? Hell, she even denies that she drinks most of the time.

"How much money does she need to get high?" I ask Claude, taking advantage of her absence to get a little more information. "Ten dollars," he says. This gives me the idea: never give her ten dollars at one time. Usually I don't, anyway, but now I have justification.

By this time, we had settled into a routine. I was part of their day-to-day life, and they came to rely on my daily visits. I even gave them rides to various places around the neighborhood, and I would bring them clothes or used furniture. I brought them a coffee maker from my house, and Claude started making me coffee every morning. Once he cooked a rabbit at eight A.M. and gave me some meat wrapped in tin foil. The following entries depict some of the dynamics of our relationship and the social context of Linda's life.

4/3/98

This morning there was a whole crowd at Claude and Linda's; not just Slim, but another couple also, all sitting around having breakfast. They got a new bed the other day and now the small bed is used by Slim, apparently. Yesterday Claude asked if I was going to drink beer with him; I said sure, but not right now. Linda tried to get her next five dollars early yesterday by telling me that she was bleeding "down there," and that she only had one napkin left . . .

I didn't give in, and today she didn't even mention it. She did try to get another five early, but I ignored her and left it alone. Claude doesn't like to beg, I know, and he'll usually back me up when I refuse. Of course yesterday she picked up a length of wood and came after me out into the hallway, and I just turned and said, "What are you doing with that?" and she laughed and put it down.

4/17/98

This morning Linda was missing and Claude was a little drunk; he said that she walked out last night and never came back. One of those little mysterious disappearances that she pulls about once a month. Claude had a dollar to pay me back for that buck I lent him yesterday; he gave it to me and I put it in my pocket, and then he asked me if he had given me my dollar yet, and I forgot that he had given it to me, and he forgot that he had given it, and so he gave me another one. It wasn't until later, after I had dropped he and Slim off on Jefferson Street, that I realized that there were two bucks in my pocket.

4/20/98

Linda was back today, as I expected. I paid Claude his dollar back plus a
dollar interest in the hallway. He acted like he didn't even remember, and
maybe he didn't. I watched her swallow the pills, watched her Adam's apple
go up and down. I was starting to think that maybe she was conning me;
maybe, indeed, she is. But the pill went in the mouth, and the Adam's apple
went up and down.

4/21/98

I see Linda and she takes her pills. Again I try to watch them disappear. I
don't see them all go in but they are all gone. What else can I do? I go, without giving the five dollars she asks for. I tell her I'll give it tomorrow, if she
goes to clinic as she is supposed to. She wants ten tomorrow. If you go to
clinic, I say. She doesn't push it beyond that. Slim asks if I can give him a
ride to the drug store where he does odd jobs. On the way he tells me how
these two women pushed him down in the mud in the park last night after
he tried to come on to one of them.

4/22/98

Linda was dressed and ready for her clinic appointment today. I brought
her in and she waited fairly patiently for her turn amongst a hectic barrage
of patients speaking Polish or Spanish or blasted on booze at nine in the
morning. She actually gained seven pounds, but it will be another nine
months at least before she is finished. "I might as well move in over there,"
I said.

This clinic visit represented a halfway point in Linda's treatment for
multi-drug resistant tuberculosis. I had been seeing her five days a week
for nine months straight. Within these excerpts, one can see the interplay
of personal and social factors as they occurred over a significant period
of time. What was more difficult in this case, the individual, or the situation? Linda was not an easy person to deal with, that is true. Two incidents recounted above reveal something of the passive-aggressive manner
with which she often confronted me. On many occasions she would talk
as though she were going to hit me with a heavy piece of wood that she
kept by the door, and sometimes would go so far as to pick it up and follow me down the hall with it. Needless to say, she never followed through
on these threats, and I never took them seriously. In the end, it became a
sort of game, where she would adopt an aggressive attitude, then abruptly
switch to an affectionate tone, asking me to bring her things such as shoes
or pants.

The other incident involved an attempt to manipulate me by telling me
that she needed money because she was having her menstrual period and

didn't have any pads. On occasions such as this, she would not let me go with a simple refusal, but would plead relentlessly, even going so far as to follow me down the hallway to the front door of the building, and calling after me from the doorway. This was not a situation that I enjoyed. Sometimes I would give in to her requests, but other times I felt I had to ignore them, although she did succeed in activating my guilt. Presented in isolation, these incidents might portray her as unstable, manipulative, immature, and violence-prone. But it's not fair to examine her behavior without examining mine, and the nature of our relationship as a whole.

I was, after all, a representative of an authority that was actively intruding in her life. I was there, technically speaking, for one thing only: to make sure she took her TB meds. To some extent, then, my own behavior was manipulative as well; my relationship with her, as friendly as it may have been, was directed toward a particular purpose. It was obvious that I had access to certain resources, and she needed me to get them. I am not saying that her motivations were pure, but they made sense from her standpoint. If anything, the variety of her manipulative techniques revealed a certain assertive spirit in her. To understand this, we must see her within the context of the street life that she had been living for over a decade. As a woman existing within this harsh environment, she was compelled, to some extent, to adopt aggressive attitudes as well as manipulative behaviors.

I also adopted attitudes and modes of conduct which I had found to be effective in the past. Patience, understanding, sensitivity—these were not only ideals, they were methods. Using them to achieve a particluar result is not a problem if you believe that your own motives and goals are totally pure. But what if you doubt the purposes of your own public health mission? The following field notes reveal some of my own misgivings about the relationships I formed with patients in the field:

10/31/97

Let's face it, this is a dirty business. And not because the patients are dirty, but because of the way that we become entangled with their lives and manipulate their day-to-day fates for our own ends. Granted, these ends may often coincide with their long-term benefit. Still, this relationship ought to be questioned more than it is. Are we always doing what's best for them?

I wonder about this as I sort through all the pills for Dana Crawley. She yelled at me for mentioning her HIV, even though it was between us and behind a closed door. She was afraid that one of her roommates might hear, and she doesn't want them to know about her virus. "You can't be talking about my business on the street!" she said. I assured her that I wasn't and that I wouldn't, but by then I already felt like shit. I felt like tossing the myriad bottles of pills on the bed and telling her to sort them out herself and then she wouldn't have to be bothered with me revealing her business. But then she calmed down and we counted out the dosages for the day. But a lot of that viral medicine is stuff that I am not familiar with and I am not comfortable distributing it. She wanted to know why I didn't know what each pill was for. "Listen," I said. "You've got to take some responsibility when you go to see the doctor, you've got to ask what all these medicines are for." She nodded in agreement but I could tell she was still mad with me. I felt like a little kid, shame-faced and sorry but unable to escape my mother's accusing gaze.

Dana Crawley was, like Linda, a "problem patient," who had been passed back and forth between our program and another local program which also did DOT. She was also very hard to keep up with, due to her active street life and drug addiction. On the occasion described here, she was living in a crowded apartment above West Jefferson Street, and she would take her medicine while I was there. Unfortunately, she had many different types of pills, tossed in a bag together in no particular order, with no written instructions, so I could not easily discern what she was supposed to take and when. She also seemed to have no idea which pills were for what. This is a common problem with HIV medicines, which often have more complicated regimens than do TB meds, and which have potentially serious side effects as well. In Dana's case, she had recurrent health issues which had nothing directly to do with tuberculosis; she was a heavy drinker with a liver disorder, which made me even more uneasy about foisting all those medications on her. Her TB disease, at this point, was not symptomatic, and it was distinctly possible that it had already been cured. The liver-toxicity of TB medicines, in this context, could make the cure more deadly than the disease.

This entry reveals some of the difficulties that arise at the point of contact, where the pills meet the throat, so to speak. In the medical mind, compliance is often seen as a simple binary: it's either yes or no, the patient is taking pills properly or she is not. In fact, as these examples show, the truth is a lot more complex and difficult to determine. In addition to this perceptual problem, there is the constant possibility of personal conflict, which can make the task even more even difficult, and the truth harder to discern.

Difficult as Dana and Linda may have been, however, there was certainly nothing monstrous about them. Linda, as noted above, was a resilient woman, whose ability to quickly recover ironically made her illness more dangerous. According to Loudell Snow, health in African American culture is measured by one's ability to perform daily tasks, to "keep on keepin' on" (Snow 69). Trusting in her own sense of her physical being, Linda found it easy to ignore medical advice once she was out of the hospital. Part of the problem with TB treatment is exactly this. It runs against much folk wisdom concerning health and illness, and requires people to obey a medical dictum which seems abstract or absurd once the symptoms have disappeared.

Linda's case, vividly reveals the importance of social relationships in bringing about desired health behavior. As time passed, and I became an accepted part of her life, losing track of her seemed less and less likely, though she would occasionally "disappear." Her trust and reliance on me also gave me more leverage in terms of monitoring her TB regimen. She was on therapy for eighteen long months, and made regular clinic visits during that time (though I usually had to drive here there). Her relationship with Claude and her trust in the doctors treating her also contributed to the success of her TB treatment. After her therapy was completed, I conducted a semiformal interview with Linda, in an attempt to learn more about her tuberculosis experience. She had been sick with the disease for at least eight years, fluctuating between symptomatic and asymptomatic states. Yet we knew very little about the circumstances of her life during that time period, with the exception of the eighteen months she spent on DOT.

Looking at her treatment record before that time, it would be easy to conclude that she was an intentionally rebellious patient. Yet, my experience with her showed that she was not inherently noncompliant, even if she was at times stubborn or manipulative. The fact that we ended up paying her fifteen dollars a week for participation in the program was probably a factor in her compliance, yet the use of cash incentives had not been successful with her in the past, so one cannot conclude that this was the sole determining factor. When I interviewed her, I wanted to know how she came to be sick with TB in the first place. From there I attempted to reconstruct both the natural and social history of her disease.

> *Linda:* But I don't know where I got the TB at . . . I guess I was around the wrong people at the wrong times. . . . I was sick, man I was so sick when I got it, I didn't know had the damn TB. I had that back since what? 1980?
>
> *Paul:* Tell me what you remember.
>
> *Linda:* I remember I was sick, I couldn't eat, it wouldn't stay down, I started losing weight, kept spitting up and shit. I stayed sick all the time, too. Losing weight, just like a damn skeleton, like a Ethiopian. That's how bad I was off, and the doctor told me I had too-berk-oo-losis. Had it bad, too. I remember, I weighed a hundred and five. Sure did.
>
> *Paul:* When was this?
>
> *Linda:* Back in the seventies, eighties—I ain't for sure. Maybe back in the eighties. In the seventies. I don't know. Anyway, between the eighties

and the seventies, I remember that. And I went to the hospital, I stayed there for two months and two weeks, I remember that. Then I got better, came out weighing 162. I went in there, but as soon as I got out, I started back to drinkin'. Then I'd take the medicine for a while, start back to drinkin', take the medicine, stop drinkin' . . . and I started back losing weight, went back into the hospital, it makes my lungs even more worser. That goddam tuberculosis. But . . . every time they let me out—well, I was coming back and forth, getting them shots and things, you know that, and take my medicine there, then I went home, waited for awhile, till I just wanted to drink, if I thought the medicine was going down. I knew I was doing wrong then. I didn't want to go on taking that medicine. See, I'd start drinking from about six o'clock, and I'd continue on . . . I didn't keep up my appointments like I was supposed to. And it came back on me again. I wouldn't take my medicine right. That's what fucked me up.

Paul: What was your health like before you got TB?

Linda: I weighed 155. I weighed 155, and more. I was healthy.

Paul: So how do you think you got it?

Linda: By being around the wrong peoples and breathing the same air. Probably got it by kissing, sleeping around, being around the wrong person, drinking out of the same bottle, somebody coughed in my face or something. Drinking out of the wrong glass. That's how I believe I got it, just being around too many damn people, breathing the same air. Everybody coughing. And the doctors . . . from the County, and other doctors I go to . . . said they don't know where it come from, said it hang in the air. But I thought doctors should know where tuberculosis come from. But they don't really know. . . . There was one doctor at the County, he said, no, they don't know. It's in the air. You been running around the wrong people, probably nasty, breathing the same air, everybody coughing, probably kissed the wrong person, drinking out of somebody's glass, or drinking behind everybody. That's how it be, how it really arise . . . That sound pretty good. Least I'm telling the truth.

Paul: So what was going on in your life at that time?

Linda: Oh, shoot, I was running around, having fun with my friends. I went out with Jack, then. I was messing around with that stuff, then.

Paul: Which stuff?

Linda: Well, I was smoking. Rocks. I ain't gonna lie. You probably smoked some, too, Paul. Shit. And, I was living all right. Until I got this here, tuberculosis. Yep . . . That shit, boy. It's a killer boy, if you don't take care of yourself. Kill you dead as a doorknob. It's your life.

Paul: How sick were you before you went to the hospital the first time?

Linda: First time? Hmmm. A long time. Yep. It took quite a while before I went to the hospital. I thought I was going through something, like it was pneumonia or something, but pneumonia will get to TB anyway, cause I ain't take it like that, going on losing weight. Til I went to the doctor: he said, Ms. Murdock, Linda, you got the TB. I said, "What is that?" He said, "a germ. That stuff can kill you." If you don't take your medicine right. Let the doctor take care of you. There's a cure for it, nothing like AIDS and all that other kind of stuff. This you can get rid of. If you take your medicine right. And now I'm done.

Paul: They told you that the first time?

Linda: Yeah. Yeah, that the stuff can kill you if you don't take your medicine right. It's not up to you, to judge, since, you think you got better since you got all your weight back and stuff, and that's what I was think-ing, since I got all my weight back and stuff, looking better, and every-thing, I thought it was right over with. But it wasn't like that. That's what, the doctor told me that, when I was taking 'em by myself. I thought 'cause I got my weight I thought I was through. Cause I didn't know anything about it. I did think that, Paul, I thought it was over with, when I picked my weight back up, I thought I was doing fine, then . . . so I took 'em by myself. So then I got my weight back, looking better, and everything, eating good, I had a tall appetite. I thought it was over with. That's what I thought. I took 'em by myself, saying, well, since I got my weight back and everything, I'm telling the honest-to-God truth, Paul, I thought I was through. Because I didn't know nothing about the TB.

In this section of interview, there are at least three consistent themes to be noted. One relates to ideas about transmission of TB which are fairly common: that the disease is communicated through kissing, sharing drinks, drugs, cigarettes, or sex, or just being around "the wrong people at the wrong times." These theories, though not strictly correct in techni-cal terms, are actually somewhat accurate in social terms. It is impossible to catch TB without being near those who have it, and social activities such as drinking, using drugs, or having sex naturally involve sharing of airspace as well.

The second theme concerns the issue of self-treatment and self-diag-nosis. Linda was evidently convinced by her weight gain that she was "over" the tuberculosis, or "walking pneumonia," as it is sometimes called. Linda explained the theory of "walking pneumonia" to me later in our interview:

Linda: It's something like you catch the TB from, the pneumonia. You didn't know that? Ask the doctor that, ask if you see my doctor, where you catch that from. From pneumonia you catch the tuberculosis.

Paul: What, you catch the tuberculosis from pneumonia?

Linda: Yeah! You didn't know that?

Paul: No.

Linda: Ask, ask, what's her name, the doctor, ask her that. Sure do, doctor will tell you. And they all don't know where they got that TB coming from. They say, it come from the air somewhere, they don't know where it come from. Shit, they should know, but they don't. . . .

Paul: What's the difference between walking pneumonia and . . .

Linda: What's the difference? Cause, you keep losing weight, you don't have no appetite, you throwing up, you paining and shit, like that.

Paul: That's the walking pneumonia?

Linda: Yeah. Straight up. You be paining with that, you be paining, in your back, your arms, you just don't feel right, you don't want to be bothered, Paul. You lose weight, and no appetite. You don't have no appetite, period. You throwing up. Let me tell you what I know, cause I done had it.

Paul: And that's when you get the TB?

Linda: That's right. That bring it on. You think I'm lying, don't you, keep asking the same question. I'm not bullshitting, I'm not.

Paul: No, I'm just trying to get it straight.

Linda: That's why, it invent the TB, you hear me! . . . Pneumonia invent the TB. . . . I'll drink on that. Pneumonia invent the TB, and bring it in to that. I ain't telling you no lie. Ask the doctor, they'll tell you. Ask my doctor, ask her. I wouldn't tell you no lie. I know what I know.

In this case, there is no doubt that self-diagnosis is tightly tied to symptoms, and especially to weight loss. If we seriously consider what she is saying, we can see that the "walking pneumonia" seems to consist of the symptoms themselves: weight loss, pain, shortness of breath, and so on. These symptoms then "bring on," or "invent" tuberculosis, which is a more abstract condition. It is abstract because you cannot diagnose it yourself, as you can with "walking pneumonia." Symptoms, both increasing and decreasing, offer the best signal to the individual that there is a persistent physical problem. Conversely, it only makes sense that one's diagnosis could be discarded once those symptoms faded and the weight returned. Many patients who are eventually diagnosed with TB enter the hospital wondering if they have cancer or AIDS, conditions often perceived as terminal. Though it is a potentially deadly and stigmatizing disease, the symptoms of TB are alleviated in fairly short order with proper medical treatment. For these individuals, physical recovery may come as a relief, and perhaps even be interpreted as occasion for celebration.

"Celebration," for an addict, often means indulgence in addictive habits, and this is the next theme to be noted. Linda's condition and the success of her treatment are both tightly intertwined with her substance

abuse. As she stated at the beginning of the interview, she feels she contracted TB as a result of her personal associations. These associations, I
found out, were connected with her drug use. She discusses this in another
part of the interview:

> *Paul:*   I'm just trying to figure out how this episode of tuberculosis fits in to
> your whole life.
>
> *Linda:* Well, see, I don't know how I got it, I was in that basement, staying with
> Claude—wait, not me and Claude, excuse me, me and Jack—and I don't
> know, I guess it's the company we kept or something, or stuff like that.
> And that's where I got it from, down in that basement, I believe that.
>
> *Paul:*   What basement?
>
> *Linda:* On the South Side, I'll never forget. I wouldn't lie to you . . . We stayed
> down there about, some months. Yep, mmm hmmm.
>
> *Paul:*   So why do you think it was down there you got it?
>
> *Linda:* The company we kept. You know what I'm saying. People come in, and
> smoking that stuff, smoking that rock, smoking that stuff, and shoot
> ing the needle. I was right around folks like that too. Now, I didn't do
> it . . . nothing but a doctor fuck with my arm . . . and during that time,
> I'm not going to tell you no lie Paul, if I tell you anything, I have smoked
> a rock before. Now I don't smoke almost none of that shit like no more.
> You know . . . but I know how that tuberculosis carry, like a germ, and
> how he kept it in the house and shit, all the people coughing and every
> thing, and blood flying everywhere, and this and that there flying, and
> breathing the same air, too. That's how it probably carry, if you kiss
> somebody or something, or the air, you know. . . . I just don't know.

Her recollections of the time spent in the basement conjure a frightening image to those who work in disease control. A poorly ventilated subterranean room, filled with addicts sharing time, air, and fluids, is nothing
short of a large-scale petri dish to the epidemiologist. What it means,
essentially, is that the seeds and soil of disease are brought together and
given a chance to germinate. This doesn't necessarily mean that she got
TB that way, but her guess is probably as good as any. It also reflects the
final theme that I would like to highlight in this interview, which is the
social substrate that underlies all of Linda's memories, and to which all
discussion of her must eventually return, and that is a condition of
poverty, pure and simple.

Linda's contact with County General began in 1991. This was not long
after she moved from the South Side to the West Side, a transition which
had definite health consequences for her. She recounted how she first
came to the West Side, and how the environment she found there contrasted with her mother's home on the South Side.

Paul: Well, how long have you been on the West Side?

Linda: I come over here in 1990, I'll never forget it.

Paul: Why did you come over here?

Linda: Cause Jack wouldn't stay over there . . . he was tired of the South Side. I said I sure don't like it over there on the West Side, Jack . . . I said I ain't moving over on no West Side, he said if I live over there, you gonna move over here? . . . I said, I don't want to stay no more on the West Side. He said, I got relatives over there, I said, yeah, you, but I don't got none over here. I ain't worried nobody fucking with me, I'll be kicking ass and taking down their names.

Paul: How was it different over here from over there? . . . I'm interested . . . You got TB on the West Side, right?

Linda: I came over here in 1990 but I got TB on the South Side. That's how I moved over here, yeah, me and Jack. But Jack was over here first. He had to come and get me. Shit, I said I wasn't gonna change my mind, but I came on, though . . .

Paul: So you were already sick when you came over here?

Linda: Yeah, that's right. I came from the South Side. Sure did. But shit, when I moved over here, I was a bitch something. I always went and took my medicine right over there on the South Side. That's right. I was in the hospital over there too. If I'd a took my medicine right then, I'd a got done.

Paul: At that time (when you moved to the West Side), you were hanging around that guy?

Linda: Jack? Yeah. I was staying . . . in a shelter at first. I went there with Jack, when Jack moved from the South Side over here, I came here from my mother's house . . . See, I had a house to go to. Jack wanted to come over here where he had relatives, shit, he stayed in a shelter when he came over here! I said, what? I stayed in one shelter, he stayed in another. I fucked up.

Paul: Well, why'd you do that?

Linda: Cause I wanted to be with my man. I did miss him. But I didn't have to do that. I had somewhere to go, Paul.

Paul: You had somewhere to go.

Linda: Back home, where I'd been staying! I was doing fine, all my money was coming in good, got my checks and every mother fucking thing, you know what I'm saying? Shit. Everything coming in good, with my mama, my two girls, her four kids, wasn't never her man there, we had ton of fun, our own selves. Never messed with the police or nothing like that . . . it was a nice neighborhood. It wasn't like this one here.

The South Side and the West Side, according to Linda, were very different social worlds. From the supportive environment of her mother's home, to the shelter where she ended up with Jack, she faced a challenge, which she acknowledges and then dismisses with street bravado when she says: "I ain't worried nobody fucking with me, I'll be kicking ass and taking down their names." Nevertheless, it is apparent that the move to the West Side represented a major change in the course of her life, one which overlapped with her drug, relationship, and tuberculosis problems. I later confirmed by checking her County General records that she had actually been diagnosed with TB before she ever came to County General.

This is important because her documented history of noncompliance essentially begins with her treatment at County General. By April 1992, she was already fully resistant to at least one major TB medicine and resistant to low doses of another. However, her initial diagnosis, according to Health Department records, was in January 1991. It is very likely that she had no proper follow-up, as this was a period when public health programs and tuberculosis-specific facilities were still in a period of decline. Increased funding for TB control in Chicago did not occur until around 1992. It is very rare that a person will develop drug resistance spontaneously, and although it is possible to transmit drug-resistant TB directly from person to person, she had no history of contact with the other documented cases of drug-resistant TB. This means that her drug resistance developed earlier, and was most likely the result of incomplete or improper treatment.

Putting her story within the context of the larger story of tuberculosis in the 1990s, we can read it as an example of the convergence of larger trends, revealed within the details of a single human life. According to Paul Farmer, there is something which may be called a "political economy of MDR TB," which means that "there are large scale forces that make monotherapy and erratic drug ingestion much more likely to happen in settings such as Haiti or Harlem . . . than in the affluent communities where MDR TB has not become a problem" (Farmer 1992, 151). This might just as easily be said about the West Side of Chicago, and in Linda's case a geographic shift in residence also amounted to an increase in health risk: between the drugs, the alcohol, the homelessness, the hit-and-run car accidents, the street violence, and the TB, it's a wonder she made it through alive at all.

She did indeed complete therapy and according to all available tests, her disease was cured. Nevertheless, the basic facts of her life did not change, and at the time I stopped seeing her for DOT, she was still attempting to qualify for Social Security disability payments. She was chronically unable to gain weight, and remained gaunt until the end of her treatment. This probably had as much to do with her drinking and drug use as it did with her TB, but it nonetheless had serious health implications. She also had pins in her knee as a result of a hit-and-run accident that had occurred years before, and this was probably her best chance at claiming disability. Tuberculosis itself, as I explained to numerous patients, is not considered a disabling condition by the state, even though it is a reportable disease.

When she completed her TB therapy, she was still residing with Claude on the West Side, in a different apartment, having been evicted from the other one due to a fight between Slim and Claude over a piece of frozen meat. I stopped by to see them occasionally, talk for a few minutes, or lend them a couple dollars. Every time I came by she asked when I would be back, and if I could bring her some vitamins or other things from the hospital. Once, on a day when she and Claude had been fighting, she grabbed my hand and told me that she missed me, and said "Nobody knows me like you do." I thought that this was an interesting thing to say, considering how tangential a relation I felt I really was to her. But this was itself a testament to the power of this relation, and how it outgrew the boundaries of its original purpose. Just by being there and listening I may have provided a form of care that she had never before had. I remembered what she said when we completed the second taped interview:

> Linda: Yeah, I talked pretty good, too, I think I did, I felt good about what I said.
>
> Paul: I think, yeah, you talked pretty good today.
>
> Linda: Yeah. I felt like that, too. The Lord can still raise me. Without Him, boy, I coulda been gone a long time ago.

Considering some of the circumstances of her life, it was a miracle that she had made it this far. How much of this she "brought on herself" is debatable, and without all the facts we could never really know. Sociologically speaking, however, we must consider not only her decisions as an individual, but the social contexts which surrounded them. In previous chapters I have discussed the necessity of seeing structural poverty, expressed within the local neighborhood environment, as a powerful determining factor in the health and illness outcomes of TB patients. Linda's life on the West Side clearly shows the consequences of street life, and the difficulty of escaping it. It also illustrates the factors that impact women in particular, and the consequences, positive and negative, of relying on men for partnership and support.

CASE 3: THE CONFUSING CLAUDIA

Unlike Linda, Claudia Carter never reached the highly disreputable rank of the multi-drug resistant. However, she did manage to secure a reputation as a terrible person. Her case illustrates what happens when the worst preconceptions about an individual are apparently confirmed by her actions, and accompanied by an image of deception and criminality. While Linda was viewed as being notoriously unreliable, Claudia was seen as a woman incapable of telling the truth, and was even deemed by some to be devious, bad, and evil. One physician had written in her hospital chart: "Patient is difficult historian, refuses to answer questions and refused to allow me to examine her." Her case promised to be a challenge. I took a deep breath and went to see her. The following excerpts describe these first interactions:

10/26/98

Made a new acquaintance today, one Claudia Carter, a "bad" patient, according to the messages I have received; all the flags are up in the charts and everywhere else; a drug-using, 28-year-old single mother of eight who has repeatedly signed out AMA [against medical advice] and refuses to answer any questions concerning her contacts; she is now locked up under authority of County Jail, and the chart describes her unequivocally as a "noncooperative patient" and a "difficult historian." I am ready for this challenge when I finally don my mask and enter the room.

I see her there, a dark figure on a bed, with an open book spread over her belly. Amazingly, it is a novel which I recognize, a book called *Rule of the Bone* by Russell Banks. I say hello and ask her how she likes the book. She turns her head, smiles warmly, and says that she can't put it down.

I end up spending the next half hour to forty-five minutes there talking (mostly listening) to this intelligent and honest young woman, who tells me openly that she wasn't taking her meds before, that she doesn't like the people from the Health Department Clinic because "they treat your house like it's their house, and they be getting into your business and everything," and she got into it several times with them, she says. She said that she is now ready to take her medicine, that before she was going through a lot of things involving her kids, her love life, depression, and her attitude was, "if the TB is going to get me, let it get me," and she had a terrible experience with TB in a hospital in Milwaukee where they locked her up for three weeks, and she says she can't stand to be confined, because she's a very outgoing and adventurous person, and that this being in the jail is eating at her and if she only knew when the court date was she could have something to focus on, and she wanted to know how long it takes to gain back weight, because she wants her butt back, her "brickyard," her "baby got back," her "chunk of junk," her butt and her hips, she wants them back so she has something to shake; she feels naked without her clothes, her nose ring, her tongue piercing.

She got locked up on an old drug possession warrant; she was speeding with a suspended license, trying to get to her daughter's birthday party when she got pulled over. Four of her kids are with DCFS and she only gets to see them once a month, but she loves them, and she loves being a mother, but she still has to take care of herself, she is only twenty-eight and she has a daughter who is fifteen.

When I leave there I almost feel like I have made a friend, and I feel good and proud about it. I stop by the Health Department offices and tell them. They are in the midst of preparing a peace offering for her, and when I tell them about my encounter, they are impressed, most of all, by her reading a novel. Helen says, "I guess I was totally prejudging her." As was I, I think; anticipating a bitter, untrusting woman whom I have to convince that I am even slightly sincere; instead finding almost instant and effortless rapport.

Obviously, I was feeling good about this interview. I thought I had made a breakthrough that would help prove some of my theories about the dangers of prejudgment. She had been defined a certain way, I reasoned, because of her attitude at a particular time in her life, and this definition had colored all subsequent interaction with her, compounding a bad initial experience with hostile follow-up. The result: medical noncompliance, repeated bouts of illness, and a bad reputation among medical professionals in two states. By putting aside all prejudgment and approaching her as I would approach anybody else, TB or no TB, I had made a chance connection (the book), which opened the door to that much sought-after rapport, and would then lead down the long hard road to medical cure. The two of us, hand in hand, me playing good cop to the Health Department's Dirty Harry. Voila. Hurray for me, another victory in the war against TB.

Alas, however, it was not to be. Claudia returned to the jail after being medically cleared by County General, then was released to the community several weeks later. She had given me an address, where she said I could find her, and promised me that she would be in touch when she got out of jail. I didn't necessarily believe that this would happen, but I decided to give her the benefit of the doubt.

My doubts would have been justified. She had given me very specific descriptions of the building where she said she would be staying. But the building that I found was a dead end; a condominium high rise near the lake, it was staffed by a front desk security guard who did not know any Claudia Carter and who would not let me go up to the apartment with the number that she had named. Either I had misunderstood her, she had not given me complete information, or she was a very clever liar. My supervisor Martha simply said, skeptically, "So, Claudia Carter is staying by the lake, huh?" In her view, Claudia's delusions of grandeur merely confirmed her status as a chronic liar.

I have a philosophy about lying: I try not to assume that anyone is. I take everyone at their word, at least at first. This may be partly due to the fact that I am lousy at detecting a lie when I hear one, and so have converted my gullibility into an ethical doctrine. Whatever the case may be, I did not give up my faith in Claudia Carter. I continued to look for her, and just about when I had given up, she found me.

In November 1998 I received a call from an official at the Health Department, informing me that Ms. Carter was at their clinic on the South Side and what did I want to do? I called the clinic and spoke to Claudia; she told me that she still wanted to receive her follow-up care at County General, and that the only reason she was at the Health Department clinic at all was because they made her sign something while she was in the jail, promising to go to the clinic after she was released. She then made her way up to the hospital, a distance of several miles, and met me there. She kept me waiting, but she did arrive eventually. After helping her get her medicine, I gave her a ride back to the South Side.

Along the way we talked about different things. She told me how she got pulled over by police and how the car got impounded and she was sent to jail; how her brother's infant child had just died in Milwaukee from a mysterious seizure (why would a child be born only to be taken? she asked. I don't understand that, she said. Nobody understands that, I said.); how she hated the neighborhood around where her mother lives, how she didn't like when all the black people were out standing around on the corners with nothing to do. She said something similar to what another patient of mine once said: "Some people don't have nothing, and they've never had nothing, and you can see this in the way they behave, because they'll take anything."

We agreed to meet again on Monday morning, between 9 and 10 A.M. Hopefully, I thought, this was the beginning of a beautiful friendship. But again, it was not going to be that easy. I was not able to find her at the address she gave me. At this point, I was close to giving up hope. I was still sending out letters and leaving messages where I could, all to no avail. I once tried to locate Claudia by bringing a chocolate cake to Ruby, the grandmother of her children. Ruby didn't know where Claudia was, but she promised to pass the word on to her. Then, about two months later, I made a spontaneous visit to her mother's house, and finally got some good information, that enabled me to find her.

1/15/99

I found Claudia Carter today, at her sister Saucy's apartment on South Miller Avenue. I had last seen her on the day before Christmas, and she had told me at that time that she was moving to Mississippi on the 15th of this month, to live with her father. So I went to the mother's house to see if she knew the father's address in Mississippi. I didn't see the mother, but her boyfriend was there, and for some reason this time he decided to tell me where Claudia was staying. 53rd and Miller, he said, and gave me a description of the building and the sister's name: Sashanda, aka Saucy.

I walked into three different courtyards checking the buzzers and finally I found a guy who knew exactly which door led up to Saucy's apartment, and I followed his instruction up to the second floor and knocked on both doors, east and west. One of them opened, and it was Saucy, and lying across a bed in the room behind her was Claudia. "Hi, Paul!" she called, then explained to her sister who I was, then shouted, "I don't have any clothes on." I waited outside the closed door until she put something on and then she let me in. We sat down on the leather couches in the living room while the two little kids carried their toys in and out and Claudia and her sister took turns yelling at them and telling them to go play.

Claudia said she had been there at Saucy's since Christmas, and hadn't left the house since New Year's. She has been helping her sister with the kids because her sister works during the daytime. She showed me the medicine, and there was quite a bit missing, and then she took her pills, "to satisfy your curiosity," though she says she usually doesn't take them until 3 P.M., because they make her sick if she takes them in the morning. I told her I would come back on Tuesday, and she said she would be there. "I'm not hiding out," she said, "I just couldn't stand to walk to a payphone." I didn't give her a hard time. I was relieved just to have found her. "Who told you where I was?" she asked, but I didn't tell her. She assumed that it was her kids' grandmother.

I was finally able to convince her to go along with a program of DOT, which meant that I would come by her sister's apartment every morning and watch her take her pills. I also asked if she was still interested in being interviewed for my dissertation, and she said that she was. So late in January 1998 we sat down and talked for about an hour. This is quite an interesting interview, so I will quote from it at some length. It covers the history of her TB disease from the time of her diagnosis through her conflicts with the health department.

Paul:	I'll just start with a general question: how did you first come down with tuberculosis?
Claudia:	Well, I know that my body was feeling funny. I was taking care of my mother, first of all. And we didn't know that she had it, until she came to the hospital. And uh, I was pregnant, during the time, with my daughter. And, the lady asked did I want to take the test, and I was, like, "No." And then they told me that I couldn't take it because by me being pregnant, if I was exposed, I had to go until I had my baby. But how I found out, because I kept feeling sick, nauseating, sweating, feverish, but I ignored it.
Paul:	So how long were you having the symptoms?
Claudia:	I had the symptoms for about 6 months. But I ignored it. You know. I didn't think, I couldn't get TB. That ain't me, I ain't got it, you know, but I was exposed.
Paul:	But what did you think you had at that time?

Claudia: Flu . . . Seriously. I thought I had the flu.

Paul: What were you doing at that time? In your life, what was going on?

Claudia: All types; I was going through a pregnancy, by myself, I was . . . having this child, by myself, trying to figure out where I was gonna live, cause I didn't want to live with my mom, dealing with my relationship, but . . . it was horrible.

Paul: How did the illness impact all these things that were going on?

Claudia: Oh, man, the coughing, everywhere I just cough, cough, cough, cough, and I got tired of coughing, and not that I didn't tell some of the people that I had it, but I couldn't be around certain people, you know, um, I felt funny cause I knew I had it but I didn't want anyone else to know I had it. It was hard, it was hard, it took a big toll on my life.

Paul: So, you said you didn't want other people to know that you had TB . . . Why was that?

Claudia: Because, I knew that it was a airborne disease, but once you mention TB, everybody got to run, you know, and stuff, and it's nothing to play with, I can tell you, but it was just like, I told everybody that I was around that I did have it, because by them being my family, you know, and stuff so, I stayed away from a lot of people, cause I was having weight loss, you know, I lost my little shape, and stuff, kept constantly coughing, and . . . it's hard, it's hard.

Paul: Now, you said your mother had TB, right? So, you had knowledge of it. But yet, even though everyone knew about it already, you were still afraid to say that you had it? You talking about your own family, or everybody else?

Claudia: Anybody. I wouldn't tell nobody that I had it. Nope, I ain't got it. I wasn't in my momma's house when they had it. You know, that's that type of attitude that I had, but I had to learn to accept it. And then, it's a airborne disease, you know, but I learned to accept it, but it took awhile for it to sink in for me. You know, I ain't got no damn TB, I ain't taking no medicine for no six months. But it was hard. You know, to deal with, cause I was in and out constantly, the hospital, cause I kept feeling sick, I was losing weight, all type of things, you know.

This section of interview deals not only with the issue of denial, which is common with serious illness. It also reveals some of the social factors surrounding this particular woman's episode of illness. Again, we see that the illness arrives at a hard time in the person's life: she was pregnant, and without much social support. Her mother had also been sick, and this was another potential source of stress. And in Claudia's case we also see the phenomenon of self-treatment and self-diagnosis:

Paul: Did you try to treat yourself, in other ways, you know what I mean, during the period when you were first getting sick, for example, self-cure. . .

Claudia: (Laughs) Shit, I went down, because at first, seriously, when I started getting sick, I was still staying with my mother, and my mother was taking her medicine, and I'm having these sweats, you know, after I had my baby, and stuff, I didn't get sick while I was pregnant with my daughter, I went to the store, I got some Nyquil, cause I thought I had a cold! Seriously. Cause, I was getting a fever, stuff like that, I got some Nyquil, some Robitussin, I was getting some pain pills, Tylenol, aspirin, and I would feel better, you understand, I did feel better . . . I stopped sweating, and everything, so like shit, I wanted this flu to leave, because, honestly, I did thought I had the flu, because of the symptoms, because some of the symptoms of TB you have, with a cold. I'm drinking hot tea, getting Vicks, rubbing it on my chest. My mama said, "Damn fool," she say, "Why don't you just go on to the doctor?" I said, "Mama, I ain't going because I ain't got this stuff," because I had seen the way, how she was, she was just disappearing before my face, and I'm just, like, "No. Un-unh. I ain't got that, I got a cold, mama. I got a cold." And then I started coughing up that flame [phlegm] and my mama said, "I'm getting tired of you, damn girl, you got it" and I said, "Mama, I ain't got this shit," you know, but I did try to do my own stuff, trying to give it up, you know what I'm saying. Shit, I kept drinking hot tea, Vicks on my chest, kept Tylenol with me, in case I got a fever, and stuff. Oh yeah.

Paul: So you didn't want to think that you could have the same thing that your mother had?

Claudia: Exactly. Something that was just making her disappear, you know what I'm saying. We small, I come from a small family, we have a nice petite size, but at this point, I'm seeing my mama, and I'm saying, I ain't got that shit. I ain't got that. I even got to the point where I was gonna take a AIDS test. You know what I'm saying? Because I thought that, you know, I knew that I didn't have it, but at this point, you're disappearing, you're losing weight, so I'm like, okay, I'm going to the doctor. . . . And then, at the time, I wasn't exposed to it.

Paul: You weren't exposed to it?

Claudia: No, I wasn't exposed to it, when I'm watching her at first. Maybe I was exposed to it, because they gave me a shot, but it didn't come back positive. They gave me one of the skin tests, with the needle, three needles, they gave me one of them, but I wasn't exposed. But later on, like a month or so later, that's when I started having symptoms.

This use of the term "exposed" indicates an understanding of TB etiology which departs somewhat from the official wisdom. Technically speaking, a positive skin test is indicative of infection, not exposure, though exposure is obviously a necessary precondition of infection, just as infection is a necessary precondition of disease. When talking to patients in the field, however, it is often easier to use the term "exposed" rather than "infected," because of the stigma contained within the notion of infection. If Claudia is using "exposed" in this sense, then she may be correct, in that a negative skin test would have been interpreted as "not infected." This interpretation provided a basis for her continuing denial, a denial which was eventually overcome by the severity of her symptoms:

Paul: Tell me about what brought you to the hospital the first time. Now, are you someone who goes to the hospital very often, or no?

Claudia: Yep, I am. If there's anything wrong with me, I'm going to the hospital. I don't care. You know. But, when I first came to the hospital, it was at night. I went to the hospital, I was burning up, my clothes were soaking wet from sweat, but I was cold, you know, but it was like, it was happening, instead of at night, it was around the clock. I said, I'm gonna take my self to the hospital, so when I went to the hospital, I told them that I think I been exposed to TB. They gave me a mask, they took chest X-rays, and my lung situation was like, gone, and I was in Milwaukee at the time. . . . And they put me in an isolation room; they told me my lungs was like shot, they could tell that I had, they knew that it was pneumonia or tuberculosis. But I come to find out it was both. So I stayed in the hospital up there for three weeks. Which I was threatening to leave, but they wouldn't let me leave, cause they told me I was society's, you know, um, something about I was society, cause I had a disease, you know, that everybody can get. So they put me under court order, with guards at the door, and I had to stay there, and it was hard, when you can't just up and go, and I took it for granted, I didn't take TB that seriously, I didn't take it seriously at all, until it really hit, they told that it messed up some of my airways, and this is what they told me in Milwaukee, okay, so I started this medicine. So then when I started feeling better, I stopped.

It was the Milwaukee hospitalization which first awakened her to the seriousness of her illness, in both medical and social terms. Nevertheless, as she indicates here, she was able to once again deny the presence of disease once her symptoms had subsided. Because of allegations I had heard relating to her drug abuse habits, I set out to ask her about the social factors which may have influenced her denial and her medical compliance:

Paul: So there was a whole year, basically, where this just went back and forth?

Claudia: Back and forth, back and forth, back and forth. The same old stuff, it just went back and forth, back and forth.

Paul: Now we talked earlier, reflecting back on how much of it was you and how much of it was them?

Claudia: I would say, 70 percent was me, 30 percent was them. Cause I just didn't want to take this, I didn't want this TB shit, you know what I'm saying? And at that point in my life I was going through a lot of depression stuff, relationship and children and stuff, recovering addict, thank God, I'm still clean been bout a year now, off and on, but I'm hanging. And then, it was a lot of personal stuff I was going through, a lot of personal stuff. So now, that I've accepted Christ in my life, I'll just go ahead and take this medicine . . .

Paul: Let's talk a little more about these other problems, not that you need to give me something specific, or revealing, but what I'm interested in was how tuberculosis, it's just an illness, it's something that you catch, but how did it become involved with all these other things? In other words, was it a worse problem, or was it secondary problem?

Claudia: It made it worse. It made my problems worse. Because I was pregnant, I was in a relationship, and I'm the type of person, if I'm with my other half, at that time, he was saying, "Claudia you losing weight . . ." "I'M NOT LOSING NO DAMN WEIGHT!" It just made my problem worse. I wouldn't take my clothes off, my clothes wouldn't fit me no more, I was disappearing, I'm already small, but I'm a small petite size, but I was just disappearing, I was losing everything, and it would just piss me off. That's how, that's one reason it made my problems, it just added on to the problems. Just getting little, just losing so much weight, didn't want to be around nobody, especially not nobody that really knew me, and stuff, it's not that I stopped taking care of myself, but it just made things worse . . . Constantly coughing, people steady asking, "What's wrong?" "I GOT A COLD, SHIT!" You know what I'm saying? Or I was with a person, then that person was like, not wantin' to get too close, and all that type of stuff . . . it was messed up, I didn't like it, I didn't like it at all.

The disease had an adverse effect on her relationships, placing stress on an already fragile support system. Intertwined with the issues of social support, denial, and the insistence on self-medication, was the problem of drug abuse:

Paul: You mentioned addiction before. Now, you don't have to go into the details of that unless you want to . . . but how did that figure into this whole thing?

Claudia: Well, like I said, I thank God, by the grace of God, I been clean . . .
umm . . . it's, okay, getting high, I was addicted to cocaine, and I
smoked weed . . . And, um, just by you doing that, alone, you know,
I mean, I could be sitting up here now, you probably couldn't tell if I
was high or not, or whatever, just by you doing that, you don't want
to take no other damn medicine that's going to affect your high! No,
because, you see, I can laugh about it now, thank God, I thank my
higher power every day for this, cause when you tooting, you on a
drain, you on a drain, and it comes down the back of your throat,
cause what don't go through your nose gonna come down to the back
of your throat. I'm taking these pills, in which they effect me being
high, it did! The pills get stuck, I can't get my fucking drainage right,
you know what I'm saying? It just messed with me, I just couldn't
deal with it. I would try to take one this hour, one that, fifteen minutes here, but it would always affect my high, and another thing,
cocaine, it had me losing weight . . . But it kept me going, that's what
basically kept me going . . .

Paul: As far as energy goes?

Claudia: Exactly. It kept, it kept me motivated, you know, a lot of energy.
And by I was constantly going, I forgot to take it. And when I did
take it, it would, you know, I just didn't feel right. My high didn't
feel right. And so, that's why I stayed, I just couldn't do it, I could-
n't deal with it, because it was messing with my high-ness, and I
just couldn't have that, so I just stopped taking it. And then, the
days that I didn't do it, not that I did it every day, or nothing like
that, but I did my share, um, and when I did take my medicine, I
would try to take it first, and then try to get high, and it just would-
n't work, so I chose, at that time, to get high over taking my medicine. It was like a mind over matter thing, well hell, if I keep this
and I'm constantly moving around and shit, and I ain't laying
down, letting this damn TB get the best of me, wouldn't take me
long to get high, and it would just constantly keep me going,
because cocaine is a up-drug, you know what I'm saying, you're
moving, and I take a pill here, and pill there, and I thinkin' I'm all
right. But then my lungs are steady getting fucked up, you know
what I'm saying, so then one day I just prayed, all I did was pray,
to where I could go see my children. And I said, I don't need this
shit. I don't need this shit. I don't need this cocaine, I don't want
this shit no more, so I'm going to take this medicine, because it
seem like I'm getting worser. So, I stopped taking it. And with
cocaine you don't go through no withdrawals, you might have a
mood swing, like, "Get the fuck away from me, I don't want you
around me!" So each day I pray, I pray, and I been praying for God
to take the taste away from me, and that's what he did. He took it
so I don't desire it no more. You know, because it was very easy

for me to get it, I didn't have to go out and get it, it was brought to me, I didn't have to worry about this kind of shit.

Again, if we refer back to the folk idea of health, the use of cocaine serves to maintain one's ability to function, to "keep on keepin' on." No doubt this is a major factor in cocaine's appeal, and that appeal is certainly not limited to the poor. However, when entangled with conditions of poverty and disease, addiction doubles the damage by making any attempt to address root conditions less likely, while at the same time inflicting harm of its own.

This is true on the community level as well as that of the individual. The corrosive physical effects of drug use are minuscule compared to their social costs, especially when one adds the toll of the "drug war." Drugs in urban communities have been a major impediment to overall social organization and empowerment, and have served as handmaiden to a whole host of epidemics, of which HIV/AIDS is only the most prominent (TB, syphilis, gonorrhea, and hepatitis would also fit the bill). The notion that drug addiction caused neighborhood poverty, as discussed in Chapter 5, is popular both inside and outside the ghetto. Actually, the poverty on the West Side predates the cocaine scourge of the 1980s, as well as the heroin epidemic of the 1970s. There is no doubt, however, that drugs make the condition of poverty worse. Illegal drugs, purchased and used by all sectors of the American population, have had a devastatingly disproportionate impact on the inner-city poor. Not only do drugs and drug violence kill and cripple countless individuals, they rob communities of their youth (through the allure of drug markets as well as rampant incarceration) and their money (through diversion of public funds, loss of economic opportunities, potential employment, and so on). As Margaret Connors has noted, when young men go to prison, women also suffer penalties, due to the unequal burdens of child rearing (Connors 107).

There is little doubt that Claudia was entangled in the drug underworld. In some respects the dynamic of her illness was very similar to that of Linda, though Claudia was younger and seemed to have more resources than Linda, both in terms of money and education. Like Linda and Ms. May, Claudia was capable of great obstinacy in the face of demands made on her. Attempts to "get tough" with her tended to backfire. In our conversation, she told me about the antagonistic relationship which developed between her and the public health agency that was originally assigned to her case.

Paul: Now, wasn't the Department of Health trying to find you at this time also?

Claudia: Yeah, they was tryin' to find me, too. But the thing is, I would not go to the Health Clinic, I always went to the hospital. And why? Because I did not want the nurses coming out to my house, I did not want them to know where I stay. Excuse me, I did not want them to know where I stay, especially one...Me and her could not settle horses . . . Just could not . . . click . . . so what I did, when I went to the hospital, they always gave me pills and stuff, even some of the doctors there that was nice, they gave me some for days, you know, a week or so, something like that. See, I never did go to the Health Clinic, I always went to the hospital, to get my pills.

Paul: So you were trying to manage your own illness in that way?

Claudia: Right, right, exactly. Instead of going to the Board of Health, or having somebody watching me take it. And that's something else I don't like, you know, they have to come and watch you take it, and stuff. I'm gonna take it, why you can't take my word for it, that I'm going to take it—but then it's like, well, you ain't taken this much. I know I'm the worst case there is for TB. You know, the worst person there is, you know what I'm saying? I'll bet they just say, this girl here, why don't she just take these damn pills, you know.

Paul: Tell me about how they first came to you with that plan, to watch you take your medicine. But you knew about that already though, right?

Claudia: I knew about it. And so, when they first came to me with that, the first thing that I was, I'm like, these people don't trust nobody, they got to see for themselves. All type of negativity popped up in my mind. Okay. So, I'm like, I'm not giving them my damn address, they ain't coming to my house. They ain't coming to my house. And uh, I didn't like it, I did not like it. I don't need nobody to tell me when to take my medicine . . .

Paul: Now, did you feel like there was something demeaning about that?

Claudia: No, I just didn't like the nurse . . .. It was the point of her attitude, and when she comes to your house, it's her house, you know what I'm saying? She just want to take over.. And I'm just the type of person, if you come here, you do your job, and leave. Don't hold no conversation with me, I don't feel like talking today. Okay? Just leave. But she would come get in your business, and all types of stuff. And I didn't have no time for that. Give me my medicine, and go. Don't come here, you know, I'm gonna treat you nice if you come to my house, of course, but once you start prying into my business or whatever, that's why I didn't like her; she was prying into people's business, wanting to know this, wanting to know that. That's not your job. You're supposed to come here, watch me take my medicine, if I let you in my door. Standing at the door, I'm gonna get a cup of juice or whatever, and you stand right here, and I take the medicine and you go. You know, but she wasn't that type of person.

Paul: When I met you, one of the things you kept saying was, "I'm not a bad person."

Claudia: I'm not. Because, they made it seem like I was the, ooh, that I couldn't be trusted...you know, because it was just they way they would talk to you. Okay, it's a way you talk to people, it's not what you say, it's how you say it, first of all. And they had down in my chart, oh she's untrustworthy, this and that, that and that. Why? Because I didn't let you get in my business? I didn't let you know about my daughter that I had? What, what? I don't like you. Don't come to my house no more, don't come to my mother's house . . . not that I tried to prove myself, or explain myself or anything to no one, they just made me seem like I was the bad guy. I was not the bad guy, because by you working in this and I'm the patient, of course your coworker gonna think this of me, because what you telling him, you see what I'm saying? And I could be the nicest person there is, but I can also be that bitch. You know, it's, cause, they just want to be able to: why she not taking this, why she walk, why? Get out of my face. This type of stuff, and they always want to be in your business, and I would always say get out of my business. And that's why I was like, when I first met you, it was fine, you know, and that's why I kept saying, "I'm not a bad person." You might think I am. And then again, maybe I was just in a good mood that day. But, it was nice when I met you, cause you can sense when a person care, and they're trying to help you, and when they're just here to do their job, it's a big difference. A very big difference. It's a big difference.

Paul: Okay, now, you said about the stuff they wrote in your chart: did you see your chart, or did they read it to you?

Claudia: I saw it. I saw it. One of the ladies, one of the ladies at the desk that make the appointments at the Health Clinic, she was like, "Oh, you Claudia Carter, you the one that they be talking about." I be like, "What you mean, what they be saying about me?" And she opened my chart, and she wasn't supposed to, I don't know if she was supposed to or not, to let me see my chart, and there I was looking, and reading, because, I be knowing her, because I used to bring my mother in to the clinic, you know, when my mother had side effects, when her feet used to tingle and stuff from the medicine, I would drive my momma to her doctor appointments. And um, she was like, "You Claudia, you don't seem like the way they describe you," I'm like, "What you mean?" And we read, and I was like, "Oh my God," they had, they just wrote down I was rude, (laughs) they just wrote so much stuff down, about me, and I'm like "Okay, they want me to be that way, I can pretend that way, I can act that way."

Fine, they don't care about me . . . but if you treat me with respect, I will treat you with respect. You can say something to a person and you will not realize what you say. It's how you say it, you know. And I'm the type of person, little stuff, I'm very observative, I sit and watch . . .

Paul: Okay, so you were talking about what they wrote in the book . . .

Claudia: They just went by that, whoever got assigned to me.

Paul: So you felt like, it was almost like another identity or something?

Claudia: No, because I felt like this: I ain't gonna kiss your ass, for nobody, for you to like me or not. All you're supposed to do is bring me my medicine—if I give you my address—bring me my medicine, or I can come in [to the clinic]. I prefer to come in. And then when I said, when they asked me do I want to come in to take my medicine, I would say yes. "Well why you don't want us to come out to your house?" You don't need to come out to my house. You're the one asking did I want to come or do I want you to come out to my house. First of all, I don't want none of y'all in my damn house. Second of all, I prefer to come in . . . Leave that alone, you just go secure my medicine, let me come in, give me a week's supply or whatever, but I just couldn't click with those people, that's all.

Again, we see illustrated here the crucial role of the social relationship in generating compliance. For Claudia, her diagnosis led to a judgment of her character: she was seen as "bad" person, a "rude" person, a "difficult" person. Such "chart lore" usually remains safely concealed from patients themselves. But when Claudia read her chart and realizing how she had been characterized, she decided to play the role that was expected of her. This bad relationship, combined with her difficult social situation and her stubborn character, made for a rough year and a half of recurrent tuberculosis. This also formed the basis of her resistance: if you want a bitch, you'll get a bitch.

I lost track of her shortly after our interview, and was never able to get her on DOT again. Her sister kicked her out of the apartment, and didn't know where she went, and she never called to tell me. Again, this was disappointing as well as befuddling, and I couldn't help thinking that the Health Department people were right to see her as just plain bad news. I didn't see her again for about three months, and it appeared that she was back to the same pattern. Again she was mired in her bad reputation.

Late in May 1999, Claudia Carter returned unceremoniously to County General, once again in handcuffs. She had been arrested for some petty crime, and the staff at the jail called me to see if she was on DOT, as she claimed to be. When I said that I hadn't seen her since February, they presumed she was still an active case, and brought her to the ER at

County General and left her there, though still a prisoner. I then got a call from a doctor in the ER and he wanted to know what the deal was. I told him that she claimed to have been taking her medicine, but that I hadn't seen her take it, and so I couldn't guarantee anything. I asked if she seemed to be sick, and he said "No, she's doing fine." Then he fetched the supervising physician, who told me, once again, that she had claimed that I'd been seeing her every day up until recently. I said, no, I hadn't seen her since the first of February.

"So she's lying," he said.

"Well, she may be stretching the truth a little bit," I conceded.

The first doctor had said that he was going to send her back to the jail right away, as she seemed to be devoid of all symptoms of active TB. So I went to the ER, thinking this might be my last good chance to talk to her before she hit the street and flew off again. I found her in an isolation room, shackled to the stretcher with a guard sitting outside. She was furious. She didn't know why she had to be there, why she had to go through all this just to get some medicine. "Look, I know I got a fucked-up attitude," she said, "but I can't stand this! I can't even wash my ass!"

A Filipino nurse came in and said she had to set up an IV. "I don't need no goddamn IV!" screamed Claudia. "Okay," said the nurse, without any attempt to explain. She turned around and walked out. "They want to stick me with an IV. For what! For WHAT?!!?" Then she started crying as she continued to rail against the system that had imprisoned her.

I stood there, leaning against the wall, listening to her, hoping she wouldn't turn her anger on me. She didn't, exactly, though she didn't seem overjoyed to see me, either. I asked, like a good snoop, "Where you been?"

"I've been in Minnesota," she said. I told her that I was only being honest with the doctors and the people at the jail when I told them that I hadn't seen her since the first of February.

"February?" she said. "I didn't think it was that long ago. What is it now, May?"

"Time flies," I said. "The last time I saw you was at your sister's house."

She told me that she had been in Minneapolis, Minnesota, staying with a friend. She said she had come back to town a few weeks ago, to be here for her son's graduation, and had fallen in with "the wrong fucking people." She told me how she had been arrested, that she had gone to her court date voluntarily, and had told the judge about her TB history, and then they took her into custody afterward.

I asked her why she hadn't called me to get the medicine for her, so I could at least vouch that she had it and was taking it. She said she had someone who was getting it for her, a friend at a hospital or a clinic that she wouldn't name, and that's why she didn't need to call me. She said she was taking the pills, and would continue to take them. I wrote my phone number on a piece of paper, and told her she could still call me if she wanted to. I told her what the doctor had told me: that they were going to send her back to the jail, and that she had a hearing tomorrow.

A couple days later, I received a call from the hospital late in the afternoon. It was a TB doctor from the Health Department, and he was at County General doing rounds and delivering a directive to Claudia. He said that she was very unreceptive, in fact quite hostile, and she kept buzzing the nurse on call button, simply to annoy people. He asked what I thought about what we could do with her. I said, "I don't know, I can't force her to do DOT," and he said, wearily: "I hope her cultures are negative, so we don't have to pursue anything." I agreed with him on that— I hoped, in short, that she was telling the truth.

On Memorial Day, I went by to see her one more time on the ward. She was a little calmer, though still quite angry about her confinement. She said she had had two negative sputum tests already. I brought her a book, *Black Girl Lost*, by Donald Goines. "Thanks for everything," she said. "If I call you when I get out, can you get me the medicine, like you did before, and leave it at Ruby's?" Ruby was the grandmother of her children, the one who wouldn't lie, not even for her.

"Yes," I said, "I can do that. If you call me."

She wanted to know about the Department of Health directive that she had refused to sign. She said she had been taking her medicine, so she didn't know why it was necessary.

"It's simple," I said, "they don't believe you. If you have been taking your medicine, and all your smears and cultures are negative, the directive will be irrelevant, because they won't be able to prove that you have active TB. If you did have positive cultures, on the other hand, then the fact that you had refused to sign it would also be irrelevant, because they would just use it as evidence against you." She had me go through the details of this a couple times. This was significant, because it revealed her desire to inform herself, for purposes of protecting her own interests later on. At some point Claudia also informed me that part of the reason that she stopped meeting me for DOT was because of her attraction to me. She said that she was very disappointed that I was getting married, and that she couldn't stand seeing me every day if she knew that she didn't have a chance with me, and so on. I found this flattering, of course, but it didn't help with monitoring her TB treatment, as she also refused to have anyone but me observing her. This left us in a bit of a catch-22 situation, and also nicely illustrated the potential dangers of too much rapport. By this time, I had basically given up on the possibility of keeping her on DOT, anyway. She swore up and down that she was taking the medicine as directed, that she was getting it from a friend in a hospital or clinic somewhere, and I decided to leave it at that.

In August of 1999, she came back to County General, this time without chains on. She had some kind of thyroid problem that possibly required surgery. I stopped by to visit her and a doctor from the medical school also came in to question her, trailed by a trio of dutiful residents. He quickly assumed the fatherly role, informing her that she needed to take her pills or she could infect others, and so on. All of this she already knew, and she said as much. And even though she had been smear- and culture-negative all year, and swore that she had been taking her medicine (which the evidence from the lab would support) they insisted on applying a definition of "noncompliant" to her, a delinquent identity that she might never overcome.

One possibility, as far as her assured compliance was concerned, was long-term incarceration. Medical compliance in correctional facilities tends to be very consistent, but Claudia was never held captive long enough for her to finish an entire regimen. In November 1999, however, I received a call from a downstate prison. They had Ms. Carter in custody there, and she had given them my name once again and told them that I had been seeing her every day for DOT. She was using this story for cover, stretching the facts to fit her own needs. I spoke to the prison nurse, who stated that she believed Ms. Carter to have active TB again. I told her that to the best of my knowledge, Claudia's TB was not active, and that her cultures and smears had been negative for about a year. I got this information from the County General laboratory computer, wrote it down, and faxed it to the nurse.

According to all our records, Claudia's last positive culture for TB had been in October 1998, when I first made her acquaintance as an inpatient and inmate. If she had been taking the medicine on her own since then, as she claimed, she was probably more or less cured. Nevertheless, the nurse seemed committed to treating her for another six months, due to her presumed dishonesty and past records of noncompliance. There is a potential for over-medicating patients, and TB medicines can cause liver problems. This did not seem to concern the nurse, however. With a two-year prison sentence for drug possession, Claudia would have plenty of time to take all the medicines that a doctor might deem necessary.

That's where my contact with her ended. As a public health professional, my obligation had been fulfilled. Claudia's imprisonment effectively closed her case, and if she didn't take her medicine now, it was not my problem. But that knowledge did not end my interest in what her story had to teach. As we can see from examining the details, there was no clear answer about her compliance. The only person who really knew the truth was Claudia, and she was not going to bare her soul in the immediate future. What's more, the facts, as I interpreted them, seemed to support her version of the truth. Outside of her reputation, there was no concrete evidence of her refusal to take meds; if anything, there was reason to believe that she had taken them, as she never again relapsed into a symptomatic state. Linda, on the other hand, had always returned to the hospital with symptoms and evidence of active disease when she was out in the street, not taking meds.

Sociologically speaking, Claudia's case reveals the ambiguities inherent in any attempt to apply preconceived ideas to flesh-and-blood biography. Here was a woman who seemed, at different times, to both confirm and deny certain stereotypes. She was characterized as a "difficult historian," and an unreliable person. I found her to be an independent and intelligent woman who would not allow herself to be placed in a box. She may not have been reliable, but "reliability" in this case was being defined purely from the standpoint of a limited public health purpose. She would simply not conform to our expectations, because she placed the demands of her own existence above our demands. Seen from a rational actor perspective, her behavior made perfect sense: she was concerned with her own health, and she valued her freedom. Her freedom to do as she pleased was dependent on her health, which was dependent on her taking the TB medicine. Therefore, it was in her pure self-interest to remain compliant with her regimen, regardless of whether or not we witnessed her actual ingestion of pills. Her resistance to the very concept of DOT is also understandable, when seen from this perspective. In fact, Ms. May Johnson was resistant for the same, very simple reasons: she didn't want strangers "in her business," and she didn't think that a "grown" person needed to be watched when taking medicines.

CONCLUSION

Claudia and Ms. May both caused problems because they actively contested the labeling process: each disputed the authority of those who sought to define them or dictate their behavior. Ms. May questioned the hospital's medical judgment, while Claudia questioned the Health Department's assessment of her character. Linda's resistance was of a different kind; she simply pursued her own interests, and followed her instincts, whether or not they conformed with those of the medical institution. By looking at these three cases together, we can see the diversity of behaviors, conditions, and meanings concealed behind the catch-all category of "noncompliance."

We can also see the social nature of compliance clearly illustrated here. When Ms. May finally did take her TB medicines, it was probably as much out of respect for me as it was for any perceivable health effect. In fact, her TB treatment did not seem to improve her overall health in any substantial way. Linda also "failed to thrive" during much of her treatment; occasionally her weight went up, but on other occasions she lost weight. It was extremely difficult to disentangle the effects of her TB from her other issues, especially that of addiction. She completed eighteen months of therapy on harsh second-line drugs, some with possible side effects of nausea and psychosis. Though her behavior was at times erratic, this is not necessarily surprising given the difficulty of the regimen, which is part of the reason that I compensated her relatively extravagantly, giving her fifteen dollars weekly for the privilege of watching her swallow pills. DOT, in this case, functioned not only as a mode of surveillance and discipline, but also as a means of advocacy and mediation, providing a crucial liaison between the medical institution and the patient, coating the unpleasant medical treatment and paternalistic oversight with a palliative layer of social comfort and financial reward.

Linda's eventual compliance, however, was not only a result of my persistence and understanding, or the patience of the doctors who dealt with her, or the weekly allowance. It also hinged directly on her social and material environment. Though she and Claude would often argue in my presence, even at times threatening each other in manner that or may not have been playful, I never witnessed any abuse taking place. This does not mean that no abuse occurred, but what I wish to emphasize here is the relative stability of Linda's social situation while she was living with Claude. While I was seeing her, she always had a roof over her head and she always had access to food. Both she and Claude would cook meals. Though the apartment was cramped and small, and much of the food was obtained through churches and food pantries, it still represented a degree of material and social stability which her life had lacked during her years on the street with Jack. As my interview with her revealed, her recurrent bouts with tuberculosis occurred within a context of homelessness and active drug use, both of which undoubtedly contributed negatively to the illness and its treatment.

Claudia's situation was a little more complex and even more obscure, at least from my perspective, because I never got a clear picture of where and how she lived. She was somewhat younger than either Linda or Ms. May; in fact, she was born in 1968 (which made her the same age as me). She was also lifelong child of the city, and seemed to have fewer of the Southern sensibilities that both Linda and Ms. May possessed to varying degrees—though she did have family in the South. She claimed to have access to plenty of money, mainly through various men, she said, and she also managed to travel a great deal: in the time that I knew her, she spent time in Mississippi, Milwaukee, and Minnesota, if her account is to be believed.

In this respect, as in many others, she was an anomaly among TB patients at County General. Most of them are quite attached to particular neighborhoods or social circles, as described in previous chapters. Her reading a book, her absolute insistence on freedom and autonomy, and her cutting criticism of medical paternalism: all of these seemed to indicate that the system had gotten its teeth into something it was not accustomed to. She was an intelligent, literate and angry poor person, who actually knew her rights. She was the object that talked back. Without making any apologies for her behavior, her case raised important questions and issues: would she, indeed, have been labeled as a "bad" patient if she had been an educated, affluent white man or woman? If she did not have eight children, all being cared for by others? If she did not have a history of drug abuse and a demonstrable degree of "attitude"? Most important of all, would her account of her self-treatment been believed if her demographics had been different?

Though stigmatized in many ways by mainstream culture, black women are also expected to be the backbones of their communities. Historically, this is the role that they have often played (Richie 289, 295). Thus, when they fail to bear this burden, they may be doubly condemned: not only by the standards of white, middle class society, but by their own communities as well. At the same time, many women living in poor environments face the prospect of sexual exploitation. Daily survival may require the adoption of aggressive, manipulative behaviors in order to guard against this or to use it for their own advantage. Certainly this seemed to be the case, to a greater or lesser degree, with Linda and Claudia. Ms. May, on the other hand, was a woman who maintained individual integrity without being dependent on men and in spite of crippling health conditions. Nevertheless, her behavior, like theirs, was interpreted as by the institution as irrational. I would argue that this also had something to do with the fact that she was a black woman, living alone, with no one to back her up or support her claims. In other words, it was her very independence, her lack of a stereotypical "kin system" that cast her in doubt.

It may be argued that much of the success of DOT in dealing with TB is due to the fact that poor individuals, in general, have fewer resources for contesting the decisions of medical institutions and public health agencies. At County General, most of our patients were poor and uneducated. Many of them had been on public welfare programs at some point in their lives. They were used to having "helping professionals" intruding in their business. Therefore, when the doctor told them that someone would be coming to their house to watch them take their medicine, they often obeyed with little resistance. From the perspective of the middle class, where personal autonomy and privacy are held as sacred virtues, the wonder of DOT is that so many people agreed to it at all. Certainly the power of a ten dollar weekly cash incentive would not have been sufficient to keep a suburban lawyer or real estate agent home, waiting for the health worker to arrive.

But even though DOT relationships were lopsided, they were not one-sided. Patients sometimes used their own illnesses as a lever against the weight of the institution, seeking to "work the system" to their own advantage. This is a tricky business, and can have negative consequences, as Claudia's case demonstrates. Because she had been judged as unreliable, she faced distrust and threats of involuntary confinement every time she returned to the hospital. Ms. May and Linda also faced varying degrees of discrimination, though their eventual participation in DOT was able to mediate antagonistic relationships with the institution. It could also have done so for Claudia, if she had allowed it. One way we "sold" ourselves and our program was by telling patients that we would keep the wolves of the state from their doors, and ease the stress of the system. In most cases, we did just that. By putting on sheep's clothing, we accomplished what the wolf alone could not. In each of these cases, the establishment of an individualized reciprocal relationship with a tuberculosis patient was a means to an end: treatment of illness and the limitation of contagion. At the same time, other important services and resources were provided, though these were often objects of negotiation, conditional benefits bestowed in exchange for desired behavior.

These three cases were some of the toughest I encountered. However, I could have chosen any number of other examples which would have demonstrated the same basic lessons. The narratives contained here show that "noncompliance" is not merely irrational, malicious or self-destructive behavior. Its motivations are often rooted in factors that lie outside the scope of the medical institution or public health agency. These examinations of "delinquent careers" raise serious questions concerning the loaded concept of "compliance" when pursued in contexts of poverty. Looking at the larger picture of these women's lives, we can see more clearly the impact of race, gender, neighborhood poverty and the growth of the drug economy, and witness how their effects were translated into personal characteristics as individuals interacted with medical institutions and public health agencies. Deviant identities were socially constructed around these ascribed characteristics. These identities, and the disciplinary behavior that followed, made the achievement of mutually satisfying social relations even less likely. We can also see how social factors complicate simplistic notions about achieving health through the successful administration of medications. Though TB was treated in each case, and the cycle of infection was eventually broken, each patient was caught in a web of factors that made the achievement of long-term health and well-being unlikely. The harsh and stressful environment of the inner city enveloped all of them, and placed distinct parameters on what they could reasonably expect to achieve.

8 Sheep's Clothing

Lessons Learned from TB in the Field

In October 2002, I visited New York City. Exactly one decade had passed since my TB training first began. Clearly, much had changed since then. But the autumn sky was blue and clear, and the city felt the same as I remembered it from ten years before, in spite of the gaping hole in the downtown skyline. The streets were full of life, and people of every possible derivation and affiliation mingled there, en route to offices, restaurants, hotels, boutiques, factory floors, flower shops, sweatshops, liquor stores, hospitals, and prisons. On the corners across from where the World Trade Center once stood, vendors hawked memorabilia of a national tragedy. Like a seasoned fighter, New York kept on punching even with two big teeth knocked out.

The September 11 morgue was directly adjacent to the city shelter where Carmela's office was now located. She was my field supervisor at the city TB clinic in 1993 and she looked much the same as she did then, a large, commanding woman with a loud, easy laugh, dreadlocks extending halfway to her shoulders. She said when the planes hit the towers, the whole city went quiet; out on the street, you could hear the whispers: "Oh my God, Holy Shit." Through her office window, she says, she watched the bodies and body parts carried in from Ground Zero.

We sat by that window and talked about the old days and what had changed. I said, "I still feel totally at home walking the streets of the city," and she responded "That's because you are." She introduced me to a couple of the "fellas" at the shelter. One had been exposed to TB in prison. One had been homeless, living in a squat in Harlem for about ten years. One had gotten kicked out of an old folks' project in the Bronx because of drinking and carrying on, and ended up in the shelter system. All of them were black men, all over forty. All had familiar stories of downward mobility, intersecting the vector of infectious disease, usually with the added help of an addiction.

Gus, another of my former supervisors who still worked for the health department, walked in the room while I was talking to Carmela. He didn't recognize me at first, but then his eyes lit up. "Paul! How are you doing, man? What are you doing here?" He looked thin and healthy, sporting a neat goatee but with the same intelligent glint and raised eyebrow that I remembered. His voice, with its musical Greek inflection, sounded familiar, as though I had just heard it yesterday. He told me to come over to his office for some strong coffee, and asked what the theoretical argument of my dissertation was. It was strange to have to defend my dissertation again on the 4th fourth of the shelter, but I did my best, talking about the social determinants of health, trying to sum up my argument without descending into academic babble.

After I finished visiting with Carmela, Gus and I walked over to a noodle joint a couple blocks away. He was impressed by the things that I remembered, like the contact investigations we conducted at a Caribbean bar on the Lower East Side and a weird little gift boutique run by a Japanese couple. "Were you taking notes, man?" he asked, laughing. "Actually, I was," I said. Over lunch we talked a lot about the social factors underlying TB and the social construction of medical facts, and the way the homeless are viewed as flawed individuals in need of correction rather than human beings living within difficult circumstances. He said they have meetings at the shelter where homeless people are gathered into groups and taught how to be "functional." Gus said, "They *are* functional, they are just regular people."

After lunch with Gus I headed downtown to see Arturo, at the Department of Regulatory Affairs, where I had worked during the last few months of my tenure with the New York City Health Department. I rode the elevator to the 22nd floor of the Broadway offices, and waited for Arturo to come out, wondering what he would look like nearly ten years later. As it turned out, he looked almost exactly the same, and as he walked up he said to me, "You haven't changed one bit."

My conversation with Arturo was more low-key than the one with Carmela. He is a soft-spoken guy, who laughed when we talked about the old days, and reminded me of things I had forgotten, such as the long hours we put in, waiting until 5:30 on Friday nights for last-minute detention requests to come in over the phone. "It's not like that anymore," he said. "We still detain people, but not nearly as many as back then." There were currently fewer than ten people involuntarily detained in New York City, and they were located on a secure wing of a city hospital, not in a separate facility as they had been in the 1990s. He believed that detention was a necessary component of disease control: that some people would not comply otherwise, and would continue to infect others. This was one of the factors behind the resurgence of the 1990s, he said, and one of the keys to fighting the epidemic was the control of the chronically delinquent.

Arturo began working with TB in the 1980s. Like Carmela, he did DOT when there were only a few people covering the entire city. He spent a lot of time in the Bowery, going to see patients in the flop houses. Like Carmela, he remembered the early nineties as an exciting and turbulent time, when the Bureau more than doubled in size and was at the center of the media spotlight. Now things seemed calm and comfortable. TB control was now an ongoing and invisible task, like maintaining sewers or graffiti removal, or HIV and homeless services, for that matter.

I had traveled to New York specifically to visit these old colleagues, to pick their brains about the lessons of the past decade. Effective fieldwork was a key component of tuberculosis control efforts in the United States in the 1990s. I have described the structural conditions and local environments that surrounded TB from the perspective of a field-worker trained in sociology. I have also related the complicated negotiation process that takes place on a daily basis between individual field workers and their assigned patients. This chapter discusses the perspectives of field-workers themselves.

But first, it is necessary to define what constitutes fieldwork and what sets it apart from other types of health care practice. This is not as simple as it sounds. After all, what is "the field"? Most people think of working "in the field" as working outside of an office, classroom, or laboratory. But many of these sites are themselves considered to be "in the field." For example, if the urban community is considered "the field," then is the nurse in the community clinic considered a field-worker? And what hospital is not, after all, located in some community or another? It is probably fair to say that anyone who is working with people in a hands-on manner is in some sense doing fieldwork. Regardless of the amount of time that they actually spend in the field, most "street-level bureaucrats" (Lipsky 1980), including social workers, health care workers, parole officers, and so on, engage in fieldwork. Within the term is captured a wide variety of roles and experiences.

In social science research the definition of fieldwork is perhaps even looser. It can be used to describe any instance where a social scientist is entering any setting at all for the purposes of studying people directly. For academics, any trip beyond the office or library can be a trip to "the field," and in this era of "virtual communities" some researchers consider themselves to be doing "fieldwork" even while seated comfortably in front of their laptops. But for the purposes of this discussion, I would like to constrict the definition of fieldwork a bit. The field-worker, I propose, is someone who spends a large percentage of their work time in an uncontrolled environment, outside of the protective boundaries of his or her employing institution, within a social terrain that is fluid and often contested. To go back to the underlying metaphor, the field is the world outside of the cabin walls, one that is open to the elements and variously occupied by plants, animals, and other people. The field-worker is out there in the rain, sleet and snow, like the mail carrier or the cop on the beat—not parked behind a desk all day. Though desk and phone duty is a big part of fieldwork in public health (as it is in police work), so are door-knocking, hob-knobbing, and sidewalk-walking.

Much of fieldwork in the social services consists of home visits; that is, going to designated addresses for the purposes of contacting clients, providing direct services, or evaluating a home or work environment. TB fieldwork often goes beyond this. We were actually tracking people down in a manner akin to that of police or parole officers. In New York, we had access to confidential data, such as addresses where welfare checks were delivered, so we were sometimes able to stake these out and nab people that way. In Chicago, we did not have the same resources, but we did whatever we could to find people and achieve compliance. We went to street corners, alleyways, local watering holes, and workplaces, as well as private homes. In practical terms, this meant that our cars were our offices, with regular visits made from the field to the institutional settings of hospital or clinic, rather than the other way around.

One of my supervisors in New York once said to me, "You love to run in the street, don't you?" I did. I was drawn back to it every day like an addict, and in this sense I sympathized with those patients who couldn't resist its pull. Perhaps, like a lot of eventual professionals from middle class backgrounds, I was trying to overcome the insulating effects of having been raised in a relatively secure environment. The street was a daily dose of reality, and it made me very aware of the invisible barriers that divided the city. It was a living sociology lesson written in flesh, asphalt, and broken glass. After almost a decade, though, I didn't feel I had anything else to prove by merely being out there. I felt little power to change the underlying factors of poverty and segregation that seemed to imprison people in the neighborhoods, and kept them running like rats on a wheel. As one of my associates on the West Side was fond of saying, "We are living in a hell of a cycle." Of course, my experience of this was primarily vicarious, and I could exit each day when I chose to do so, unlike most of the patients that I saw. In time, I left the street behind.

Chicago rents were climbing throughout the 1990s, and though mine was stable, my salary also stayed pretty much the same. I loved my job, or I would not have been there that long. But it was also getting to be a bit of a grind. I would be sitting on a patient's couch, watching him swallow pills and making small talk while taking in reruns of *Hunter,* or *The Andy Griffith Show,* and I would ask myself: What am I doing with my life? I had developed a fairly consistent pattern: I would work from 7 A.M. to 3 P.M., go home, take a nap, then get up and write field notes or dissertation chapters until midnight or so. Then I would go to sleep, get up and do it again.

I also took out time to play soccer, go to movies and clubs, and just hang out. Day by day, the writing accumulated, and I was able to finish my Ph.D. within six years of beginning. When an opening came along that happened to fit my credentials, I decided to try the professor thing for a minute or two. By the summer of 2000 I had accepted a two-year teaching position at a small liberal arts college in the middle of Iowa, and in mid-July I finally left my post at County General Hospital, after nearly seven years.

But I never stopped thinking of myself as a field-worker. When I returned to the city, which I did about once a month, I made a point of catching up with some of my "fellas" on the West Side, checking if they were still alive. Each year there were fewer of them to see. In the fall of 2001, about a month after the September 11 attacks, I gave a presentation to the Chicago Metropolitan Tuberculosis Coalition. For me this was a chance to speak directly to TB field staff from across the city, and also to do some justice to their work in front of the doctors and administrators who supervised them. I wanted to articulate an ethic, a method and a rationale for the role of the field-worker in the health care system, even beyond the field-worker's obvious importance as an agent of medical supervision in TB control. Ethnography provided a means of doing so.

In traditional ethnography, the ultimate (and somewhat illusory) goal is to capture and transmit the "insider's perspective," usually through the mechanism of written description. While actually interacting with people, participating in their lives as well as observing them, the ethnographer must exercise keen discretion and refrain from making judgments based on external criteria. Some interpretation of social phenomena is both desirable and inevitable, but it must be carried out with utmost regard for the beliefs that people themselves hold. According to Van Maanen, "the trick of ethnography is to adequately display the culture (or, more commonly, part of the culture) in a way that is meaningful to readers without great distortion" (Van Maanen 13). In other words, one's interpretation of another's situation should not violate the perspectives of the subjects themselves. I would argue that intervention in social reality is another inevitable result of inserting oneself into a cultural milieu, whether you want it or not. From an ethnographic standpoint, this intervention should be cooperative, not coercive. As my discussion of DOT has shown, cooperation and coercion are not necessarily mutually exclusive. Nonetheless, the researcher must be extremely cautious about manipulating observations to fit desired conclusions and blatantly interfering with the lives of others. In ethnography, this amounts to colonial domination, and is not consonant with the fundamental ethic of respect that allows one to enter the field.

There are many parallels to be drawn between the ethnographer and the TB field-worker. Like the ethnographer in the field, the field-worker may seek to present him or herself as a sort of "marginal native"—hence the logic of employing the "indigenous" field-worker (Van Maanen 2). Also like ethnographers, however, field-workers may be perceived as "Meddlesome busybodies, Hopeless dummies, Management spies," or "Government dupes" (Van Maanen 2). This is because patients, like research subjects, very accurately detect that those who seek to walk among them often serve other agendas. Effective field-workers are those who successfully balance their institutional agenda with a genuine concern for, and commitment to, the patient, which is something that people can also detect. As I have already shown, this is a task which is superficially simple but complex in practice. Even "indigenous" workers have to manage their image in the field, because now they are working for an institution that some may perceive as unresponsive or even oppressive. This often means obscuring one's connection to authority. Unlike the uniforms of police, which are designed to impress and even to intimidate, the "uniforms" adopted by field-workers allow them to "blend." Most field-workers dress in a manner that is both acceptable in the street and in the more professional environment of the clinic or hospital, trying to stand out somewhat, but not too much. They need to convey their special status as institutional emissaries and representatives of the state, while at the same time appearing to feel at home in the communities where they carry out their work.

These are some of my own observations and assertions, based on years of experience going into the field and working with other field-workers. Again, fieldwork was like a drug for me, not just because it was a habit, but because I found it to be a mind-altering experience. It took me outside myself and made me look at the world in a new way. In talking to some of my colleagues from tuberculosis control, among whom the amount and intensity of fieldwork experience varied greatly, I sought to understand what the experience of fieldwork meant to others, besides myself, who had engaged in it. For this purpose I conducted tape-recorded interviews with six people: four of them were present or former tuberculosis field-workers, and two of them were supervisors responsible for hiring and managing field staff, who had also done extensive fieldwork themselves. Three of these individuals were in Chicago, and the other three were in New York.

Martha, a black woman in her late thirties or early forties, was my field supervisor for six years in Chicago. She described how she first came to do fieldwork in public health:

> Prior to coming to Chicago I basically worked in a clinic, and that setting
> was very comfortable for me in the beginning, because you just, you weren't
> out there, I felt very secure and we always had a security guard there in case

there were any problems, but in the field you clearly realized very early that you were on someone else's turf, so I had to eventually take a job working in the field and so that prepared me for my role here.

Stated very clearly here is the central difference between the institutional and the field environment: between the "comfortable," "secure" clinic and the uncertainty of being on "someone else's turf." Awareness of that turf was a major theme in the discussions of fieldwork. Carmela is also a black woman in her forties, and she was one of my field supervisors in New York City. She oversaw the Return to Supervision unit, the "SWAT" team that I worked for in the early 1990s. I asked her what her advice would be for someone going into the field. Her answer reflects the safety concerns that permeate this type of work:

> Well, a good field-worker definitely has to be organized, plan her day correctly, and try to cluster your field stops, don't spread yourself out too much, be street smart, read sign language and body language, know your surroundings, go to your area before you go to work so you get a sense of where you're at and the population that you're dealing with, if it's drug infested, and you see a lot of drug activity, you know that's dangerous, and maybe you need to go with another worker. Don't wear anything you can't defend, if you're a jewelry-wearing person and you can't defend yourself, don't wear it (laughs). Keep a lot of quarters on you, if you have cell phone make sure your battery is charged. Know who you're going after, don't go there guessing and babbling and reaching and pulling for stuff, have everything in your hand, travel light. Get in and get out quickly. I remember one time I got caught up in a drug sweep.

In the 2002 film *Training Day*, Denzel Washington plays a veteran narcotics detective who takes a young cop into the field to show him the ropes on his first day. While cruising around in the car, pointing out the vicious characters that prowl the urban jungle, he tells the rookie to roll down the window, saying, "You got to hear the street, you got to smell it, you know, taste that shit, feel that." Later he imparts this wisdom: "To protect the sheep you got to catch the wolf, and it takes a wolf to catch a wolf, you understand?" Though Washington's character turns out to be quite violent and corrupt, he expresses a commonly voiced sentiment: if you are entering a dangerous environment, you need to be dangerous yourself. This might work in some professions, but it is exactly the wrong approach to field work in public health. Rather than being a wolf, the field-worker who wants to survive and succeed needs to don garb that conveys neither threat nor fear. At the same time, as Carmela explains, she has to know how to "read" the signs that are available in the field; this necessitates some understanding of the local cultures that one enters. "Street smarts" may be seen as roughly equivalent to ethnographic awareness—not knowing it all, but knowing enough to pass muster, get by, survive.

Randall is an African American man in his late thirties; he is a native of Chicago's South Side and would probably be considered "indigenous" in that sense. Most of his clients were located in South Side neighborhoods that he knew. But he also had to regulate his own conduct and demeanor in the field:

> *Paul:* People might say to you "Aren't you afraid to go into these neighborhoods, these different communities and stuff?" What kind of advice would you give to somebody, what kind of response would you give?
>
> *Randall:* You live in those same communities all your life, or you know, these are people just like you and maybe have not had the opportunities or maybe have not taken advantage of those opportunities to make things better for themselves. You know, I've found that going to these projects or these places where people are selling drugs most of the time, they normally don't say a word to you. Or do anything to you, because they know that you are not from there. They know that you have to be a police officer or a health care worker or something to be coming through there, so they normally don't even bother you. Because you're not bothering them. I have no fear of going into these places, as long as I'm not being bothered I have no fear of going into these places. I don't think anyone should really have any fear of going anywhere at any time.
>
> *Paul:* So what would you tell people about conducting themselves? Are there any guidelines or anything like that?
>
> *Randall:* Oh, there are, definitely. Mind your business. Go in there for what you're supposed to be going in there for and leave when you're supposed to leave. Make acquaintances or friends (laughing).

Again, the first thing is to show you mean no harm. Beyond that, cultivation of positive relations is the best way to protect your own safety. Rosa, a Latina field-worker in her forties, gave some similar advice about life in the field:

> *Paul:* What kind of advice would you give to other people going out to do fieldwork, even if it's not necessarily TB?
>
> *Rosa:* I think they have to be, how do you say that, humble, they have to understand that there are all kinds of people, and they also have to understand that we're all the same. There's nobody that's more than you or less than you no matter who they or what they are, and once you're there, then you see people the same, everybody, and you will be able to treat them better.

She also had a story that illustrates some of the problems that women may confront in the field. It involved a visit to one of Chicago's many low-income housing projects:

This lady in the projects here on ____ Street, and I've never been into the projects, not those, I mean I've been to Cabrini Green, that was fifteen years ago, twenty years ago, not after that. I said, well I want to try it, I don't mind checking it out, so I went there the first time, and there was no problem, I went looking for this lady, she never opened the door, so I came back empty-handed, so I tried the second time, and the second time that I tried I got on the elevator and this young man got into the elevator with me and we're moving, going up, I was like looking the other way and I'm trying to not look at him just in case, and all of a sudden he goes, "Hey" and when I looked at him he was masturbating himself. And then he looked at me like this, and I kept my eyes straight . . . because I figured if I turn my face he's gonna say she's scared or something, so I just looked at him like, he looked at me, he started smiling, and then the elevator opened he came out and he started cracking up and he said, "Next time, next time." That's all. So I went up there, I came back down and I told her, I'm not going back. (Laughs) But that's the only bad experience I've had, everywhere else has been okay, I've been to the West Side, far north, you know.

This experience, however, didn't change her basic rules of conduct in the field:

The first thing that I do is check the neighborhood, go around once in the area to see, like I had two patients that were in two very big drug places, so when I went there the first time they saw me going by there, and these were black neighborhoods so they see this white woman they think that she wants to buy drugs, when they stop by there they came down so I grabbed my notebook and I said "County General Hospital," and they said "Okay," and then I say hello to them, always, good morning, good afternoon, and it turns out that eventually they, they don't bother you if you don't bother them, and so far nothing has happened. As a matter of fact, they come and they treat me with utmost respect, hello ma'am, how are you? But mainly, see the neighborhood beforehand, go around once or twice and make sure that you feel comfortable.

Here we see the balancing act again. The paradoxical position of the ethnographer is that of being both inside and outside. "Learning the ropes" means not only finding one's way around, but becoming comfortable on someone else's turf. This requires more than adherence to rules or method; it also requires a certain state of mind. In Rosa's words:

Yeah, you have to be patient, and you have understand them, and maybe I think the most important thing is you have to like people, love people, because if you don't, then you're not going to make it. Because you're gonna always find something wrong with somebody.

Refraining from judgment and exercising empathy were hallmarks of the fieldwork experience, but these do not necessarily come naturally. The environments encountered by field-workers often challenged them at a basic human level, and they had to find a way to respond. Spanner, a black man now in his mid-thirties, worked with me in NYC when we were both in our mid-twenties. I asked him what he knew about tuberculosis before he became a Public Health Advisor (PHA), and what he learned from working in the field:

> Well, I'll be honest with you; when I first started I had no clue, really. I mean, you knew it was the coughing disease. I was really ignorant about it, you know, I was fresh out of college . . . I remember I went there with a shirt and a tie my first day, and . . . they teamed me up with some guy, and we went around, and we went up to Harlem, and this is when it first struck me. I went up to Harlem and he was this nice guy, but he was, you could tell he was slow, he had mental problems and stuff, and he was a really nice guy, and I was really struck by this, and this guy had, he was HIV positive, and the reason he was HIV positive is because he was abused, sexually abused as a child, but now he was a father, he was a father himself, now, he had a kid himself, and he was such a nice guy, and the fact that—again, I was really ignorant about HIV also, at that time, too—but he was HIV positive, and I remember when I came home that day, I just came home and I cried. . . . I grew up in a basically a near-suburban environment in Queens, it was in New York City, but it was in Queens. And I had never seen anything like that, I didn't even know anybody who was HIV positive, and I meet this guy and I came home . . . I was crying because I thought, this guy is gonna die. And that was like my first introduction to TB, like, I'm dealing with life and death matters here. And I kind of like, I think after seeing that I kind of decided, you know what, this is something I'm going to take serious. Also I was still very idealistic too, and I think that's what also helped too, that, that, why I went into that job with the passion that I did, and I still have a lot of love for that job, because of what we did.

Isabel, who also worked with me as PHA in New York in the early 1990s, reflected on her fieldwork experiences and how they informed her views of people with TB:

> Well, one, I have to say I really miss the autonomy of it, you know, just like, going out on your own, and being able to, you know, if you have a caseload, you get to choose where you are on a particular day, which I really miss. But um, you know, going into peoples' homes and finding them where they are is, I think, essential, especially in that kind of work, because if somebody should happen to show up at a doctor's office, you don't know how that per-

son lives, you don't know what their daily trials are and getting to know a person in their own environment gives you a different perspective, and a different appreciation for what somebody has to go through, to get what needs to be done done, you know, as far as medication, even filling a prescription. You know, most people who needed DOT or who needed to be returned to supervision were not, you know, didn't have a lifestyle where they have their prescriptions filled . . . that wasn't the first thing on their mind, you know, taking their medication is secondary to the business of survival, and not having seen that first hand it's easy to say, "oh, why don't these people take their meds," and you know, "it's being provided for them so why don't they do A, B, and C?" Whereas, you get a different appreciation for it if you actually see how people live and learn what's important to them.

Here we see clearly the empathetic response, a recognition of the necessity for seeing the world as another sees it. Beyond that, though, there is a learning process taking place which is implicitly sociological, because of the recognition of material forces that shape peoples' cultures and their actions. Both Spanner and Isabel were life-long New Yorkers, but each of them came to see their city, and American society, in a different way as a result of their TB fieldwork:

Well, when you're working in the field, it's, you see different parts of the city that you normally would never see before. Like I told you, I basically lived, I grew up in Queens, with mom and dad, so I, they did a good job of keeping me from shit. But the very first time I ever walked into a crack house was when I was a field-based PHA. And that was a harrowing experience, in that, you just don't see that. But that was my job, and I went into crack houses, I went into projects, you know, places that I never went to, never would want to go but that was my job and I went there, and you saw different parts of—you saw New York City, warts and all. You know, I remember going into a real upper-crust neighborhood once because somebody came up positive, and I remember going into some of the skeezy [areas]—so you saw the spectrum New York, man . . . I'd go to clinic, which is what I remember the most. In clinic you kind of saw those same people, but you saw them coming to you, you kind of saw the dregs of society coming into the clinics and stuff like that, you know, you saw people coming in really sleazy looking, and part of you wondered if they were coming in there for medical treatment, if this was their free medical clinic facility and stuff like that. But what you saw there was basically what you saw in the field; you saw a lot of poor coming in.

Isabel's response was very similar. She also felt that fieldwork was an education in social reality:

Isabel: I probably learned a whole lot more about this city being a field-worker than I think I ever would have had I just taken like a corporate job or an administrative job.

Paul: Even in public health?

Isabel: Even in public health, yeah sure, because you don't get to see how people live. Do you remember K____? He was an Asian guy [a fellow fieldworker] . . . we went to the projects, and we were going to test this family that had like fourteen people living in an apartment and we woke them up at about 11 o'clock in the afternoon, well, the midmorning. It's like 11 o'clock, we go and knock on the door and wake them up, and he was entirely flabbergasted that people could live this way, and he's like, "I can't believe people live this way, this is like a television show." Or something like that, and I just remember thinking, wow, that's pretty, I don't know if it's ethnocentric, but you know, he was just . . . he kind of thought, you know, people don't live like this, this is not part of his existence.

Paul: Not in America . . .

Isabel: Yeah, not in America, not in New York City, not, you know, it just didn't seem feasible to him, and I mean, that's what struck me, is that, he was completely incredulous that people could live like that . . . So I think it opens your eyes to a lot of things, and those are one of them. I mean, shooting galleries, I remember going into a, going to find a delinquent patient that lived in D____, or K____ Street . . . and I happened to know people that lived right [there] so I was like in an area where I knew people but I was kind of afraid to go upstairs, and when I went upstairs the door was wide open, and there was a woman, very nearly completely naked, with a needle sticking out of her arm, and she was like, she had just shot up, and was laying, you know, completely out of it, and she was my patient. And I had to get a sheet, cover her up, say, "I need to talk to you, I need to talk to you right now," and that's like a situation that you don't find yourself in, like in normal circumstances. So yeah, I mean, it kind of like opened my eyes to the realities of society.

Like many of the other examples already given, this anecdote provides an illustration of the interlocking factors that often surround tuberculosis, most notably poverty and drug addiction, but also race and gender. The experience of going into the field, by enhancing understanding of such underlying social conditions, also improved relations with patients who came into the institution. Martha, who went into the field occasionally, worked most intensively with patients when they came into the pulmonary clinic for monthly examinations. She emphasized the impact that her fieldwork had on her clinical role:

Paul: What do you enjoy about your job?

Martha: I enjoy meeting the patients in clinic; I get to talk to them about their conditions, and also when I go out into the field I have an appreciation of their environment and when I meet a patient in clinic I feel like I have a real good understanding of their environment, and I feel that I have a good rapport with the patients, I communicate with them, and they seem to be appreciative of anything I can do for them.

Paul: So you find that going into the field yourself helps in terms of relating to the patients?

Martha: Absolutely, that's very important. I mean, even, you know, just if you have a patient that's chronically late, and you happen to make the home visit and you realize that this patient lives a distance from the bus line, or there are so many obstacles that they have to endure in just trying to make it to the clinic, you really have an appreciation of what's going on in their lives, and being in their home environment oftentimes you really get to see that our patients really don't have a whole lot, I mean that any little thing we can do for them they really appreciate it, because, I mean a lot of them are making it on social security or welfare and you clearly see that that's not enough.

Beyond the greater understanding of a patient's plight that fieldwork can foster, seeing patients in their social context can engender a greater appreciation of them as individuals as well. I remembered something that Carmela always used to say, that our patients "had PhDs in the university of the streets," and I asked her what she meant by that:

Carmela: They can tell you where to get the best meals, where to get the best clothes, what drug programs you can go to and get your [commercial driver's] license, or get a chef's license. I mean these homeless people that live here have taught me so much. I'm re-educated every day, because some cat up in here has something new to tell me, and it's really profound, but you have to take the time to listen to them. I have medicated a professional photographer, I have medicated a professor, I have medicated a doctor, I have medicated preachers, teachers, carpenters, plumbers. These are people like you and I, who took a nose dive in life because of substance abuse.

Paul: Is that a factor with a lot of them?

Carmela: Yes, most of them. Substance abuse. Which opened my eyes to something else. I was so blinded, I didn't see that. People don't become junkies because they're junkies. People become junkies because they had the money to buy the junk. Now they don't have the money to buy the junk because the junk has taken over them, possessed them. Wherein, right now, we're possessed by our job, by our employment, we know we have a responsibility to get up every day and go to work, pay our bills, in order to keep a house, roof over our head. These people at one time were the same way, and they thought they could handle addiction, and soon addiction took over them, and this is why they lost their jobs, they lost their homes, and they lost their cars, and they lost anything that made them whole at one time, and what I learnt, that because you are who you are is no guarantee if you start dippin' and dabbin' in drugs, and in alcohol, you will take a nose dive, you will spiral, and this is somethin' I learnt working with this homeless population. So now I open up, because when I heard their history and their family, and they talked about their family, and how their family turned their backs on them, because they didn't want to be a part of them, and what they did. You know, it made you rethink, you know, I'm no better than them, it's just, I just don't have that problem, but anybody can be an addict.

Most physicians see patients solely in institutional settings for very limited periods of time, and they may not be aware of what a patient faces at home or in the street. They may not know the "back story" in the sense discussed by Carmela. The patient may tell them about these things, if the physician takes time to ask, but there is no guarantee that the patient will answer honestly or that he or she will be believed. The field-worker, as an intermediary between the institution and the local environment, who spends significant amounts of time with patients, can play an important role here on a several different levels: providing the patient with a voice, providing legitimacy for their claims, and also providing the institution with a face. Randall's comments below express these closely related functions of the field-worker:

Paul: Do you feel like the field-worker had something to contribute to the medical system?

Randall: Indeed. Yes, I do. I feel that we should consider ourselves a branch of County General Hospital. County General Hospital walking around in the street. I know that we're not qualified to be any doctors or nurses or anything like that. But I feel that what we provide, and it's free[for the patient], and what we can give them can actually help them ease the process of the paperwork or the time that you can spend in County Hospital. Some things that we can do can really lessen that amount of time that a person can really spend in County Hospital. Bet you can come in here and spend 4 or 5 hours sometimes, and just being here for a clinic appointment or waiting for prescriptions, for getting a referral to see another doctor, just trying to find out what's going on period. I think we really lessen that blow. The amount of time a person has to spend, they can spend, sitting around in those clinics in County Hospital. Or we can try and find out who their doctor is and what their doctor is trying to do. Or help them out, like I said with referrals to other clinics, or prescriptions. We both know that that's a big thing to people. The amount of time to wait for a prescription is normally two to three hours or something like that. We can pick up their medicine and maybe bring it to them. That's the way we can help. I think the field-worker doing their job, the way they should do it, is really good for the community. It's like an outreach portion of County Hospital.

In addition to "lessening the blow" of the institution upon the individual, reaching out to the patient as an individual and giving the hospital a human face, the field-worker also serves as an advocate for the patient, giving voice to their conditions as well as their complaints. Randall, who had previously worked as a professional radio disc jockey, was very aware of the importance of communication, and so I asked him about this:

We can be their liaison between ourselves, the patients, the doctors, the nurses or whatever the case may be. Since we're out there we see them every-day. We know what they go through. We see how they're living. We know them—I would say 50 percent of the patients that I've worked with they don't have phones. They don't have enough money most of the time for transportation to and from the hospital which you need a car for that. We go back and forth for referrals or to the pharmacy early and then we'll come back later in the day. But most importantly, like you were just asking me about. Talking to doctors. I think when there's a problem or they've lost their medicine, they ran out of medicine, or they need to talk to their doctor about something that they're not sure about their medicine. I think we represent them well, and that we can represent them well. Because we know most of the doctors that are on staff here . . .

When there is a cultural or language barrier, this situation becomes even more complicated, though sometimes it is the physician who helps bridge the gap between patient and institution, as revealed in the following story from Isabel:

Isabel: [I had] a Creole-speaking patient who was very irate, didn't want to be in solitary, you know, didn't want to be in an isolation room, and would not answer my questions, and basically threw me out of his room, and I went to go get a doctor . . . And I went and I told him, you know, I can't even interview this patient, because he basically threw me out of the room, and I said, I don't understand what he was speaking, and he asked me, you know, what language he was speaking and I said he was Haitian. And I walked back into the room with [this doctor] and he started speaking Creole to him, and the patient's face just completely changed, and he was welcoming, and it was like a night-and-day kind of thing just because of the language barrier.

Paul: So [the doctor] spoke Creole?

Isabel: He was actually, he's of Lebanese descent and he was born and raised in Haiti, which was a stroke of luck in that patient's case, but just really kind of blew me away how a language can make that much of a difference. But also other things that have to do with culture and cultural differences, because the third patient I'm thinking about was West African and would not talk to me and not tell me any of his contacts—because at that time that was my primary concern was eliciting contacts—would not tell me any of his contacts until I found him fou fou, so I had to search and find a West African restaurant that would make fou fou and bring it to him. (laughs) And you know, so, one, bribery works, and also people, you know, especially in circumstances where they're stressed or you know, a crisis kind of situation which most people with TB find themselves in, having been diagnosed, they kind of want the comforts of home, and it kind of stressed that point to me by having to go find fou fou.

Here again is the negotiation (or "bribery") process, through which rapport is built (or bought), and in this case the parallels to ethnography are quite apparent. The field-worker must actively learn about the patient's culture in order to accomplish her task. In some cases, it may be that the cultural differences affect medical care in unanticipated ways. For example, Rosa describes how some of her patients have such a degree of deference toward doctors that it sometimes creates problems of its own:

Well, there is somewhat of a culture problem, but that's not the main thing, I think the main thing, the main problem is basically the language, and the only different thing cultural wise that I see is that a lot of the Mexican people, or Latino people that we go see, they're mostly poor-paying people, they work at poor-paying jobs, so they're poor people . . . they're not fighting for their rights or whatever, so when you go and see them, they're very scared of you, and they don't want to contradict you in any way, and I'm sure that's the way they do it with the doctors or anybody else, and then when you come and see them they have a lot of questions for you, some that you cannot answer, so you got to go back to the doctor and ask them, so what I do is tell them, look, the doctor is there to see you, to understand you, to know what your questions are, you got to tell them. But they don't understand you, they say, well ask for a translator and they'll give it to you. That's the only thing that I've seen aside from language, the fact that they don't try to come to the doctor because in the Latino culture it's like the doctor is the boss, you know. You go see the doctor, he knows what he's doing; you don't question the doctor, you know.

In this case, the problem is not necessarily one that leads to noncompliance, but it can lead to inadequate treatment if the patient does not raise important issues with the doctor. The field-worker here acts again as an intermediary, someone who the patient is not afraid to ask questions of. The field-worker, in turn, can articulate those questions to the doctor or encourage the patient to raise them in the clinical setting. What the field-worker provides is not only a person who speaks the language and understands the culture, but someone who stands at a social level closer to that of the patient. The distinction is important because a field-worker can fill the latter role, even if she does not fully understand the language and culture. By being in the house every day, becoming a part of the patient's routine, the field-worker can become a sort of confidante. This is one of the beneficial side effects of rapport-building. The relationship may begin as a means to an end, but once established, it may influence other aspects of the patient's life—and that of the field-worker as well. Carmela hit on this when she explained how the City of New York, with CDC guidance, altered its practices in the 1990s and achieved both better patient relations and better results:

> So bringing in the federal staff really enhanced the City of New York at that time, because we were re-trained; we learned about the new medication, we learned about the side effects, we learned new techniques on interviewing skills and how to ask open-ended questions and really sharpen the worker to really deliver the goods we had to deliver, but I believe the reason why—you were asking me earlier about the population—the population changed because of the information we were giving them, to wake them up. They never had anyone speak to them in that manner, and giving them that much information, you can get a better response . . . Prior to that we weren't getting the right response from the patient—this is my opinion—because we weren't really giving them enough to respond, and it wasn't being delivered in their language, so they really didn't understand, and that's when the language banks came out, and a lot of other educational tools came out, which were enablers for the worker as well as the patient. We were able to retrieve more from them, because we were asking them the right questions, and asking the questions in their language where they can understand really helped to get the right exchange, so that piece was very good.
>
> And I believe in any field you have to educate the population that you're working with in order to get the best response from them . . . Why I say that, because, it's interesting, when they told us we had to speak to homeless people or people who lived up under the highways and byways, I just didn't get it, I couldn't see where that would help someone that's so wasted, that's out there, but (pause) a lot of times people just didn't take time with this population because they felt they were just goners, and when I started working with the homeless population, I saw where these people were highly educated people, but because substance abuse had brought them to their knees, and the families turned on them, because at one time they were important individuals, and they took a hard fall in life, and people just turned their back on them. So it made me very sensitive; I became sensitive. I wasn't so sensitive when I first started.

These statements are useful because they place the changes within a system and the changes within an individual side by side, so that we may see the connections between them. Carmela, as a worker, was directly affected by policy changes that were implemented in order to make the public health system more responsive to the needs of patients. These changes were not mere rhetoric; they were backed up with substantial training and material support. For those who disparage the public sector, declaring that bureaucracies cannot change, and that "throwing more money at a problem" does nothing about the problem itself, the example of tuberculosis control in the 1990s can be held up as one response. More money was put into TB, but it was not just "thrown" there. Strong leadership, practical training informed by solid research, and perhaps most importantly, more people engaged in the problem on the front lines, in the hospitals, clinics, homes, and streets helped bring the much-hyped TB resurgence to a standstill in less than a decade. I asked Carmela to talk about the TB of the 1990s and how the city had responded. Her account is a useful summary of those events as seen from a field-worker's perspective:

> *Carmela:*   When the epidemic hit New York City, most of the spreads were in the hospital, and a lot of physicians and public care workers were being exposed to this at a very rapid pace, and the bureau had to be revamped, and they sent in big guns from the CDC, to target this epidemic, and I remember vividly that they wanted all senior public health advisors to work at these facilities, these hospitals, that had the nosocomial spread, and I was one of them, that was placed at _____ Hospital, which was really a HIV hospital, but a lot of the patients there were sick . . .
>
> Anyway, that kind of frightened me when I actually went into the facility and saw a real live TB patient; I mean, they were thin, they were *very* sick. You know, I never was exposed to that, individuals that looked like that, because most of the people I worked with were people who were either just PPD infected, they were in treatment preventively, or if they had TB disease, they still wasn't that sick; you know, they had abnormal cavities in the lung tissues, but they weren't really broken down to that degree, as when I went into the hospital facility and saw real live TB patients, which was frightening, and you could see how death was just . . . you know, the eyes were sunken, their body weight was very low, and they couldn't eat, and I just saw them laying there, just dying . . . . and that was very frightening.
>
> That was in the nineties. '92, '93, '94. And that was scary. However, you know, some of them pulled through, some didn't. After that episode, TB kind of leveled off, I think its maybe 1,200 cases a year now, where at that time it was anywhere from 6,000, 10,000 cases a year, and with the new administration and these experts that

CDC sent into New York to combat this infection, we were able to get it back under control, and it was a lot of money involved, but it was worth it, because we didn't totally eradicate it, but we did slow down the process.

Paul: Tell me a little bit about what was done, and how it affected you, and your role.

Carmela: I noticed they hired numerous people, to do fieldwork, to do hospital work, people were placed in the shelter system. I don't know how much it cost to put a sputum induction machine in the shelter, but they did, just to deal with the homeless men here. The SROs, started to come about, around that time, and they put public health advisors in the SROs and that time there were no public workers working in these areas, you know, most of the people would come into the clinic to be screened, and treated, but with the epidemic, they had to put people directly into these facilities to control the population and the spread of tuberculosis. Also, they never had units in the field, maybe one or two people would cover a borough, but at that time they had anywhere from ten to twenty field-workers going out doing DOT, so it was a lot of money dumped into the city at that time to combat this infection, and there were more educational pieces being done to educate people on TB because they thought TB wasn't that serious, and the educational pieces were done in different languages, because we had a lot of immigrant population coming in; we also had public health advisors at the airports now, so once they come into the city, they're now being screened and being followed by the Department of Health, and before then, they didn't have these things in place, and so this contributed to controlling the TB epidemic in New York at that time.

By 1995, Frieden, Fujiwara, and Hamburg were able to write about turning the tide of tuberculosis in New York City (Frieden et al. 1995). Workers at all levels contributed to this effort, and many of them felt that they were a part of something important, as these comments by Spanner and Isabel show:

Spanner: Like I told you before, that's like, that is still the best job I had ever had; it's the one job that I felt that I actually did, I did something positive, I did something good. Well, actually we, I don't want to say I— when I say "I" I mean "we"—us, who worked in TB during that time, because it's the only job I ever felt, that I actually felt I was saving lives, that I was making a difference, and like, every once in a while I'll hear a report on the news or something like that, they talk about TB's going down in New York City, and you know, I take pride in that, that I know that us, that group of us in the nineties, we kind of started that, you know, we worked really hard, and I take a lot pride in that, what I did during that period of time. It's still the best job I ever had.

Isabel: Well, that was real disease intervention. You know, you were stopping the spread of a disease, whatever intervention you did, whether it was testing people and letting them know they had, were infected with tuberculosis, or getting people back under treatment, or uh, you know, helping to actually diagnose somebody or get them on the right meds or whatever it was, it was actual disease intervention, which I haven't really done since then. I've done more education, or counseling or testing around HIV, which really isn't disease intervention the way it's practiced here. So, it was the one job that I had that actually tried to stop a disease in its tracks.

This accomplishment, significant as it is, must be qualified on at least two counts. Concerted TB control efforts, based on aggressive fieldwork, did indeed stop TB "in its tracks." TB rates were rapidly arrested in the early 1990s and then decreased for several years running, bottoming out at record-low levels in Chicago and New York by the late 1990s. As cases declined, more resources were devoted to providing DOT for preventive therapy (called DOPT) to keep newly infected individuals from progressing to active disease. This is a highly labor-intensive means of smothering the disease *before* it can flare up in new bodies. But the underlying factors of poverty, drug and alcohol addiction, substandard housing, and residential segregation are left largely untouched by these approaches. As one of my former supervisors in New York told me, TB rates were down to about 1,000 new cases per year by the end of the 1990s, and the city didn't expect them to go much lower, because of "existing reservoirs" of disease. In other words, aggressive public health efforts had driven TB back into the impoverished cavities of the city—the ghettos, the housing projects, the overcrowded immigrant neighborhoods, the single room hotels, the homeless shelters, the drug dens—and contained it there, assuming all other factors stayed the same. Like old cases of disease, arrested by the immune system, these reservoirs are harmless to the rest of the body until some environmental assault weakens those defenses and allows the germs to spread once again.

The threat that TB posed to the American population as a whole was not great, even at the peak of the resurgence. Because of those very same factors of inequality and segregation, its spread was largely limited to the urban cavities inhabited by the poor. Therefore, the lesson that tuberculosis should have taught—that inequality and poverty have a price—was not learned. Or rather, that price was seen as acceptable, compared to the much larger cost of pursuing equality and social justice, both essential elements of community health. The success of the fight against TB was at best a partial one, because it did not address the roots of tuberculosis and the soil in which they grew.

The second qualification is closely related to the first: the TB control efforts of the 1990s, like most public health achievements, were promptly forgotten. They were not forgotten by those who worked in TB control, many of whom were victims of their own success, finding it harder each year to maintain funding for a problem that was no longer high-profile. But the success of TB control, and the implications of that success, never garnered the attention that the TB crisis had gotten. I was reminded of this every time someone would say to me, after I told them I worked with TB: "Oh, that's on the rise, again, isn't it?" This reaction persisted throughout the 1990s, even though the rates were continually dropping after 1993. The explanation was simple. The TB *scare* had made an impact on peoples' minds. The *control* of TB did not. One merited a five-part front-page series in the New York Times, the other received a paragraph. Like the terrorist attacks that never take place or the fires that never start, cases of disease that are systematically cured or prevented do not receive much airplay in the era of short attention-spans. As a result, the work of Spanner, Isabel, Carmela, Martha, Rosa, Randall, and hundreds of others across the nation went largely unnoticed, except by those who were in the know.

I do not wish to argue that these individuals deserve attention and honor for themselves. Rather, I would like to see their work honored, and their wisdom applied. I have tried to extract some of that wisdom and frame it here. It is the wisdom of sheep, not of wolves. In the movie *Babe,* the talking pig of the title has to earn the trust of a flock of sheep by proving that he is not a predator, and that he is not seeking to control them through fear, as the dogs in the movie do. In order to accomplish this, he learns some of the sheep's language, and their secret phrase: "Bah, ram, ewe, to your flock, your fleece, your breed be true." Even though he is undeniably "other," he achieves a sort of sheep-hood, in the same manner that an ethnographer or a field-worker seeks to become a partial insider. In the end, the sheep identify his interests as their own, and by working together, they achieve goals that are mutually beneficial. He is not sent to the butcher, and they are not terrorized by dogs pretending to be wolves.

I risk trivializing the role of field-workers by comparing them to pigs and sheep, but we are not used to being high on the totem pole anyway. We are the ones who just want to get along with others, not to threaten, control, or conquer them. As Randall said, we seek to "Make acquaintances and friends." In Rosa's words, we try to see "all people the same, everybody." In an era where "personal responsibility" is sometimes used as a justification for withholding basic necessities of life, the idea that people deserve help simply because they are human is not one that is trumpeted loudly. Nonetheless, I believe that this humble doctrine is the one that ties our society together, and prevents it from falling into a tumult of warring tribes. It is the one that allows the firefighter to enter any neighborhood unarmed, with confidence that he will be recognized as someone who seeks to serve, not harm. It is the one that gives the teacher the resolve to return each and every year to face a room of blank and hostile faces, seeking to plant a thought in a resistant mind. It is the very foundation of public health. As expressed in the words of Louis Pasteur, engraved on an old statue, now splattered with pigeon shit and surrounded by benches favored mostly by vagrants, located between County General Hospital and a roaring eight lane highway:

> One doesn't ask of one who suffers, what is your country and what is your religion? One merely says, you suffer, that is enough for me, you belong to me, and I shall help you.

By entering the domain of another, field-workers carry this implicit message. Their very presence says we care, we want to help you. No matter where you live, how much money you have, no matter the color of your skin, or what drugs you take, we are here because your fate matters. The doctor in the clinic may skip you and forget you if you don't show up, but the person who comes to your door and says your name is there *because of you*. The field-worker proves this by learning from you, by respecting your home, your beliefs, and your fears. That very basic fact makes a difference, regardless of all other complications.

Conclusion

Implications of a Marginal Epidemic

Such, and so magnifying, is the virtue of a large and liberal theme! We expand to its bulk. To produce a mighty book, you must choose a mighty theme. No great and enduring volume may be written on the flea, though there be those who have tried it.
—Herman Melville, *Moby Dick*

THOUGH MUCH smaller than a flea, the tuberculosis bacterium has wreaked more havoc on the human race throughout history than any white whale, hurricane, earthquake, flood or war. Tuberculosis has cut down millions of people in the prime of life, and continues to do so. The story of this illness, therefore, encompasses many great themes: suffering, struggle, perseverance against great odds, and also real death, real loss, real tragedy. This tragedy is twofold. On one level, tuberculosis, like all other manners of natural illness and disease, forces us to recognize our mortality and confronts us with existential dilemmas of meaning. When a stray bullet strikes a loved one, a car accident ends a young life, or cancer claims another victim, we must face the void, and somehow endure. The same may be said of the individual stricken with illness, forced to adapt and transcend the limitations of the physical. I have not focused on TB's essential deadliness or the physical misery that it causes, but on the disease's social dimension. This is shaped by the particular structure and orientation of our society. It does not result from any inherent characteristic of the microbe.

I have presented this perspective on "America's first preventable epidemic" in an attempt to provide a glimpse of that part of the American urban experience which tuberculosis helps to illuminate. Tuberculosis does not discriminate—at least not among the poor. Tuberculosis selects a fairly randomized sample of the marginal classes: the addicts, the alcoholics, the homeless, the brutalized, the wounded, the impoverished, the imprisoned, and the underfed. Among them, it carries on a regular trade. When it starts to cross the boundaries, entering the realm of the empowered, only then comes a response. The torches are lit and the troops are

255

sent into the caverns to chase the bugs back. I have been in the caverns, and I have something to report: there are people living with the bugs, every day, and they aren't going away. As a TB field-worker for the better part of the 1990s, I wandered up and down this strange middle terrain, patrolling the border between the social world of modern medicine and that of the poor inner city. Here the two worlds met, and a struggle ensued, however subtle its form. In many cases it was not subtle but straightforward—one will against another, the individual versus the institution, or vice versa.

As I have tried to show, this clash is not necessarily any less severe because one party is trying to "help" another. Doctors and nurses don't often see themselves as playing a role akin to that of police and prison guards, but there are definite parallels in the minds of patients. One hospitalized man stated outright to me: "This is just like being in jail." Another, having escaped the hospital and returned to the street, said: "I'm sorry Paul, but it was so goddamn boring up in there. I just couldn't take it any more." Faced with a choice between "health," as communicated through strictly prescribed rules and boundaries, or the much riskier proposition of life on the street, characterized by violence and betrayal as well as sociability and solidarity, many have chose the latter.

I have tried to make sense of their decisions, and to communicate their perspectives, relying on their words and meanings as well as the behaviors I saw. At the same time, through recounting their stories, I have tried to convey the very real impact of a daily existence within social conditions as dangerous as those of a coal mine or war zone—other places where human beings have persisted, desired, survived, and died for no good natural reason.

I do not mean for these portraits to give the reader an exceptionally pessimistic outlook on this problem, although I recognize that they have this potential. Rather, I would hope that this study would encourage a more holistic and humanistic approach to illness and disease than that which currently prevails in either American medicine or public health. Sociology, as a discipline, encourages us to look at individual struggles within the broader contexts—history, culture, politics, economics—that shape and constrain human lives. Ethnography, as a practice, provides a means of discussing the internal dynamics of everyday life-worlds, the local and specific places where individuals experience those struggles, and find meaning within them. I have examined the disease called tuberculosis as it was manifested in certain cities in the United States of America at the end of the twentieth century, and described how the experience of that disease affected particular individuals who lived in those cities.

Behind these stories of tuberculosis and tuberculosis patients lies the larger untold story, of struggle and survival on the harsh margins of the wealthiest society in human history. If successful, these narratives of experience will draw attention to the persistent connection between poverty and disease. They will also inspire some reflection on the role played by medical and public health practices in negotiating and maintaining the borders between social classes. The particular conflicts that occur between individual medical practitioners and individual patients, imbued as they are with myriad prejudices carried over from the surrounding society, may be less important than the inability of the biomedical model to grasp those dimensions of human experience that fall outside its analytic categories, or that resist detection by its standard tools.

It cannot be left to medicine to correct this institutional myopia on its own. In the same way that economic markets must be constrained and regulated by a conscious and consensual exercise of social control, so too must the institution of medicine be circumscribed by a vision of health and well-being that is articulated at the social level as well as that of the individual. Sociology provides a language capable of connecting "subjective" concerns about things such as "health" and "quality of life" to the larger social context which surrounds and produces the relationships both within and outside the walls of the institution. I recognize that criticizing these relations is one thing and changing them is quite another. Nevertheless, this research does suggest certain general policy goals which stem directly from my observations.

First, the social history, oft-neglected in medical and public health practice, must be regarded as a fundamental aspect of health care, even if it is not always crucial to the process of medical diagnosis. Those who gather social histories should ideally be trained in something akin to an ethnographic method. This entails a good faith effort, on the part of the institution, to understand and articulate the perspectives of patients, not just to itemize their problems. This task need not fall to doctors themselves. Social workers, field-workers, nurses, or medical students could also be empowered to represent the interests of patients, and to balance the need for medicines and tests with the need for food, shelter, adequate drug treatment, employment, or empathy. Whenever possible, continuity of care should be preserved, so that patients may be treated consistently by the same doctors, and hopefully seen as complex individuals rather than "cases." Along these same lines, poor patients should be given the means to challenge and change their doctors as well as their social workers.

The second recommendation is that the environment of the hospital must be transformed. Models of conviviality should be pursued, whether they are drawn from history or from other societies, in either the First or Third Worlds. "Conviviality," as defined by the late social critic Ivan

Illich, is ". . . autonomous and creative intercourse among persons, and the intercourse of persons with their environment; and this in contrast with the conditioned response to the demands made upon them by others, and by a man-made environment" (Illich 1973, 11). Most hospitals are still based on a factory model, with patients grouped and treated according to their primary diagnosis, in the interest of technical efficiency. But hospitals are social places that treat social beings, and the process of healing cannot be separated from the environment that surrounds it. All of us, including those trained in the methods of biomedicine, belong to cultures, and we all experience suffering, though we may do so in subtly different ways. The practice of medicine only complicates its own ends by overlooking this fact. When a patient can see the hospital as a place that only seeks to "suck her blood," the shortcomings of the biomedical model become apparent.

The medicalized model is currently being questioned on many fronts; in hospices, nursing homes, and maternity wards, spaces are being redesigned for people rather than for doctors and technical implements. The emergence of holistic medicine as a valid component of institutional health care offers many possibilities for useful reform, by creating a space where issues of mental, spiritual, and social health may be discussed and taken seriously. This questioning and revision should be pursued in public health institutions with even greater vigor, for their patients need respite and regeneration of a social as well as a physical kind. Qualitative methods such as ethnography could play an important role in this process. As long as poor people are seen as supplicants of medical largesse and objects of medical practice (in the sense that "practice makes perfect"), hostility and suspicion will persist and health outcomes will suffer.

The final recommendation is that the medical community should learn from the work of both ethnographers and public health and social service field-workers who traverse the boundaries between social worlds as a matter of daily course. The rules that guide these occupations are essentially similar. Each demands a degree of patience, empathy, and tolerance for the different ways and beliefs of others. All are also based on a fundamental concern for the welfare and dignity of all human beings, no matter how poor or marginalized they might be. Ethnography, as I see it, is not only a set of methods for doing research. It also constitutes a particular approach to the study of social phenomena, which has a strong ethical component at its core. What distinguishes ethnography from other modes of social research is its fundamental concern for the meanings that people find in their own everyday lives. The ethics of ethnography rest in its obligation to represent people truly, and to take their perspectives on their own lives seriously.

The same dictum might be applied to the work of public health. Its mission is to identify and advocate for the needs of local communities and the people who live in them. Too often, public health is reduced to a one-way process of imposing abstract standards on people, or disseminating medically approved information amongst populations who are presumed to be ignorant.[1] For those trapped in the tightening net of social circumstances that results in incarceration, homelessness, addiction, or terminal disease, we cannot expect that the fatalism which Freire calls "the fruit of an historical and sociological situation" will fall away just because we walk up and shake the tree. We cannot expect that a forty-minute "behavioral intervention" will achieve a revolution of the self, much less society. "Health" may be a meaningless goal to a man or woman caught in a perpetual material and existential crisis, who might simply ask, "Health for what?" This is a sensible response when one seems to have no visions of life beyond tomorrow. Nonetheless, if we are really concerned with transformation, both of individuals and of society, we must approach people with a view toward this end. Even in a situation of captivity, one can feel ownership of one's own body. Health, as a universalizing concept based in bodily experience, can possibly form the foundation for exactly the type of concrete problem-posing that Freire discussed.

This brings us back to the role of the public health worker who is engaged "in the field." In the field, as I have shown, one sees health problems in their proper habitat, influenced on all sides by social factors that will shape outcomes, for better or for worse. The health worker thus sees public health as an embodied, socially embedded practice, and not as an abstract, technical, or intellectual endeavor. In the tuberculosis control program at County General, meetings of field-workers often spun off into extended narratives of our patients' social lives and circumstances. We also communicated information through stories, the details of which were often quite relevant to the health of the patients, even if they didn't directly affect the treatment at hand. If incorporated into practice, such stories can allow us to see the objects of our actions as autonomous beings, as participants in the process of healing, rather than mere recipients of "care" or "education." They also provide insight into the social relations that mediate between institutions and individuals.

Patient-based stories do not have to be seen merely as amusing or confusing by-products of public health practice. They might instead be viewed as valuable resources for identifying both individual and community needs. As much health care shifts away from the centralized, medicalized environments of large hospitals and into the homes of patients or community-based clinics, the role of the field-worker might be incorporated into a more sociologically informed model of what health care is—and is not. The field-worker, as a professional boundary spanner, is a transmitter of texts and narratives in both directions, and is an active part of this process of mediation. Many field-workers come from backgrounds and communities that are very similar to those of the patients that they serve. This does not necessarily mean that they will be more empathetic toward stigmatized patients. However, it does often place the field-worker in a sometimes ambiguous position relative to the medical institution. The field-worker is just as likely to be treated as a social peer by the patient as he or she is by the physician. The field-worker, therefore, may be more likely to grasp and communicate the patient's point of view—indeed, may find it necessary to do so—while at the same time attempting to carry out a medically defined mission in a socially contested terrain.

In a lecture entitled "The Birth of Social Medicine," Foucault stated that the innovation of the English health care system lay in its "creation of three superimposed and coexisting medical systems: a welfare medicine designed for the poorest people; an administrative medicine responsible for general problems such as vaccination, epidemics, and so on; and a private medicine benefiting those who could afford it" (Foucault 1974, 134–156). This description might also be applied to the contemporary United States, where public hospitals and public health agencies bear the brunt of caring for the poor and for monitoring health at the level of population, while private doctors and hospitals concentrate on treating the insured and the employed on an individualized basis. As an airborne infectious disease, TB potentially traverses all sectors of the population and all of these systems. In reality, however, it remains largely confined to poor urban minority populations. Tuberculosis, read as a text written across populations and individuals, makes these fissures visible, like a stain on a microbiologist's slide. After the disease is treated, the divisions remain.

The control of TB, in the past, has had a particular purpose beyond that of treating individuals and limiting the spread of disease within communities. It also served to patrol the border between segregated communities and to contain tuberculosis within these socially constructed reservoirs (Acevedo-Garcia 2000). While effective as a practice that establishes trust and compliance through bridging social boundaries and extending institutional power into local contexts, DOT may also be seen as an instrumental relation, aimed at controlling threatening bodies, not repairing communities. Rather than serving as a palliative for the damage wreaked on poor communities by years of political neglect, economic disinvestment, drugs, violence, and other all-too-familiar social ills associated with poverty, health care systems might provide a means of illuminating the proper direction of future public policy. Instead of investing millions in marketing and consultant fees, while placing bandages over broken bones at the bottom of a growing cliff of social inequality, these systems might point us toward more effective preventive strategies and long-term community development. TB might be seen as guide, an indicator of the societal factors that underlie many nested and overlapping health problems (Jaramillo 1999).

New York City lowered its crime rates significantly throughout the 1990s through a data-driven system called Compstat, which sought to identify and control emerging issues before they blossomed into crises. Such an approach can only be called epidemiological, and the parallels to the TB control campaign of the 1990s are apparent. For each to be successful, they required adequate resources and flexibility to move beyond the stage where systems were merely reacting to yesterday's tragic deaths. But confining surface phenomena such as crime and disease within socially acceptable borders of race and class should not be enough. Recent efforts at treating asthma among poor families in Harlem have sought to extend the reach of public health outside of the hospital and into the community, even going so far as to modify social and physical environments to make them more healthy (Pérez-Peña 2003). These approaches not only seek the consent of those being treated, they require their active cooperation. TB control programs in countries such as India, China, and Peru have adapted the DOT model to fit local cultural and historical contexts, and the treatment of HIV/AIDS in Africa will necessitate field-intensive public health campaigns. While precedents for these efforts exist, and templates may be borrowed from other areas, each new venture into the field brings its own lessons and challenges, just as each patient is unique in their particulars. It is incumbent on health systems, and those who work in them, to build on what they learn in the field, and to consistently raise hard questions that must be addressed at the level of society.

My grandfather's story, related in the Introduction to this book, may be read as a reminder of our own collective susceptibility. His body carried within it the living scars of his history. He was originally infected at a time when TB was endemic. Though he recovered his health, the disease persisted, contained in a cavity inside his lung. When his body was weakened with age and abuse, the germs revived. Human beings are connected to the past through our own biology, and what has stricken us once may strike us again. The same may be said of societies: they contain within them at all times the records of past plagues and the seeds of new diseases. In 1959, Rene Dubos prophetically wrote that there is no utopia free of maladies that awaits us, in the near or distant future. But no matter what the next affliction may be, we can do no better than caring for the commons. Those consumed in the cities cry out to us. Tuberculosis, a persistent reminder of the poverty we allow to fester, points us back to the neglected pursuit of the public health.

Epilogue

Back on the Corner, Chicago, 2002

BACK IN Chicago on academic business, I set out to see two guys whom I knew from my TB days. Rick was now living in a secure building on the South Side, and Isaiah was in a nursing home somewhere, the last I heard.

Rick was a tough, aging thug with one eye and an attitude. When I first met him he was homeless, and I used to find him every morning, sitting on a bench in front of a low-rise housing project on the West Side. But we hit it off, and after he finished his TB treatment, he asked me to help him manage his monthly disability check. I agreed, and we got him a room in a nearby hotel. Then he was arrested for threatening a convenience store clerk, and because of his long criminal record, he agreed to a plea bargain and did several more years in state prison.

I kept in touch with him by mail, and he let me know when he finally finished his sentence and secured his own apartment in the city. I decided to go visit him there. Shortly after I arrived at the building he walked in the front door, and said, "Hey, Doc." He didn't seem the least bit surprised to see me.

We went up to his room and talked. He told me how he was doing, and we discussed the building, and the neighborhood. He said he tried talking to people on the corner to get them to see what they were doing with their lives, but he believed that people who are addicted can't be helped unless they want to help themselves. A long-time alcoholic, he no longer drinks at all.

I took him to lunch at Valois in Hyde Park, an old cafeteria-style restaurant immortalized in Mitch Duneier's *Slim's Table*. He had never been to that neighborhood, even though it was quite close to where he was now living. We each had the chicken cacciatore, and he took his left-overs home with him. He said that he usually cooked for himself, though sometimes a woman in the building prepared some of his food for him, and he paid her for the service.

When I dropped him off I told him how good it was to see him doing well, to be able to hang out with him and talk and not have to worry that he's going to squeeze me for funds or play some kind of game, which was always the case when he was living day to day in the street.

263

The next morning I went to the West Side to sniff around for Isaiah. In late May I had looked for him in the neighborhood, and I was told that he had a stroke, was taken to the hospital, and from there to a facility in an unknown location. Billy had passed away in November 2001, right after Thanksgiving. He had been transferred from Maple Grove to some city nursing home. One morning they found him dead in his bed. His family suspected negligence, but they couldn't prove it. So I didn't expect good news about Isaiah, but I was pleasantly surprised when I walked into the neighborhood lounge and asked if anyone had seen Isaiah's cousin, Hank. Hank usually knew where Isaiah was. The guy behind the bar recognized me and said, "You're Isaiah's guy, right?" and I said "Yeah," and he said, "he's around the corner."

"In that empty lot?"

"Right there."

So I went around there and found him sitting on a chair under a tree, with Mr. Smith and another old man whose name I didn't know. He looked up and said, "Hey Paul, long time no see." He also did not seem surprised.

He told me how he had been placed in a nursing home down by the jail, and how he walked out because the place was like a jail itself. He said, "I don't care if it's a coon, or a dog, or a bird, don't no animal want to be kept in a cage." Suddenly it occurred to me that this might be the same place where Billy went, and where his life ended.

Isaiah didn't know about that, but he didn't have anything positive to say about the place. They started processing him for disability but by the time he left he still hadn't gotten it, and so once again he was doing without it. Now he said that the shelter didn't want him.

But it was good to see him, to know he was still the last dinosaur. I said this to him, and he laughed: "I almost wasn't, either."

Before I left I took him over by Richardson's, because he told me that Mitch was back over there, and we did find him there, sure enough, along with Henderson, Ethel, and the usual cast of characters. Even Geronimo showed up, after I showed some pictures of Billy with his leg amputated that I took down at Maple Grove when I visited him there last summer. Ethel took one of the pictures and showed it to another guy, who came over and shook my hand, introducing himself as Ace. When I used Billy's old line, "Straight up, no chaser, and all jokes aside," he and Henderson both laughed out loud, and Henderson said, "Billy was my buddy," and Ace said, "You see, that just shows he's still with us, you just brought a little bit of Billy to us, that shows that a person's spirit lives on." Another man came over and said that Billy gave him his first black eye. "Billy could fight," said Henderson, "he was a hell of fighter, he'd hit you with that left, bam, bam, quicker than you could see." Geronimo took the photo upstairs to show it to his wife. When he brought it back he said that it made her cry to see it. Geronimo thanked me for all that I've done for the guys around there, picking them up, taking them to the hospital, giving them something to eat. He made it sound like I did it everyday, like I did it because I had a holy mission, and not because it was my job. But I did not argue with his praise. It felt good.

All of these guys except for Geronimo, Ace, and Isaiah asked me for money. I gave one five spot to Mitch and Ethel, telling them to split it with Henderson, who Isaiah said is "like a Timex, he takes a licking and keeps on ticking." While we were all standing there I saw one patrol car and an undercover cop drive by. Mitch said, "You want to get caught up, just keep talking to him," indicating Henderson. Isaiah was also ready to leave at this point, and so he and I got in the car. I fended off the last request for money, which came from a skeleton-thin woman who already had a bottle in a paper bag. She said she needed to get something to eat and wanted to know if I had a sandwich in my car. She said she knew me from the alley where I used to see Uncle Jesse, who she said was in the hospital with a bleeding ulcer. I would have given her a dollar or a sandwich if I had it, but I didn't, I had one five dollar bill left and it was going to Isaiah.

I left him back at the corner where I found him, gave him the five dollars, and had Mr. Smith take a picture of us on the street, the latest installment in a series dating back to 1997. I prayed that he would be preserved until the next time I passed through.

Notes

Introduction

1. Ivan Illich, in *Medical Nemesis* (1976), made a radical and compelling argument that modern medicine does more harm than good: that it does actual physical damage, that it invents illness, and that it deprives communities and individuals of the capacity to heal themselves and experience suffering in a meaningful way. Sociologist Irving Zola made a similar claim when he wrote that ". . . medicine is becoming a major institution of social control, nudging aside, if not incorporating, the more traditional institutions of religion and law" (Zola 379). Both Illich and Zola saw the "medicalization" of society as a dangerous development, and some people in the medical professions have embraced aspects of Illich's argument. For example, David Thomasma of Loyola Medical Center has written: "Of the main evil results that Illich detects, I agree with his perception of the cultural effect of overreliance on medical professions as a symptom of the dependency of man in an industrialized society. . ." (Thomasma 43). Robert Mendelsohn, physician and self-proclaimed "medical heretic," even declared that ". . . more than ninety percent of Modern Medicine could disappear from the face of the earth—doctors, hospitals, drugs and equipment—and the effect on our health would be immediate and beneficial" (Mendelsohn 13).

2. At the same time, these critics tend to see medical discourse as imperialistic, constantly extending its reach far beyond the borders of clinics and hospitals and into more and more aspects of daily life. For example, Waitzkin observes that " . . . doctors communicate explicitly or subtly a message that work is preferable to idleness" (1989, 222). Referring to the theories of Lukacs and Gramsci, Waitzkin argues that medicine in practice contributes to the reification of hegemonic ideas about work and family: "In this sense, medicine exerts ideologic effects that parallel those of such institutions as schools, churches and the mass media" (1989, 223). In focusing their attention almost exclusively on personal troubles rather than social issues, doctors work to deny the validity of the "lifeworlds" of their patients (1989, 232). Thus, according to Waitzkin, the social determinants of health—social class, race, gender, poverty—are *systematically* denied or ignored for two reasons: (1) they are simply not amenable to the technical solutions available to the doctor, and (2) they lie outside the standard analytic framework permitted by the dominant ideology of capitalism. They are translated into purely personal problems to be solved through some kind of therapy or individual intervention. This ideological, context-denying element of medicine, coupled with the expansion of medical expertise into new areas, works to broadly suppress the political and economic implications of health problems.

3. Kearns and Joseph (1993) have argued for a synthesis of humanistic inter-
pretations of place and socio-spatial theory, emphasizing the dynamic relationship between health and the particularities of social as well as geographic location.

4. Rodrick Wallace, for example, has examined the linkages between violent
death, drug abuse, AIDS, and a process which he calls "urban desertification."
This process, he argues, is ". . . directed against African-American and Hispanic
communities, and implemented through systematic and continuing denial of
municipal services–particularly fire extinguishment resources–essential for maintaining urban population density and ensuring community stability" (Wallace
801). Using evidence gathered in Harlem and the Bronx, Wallace concludes that
loss of population and destruction of social networks in inner city areas ". . . is
closely and causally associated with a broad spectrum of pathological outcomes,
including raised death rates from homicide and substance abuse, and the distribution of the AIDS epidemic in both geographic and social space" (Wallace 801).
Wallace's synthesis of spatial and social analyses points the way toward a critical
epidemiology of disease in urban neighborhoods.

Chapter One

1. Concerning diagnosis, Phil Brown has stated: "For socially powerful groups
and institutions, diagnosis can be a tool for social control, such as the medical
labeling homosexuality as a mental illness . . . Diagnosis is central to such social
control, since *giving the name* has often been the starting point for social labelers
. . . Diagnosis locates the parameters of normality and abnormality, demarcates
the professional and institutional boundaries of the social control and treatment
system, and authorizes medicine to label and deal with people on behalf of the
society at large" (Brown 39). In the doctor's eyes, the human suffering may in fact
merely provide the occasion for the diagnosis, and the diagnosis may itself be mysterious to the patient who is actually suffering (Frank 1998a, 341).

2. Herman Melville, *Moby Dick,* Modern Library Edition, New York, 1926,
p. 282.

3. Foucault repeatedly stated that wherever there is discipline, there is resistance, though he did not detail its forms (Lupton 102). But Foucault's theories,
while indispensable to the understanding of disciplinary surveillance, do not
always account for the humanity, the subjectivity, the agency, of those who are
regulated or of those who do the regulating. The state-ordained right and responsibility of the surveillance worker to monitor and regulate the lives of others as
though they were merely "bodies" while knowing, at the same time, that they are
people, can result in complex relationships of give-and-take. Sometimes, as people are prone to do, the objects of medical scrutiny talk back to discipline when
it confronts them. This is one way in which the individual demands recognition
of his or her particularity, and this was another fact I had to face. Just as the utopia
of the "perfectly governed city" remains the stuff of dreams and not reality, the
practice of health surveillance is everywhere fractured and incomplete. It is exactly

in this sense that the panopticon of public health is myopic. In spite of its fractured vision, however, the public health system is panoptic in a crucial sense: it is capable of exerting power over individuals.

4. For details on the revision of the health code governing the use of coercive measures to control TB, see "Developing a System for Tuberculosis Prevention and Care in New York City," in *The Tuberculosis Revival: Individual Rights and Societal Obligations in a Time of AIDS,* a report by the United Hospital Fund of New York, written by New York City Tuberculosis Working Group, 1992, pp. 51–58. For critical discussion of detention policy, see Barron Lerner, "Catching Patients: Tuberculosis and Detention in the 1990s" in *Chest* 115:236–241, 1999.

CHAPTER TWO

1. In many other areas of the world, TB was, and remains, quite widespread. In 1993 the World Health Organization declared TB to be a "global health emergency," estimating that one third of the world's population was infected with the tuberculosis bacterium, and that the disease killed about three million people every year.

2. "In the context of the Progressive Era, the TB menace had a unifying as well as a fragmenting effect on a diverse society: the yardstick of health morality could be used to compare different groups and chart the path of their reclamation, both in personal and social terms" (Tomes 286).

3. Of special concern to Patton is the way in which pre-existing stigmas were preserved and reinforced by "scientific" AIDS language: "The effectiveness of science-logic in policing society has both reified science-logic and inured us to science's inability to solve the problems it sets for itself. The categories of science, especially the conjuncture of virology and epidemiology, have placed a barely invisible cordon sanitaire around minority communities, "deviant individuals," and around the entire continent of Africa" (Patton 99).

4. Wallace postulates that the process of "urban desertification," which he defines as ". . . systematic and continuing denial of municipal services—particularly fire extinguishment resources—essential for maintaining urban levels of population density and ensuring community stability," is closely and causally connected with patterns of cirrhosis, homicide, and AIDS deaths, among other things (Wallace 801). Although Wallace focuses on fire services in particular, the same might be said of the process of deindustrialization and, to a lesser extent, of gentrification. These processes all have potentially devastating effects on poor and working communities (which soon become poor when the jobs disappear), as they are either plunged deeper into poverty, or are dislocated by rising housing costs.

5. According to Stuart Hall and colleagues, the petty bourgeois classes live in a state of perpetual anxiety: deprived of either wealth or solidarity, the only thing that they have to distinguish themselves from the profligate upper classes and the indulgent lower classes is their moral superiority and their "common sense" (Hall et al. 163). Their anxiety, in turn, exudes a sort of paranoid fog which obscures

the social and economic structures that manufacture and maintain class and race differentials.

6. Gandy and Zumla (2002) claim that the three factors that characterized the epidemiology of the "new tuberculosis" were: "the emergence of drug-resistant strains of TB; the prevalence of co-infection with HIV; and social and economic developments affecting access to medical care."

7. However, as Gandy and Zumla have argued, "The DOTS strategy is approaching the limits of what can be achieved without more fundamental changes in public health policies as part of a wider programme to tackle poverty and social inequality" (Gandy and Zumla 389). They, like Farmer (1999), call for a "rethinking" of the epidemiology of infectious disease. This would entail an integration of biomedical approaches with historical analysis, social science research and progressive public health. They likewise maintain that the phenomenon of tuberculosis in the 1990s, the so-called "new tuberculosis" or "tuberculosis resurgence," cannot be understood without an understanding of the social and economic circumstances that surrounded it—what Farmer calls a "broad, biosocial view"—and that the problem of tuberculosis in today's world cannot be addressed with strictly medical means.

Chapter Four

1. In 1949, the United States Health Service conducted a study of TB in Chicago. This was before the development of effective antibiotics, and the disease took an enormous toll in terms of both death and prolonged suffering. The study calculated a TB death rate of 62.4 per 100,000 in the years 1939–1941; in 1940 there were 4,942 new reported cases of active pulmonary tuberculosis in Chicago. To offer a point of comparison: fifty years later, in the midst of a much-publicized resurgence of the disease, there were only 705 new reported cases.

2. The number of documented tuberculosis cases in Chicago dropped from 1982 (1,069 cases) through 1987 (649 cases).

3. According to Kearns and Joseph, ". . .the inhabitants of specific localities are more or less prone to illnesses for which the aetiology is embedded in their lived environment" (Kearns and Joseph 712).

4. The main difference between the ghettos of yesterday and today, as William J. Wilson has pointed out, is the absence of work (Wilson 28). Certainly there is a great lack of financially rewarding employment in many poor neighborhoods. That does not mean, however, that people don't do anything, or that they don't, in fact, work.

5. According to Singer: ". . . the inner city health crisis . . . is characterized by a set of closely interrelated endemic and epidemic conditions, all of which are strongly influenced by a broader set of political-economic and social factors, including high rates of unemployment, poverty, homelessness and residential overcrowding, substandard nutrition, environmental toxins and related environmental health risks, infrastructural deterioration and loss of quality housing stock, forced geographic mobility, family breakup and disruption of social support networks, youth gang and drug-related violence, and health care inequality" (Singer 933).

6. *The American Journal of Public Health* devoted an issue to urban health in June 2000. Several of the featured editorials highlighted the importance of recognizing both broad structural forces and local ecological factors as powerful determinants of individual health and illness. According to Geronimus, ". . . evidence of important interactions of race, poverty and locality in influencing health is growing, but social epidemiologists more often look at general patterns of the relationship between socioeconomic position and health . . .Stepping up research on variation among local poor populations may prove beneficial to those hoping to remedy the effect of urban life on health" (Geronimus 870).

Chapter Five

1. The neighborhood is perhaps the most familiar urban example of what Kleinman has called a "local social world"; according to Kleinman, these worlds "are particular, intersubjective, and constitutive of the lived flow of experience. They are not simply reflections of macro-level socioeconomic and political forces, though they are strongly influenced by such forces" (Kleinman 1992, 172). Private geography, local social world, "place" as opposed to "space"—this is where illness occurs. Only later does it enter the doctor's field of vision—what Foucault called the "medical gaze"—where the mercurial experience of "illness" is translated into the stable category of "disease" (Foucault 1973, 9).

2. In radical black thought, the prevalent sociological notion of the ghetto as *deviant subculture* has been contrasted with the metaphor of the ghetto as *oppressed internal colony,* a strain of thought commonly associated with Frantz Fanon. For instance, Fanon writes: "The colonial world is a world cut in two. The dividing line, the frontiers are shown by barracks and police stations. In the colonies it is the policeman and the soldier who are the official, instituted go-betweens, the spokesmen of the settler and his rule of oppression" (Fanon 31).

Chapter Six

1. Simon, David, and Edward Burns. *The Corner.* New York: Broadway, 1997.

2. Abraham, Laurie K. *Mama Might Be Better Off Dead: The Failure of Health Care in Urban America.* Chicago: University of Chicago Press, 1993.

3. As Wright and Fife have argued, "self concepts of stigmatized persons are constructed over time through social interaction," and Jeremiah's case provides a clear example of the circularity of this process (Fife and Wright 64).

Chapter Seven

1. March 24, the day when Robert Koch first announced his "discovery" of the tuberculosis bacilli.

2. Although there are cases where permanent cure is not achieved despite of medical compliance, and there are also cases where noncompliance does not result in recurrence of disease.

3. In the context of DOT, "compliance" was defined as cooperation with the goals of the program: the ingestion of prescribed medicine in the presence of an assigned worker, attending monthly clinic visits, and obeying infection control guidelines, such as wearing a mask or staying away from congregate settings, as long as this was deemed to be necessary. Once chemotherapy began, infectiousness was usually reduced rapidly, and within a month most TB patients no longer needed to wear a mask or avoid sharing airspace with others. Patients who were compliant with medications could avoid other medical restrictions on their behavior, and the DOT worker was assigned to both verify and enable medical compliance.

4. Two publications of the CDC, "Improving Patient Compliance in Tuberculosis Treatment Programs" (1989) and "Improving Patient Adherence to Tuberculosis Treatment" (1994) both emphasize that responsibility for compliance must be shared by the patient and the health care provider. The latter article, which is a revised version of the former, additionally highlights the multiple individual and social factors that can influence compliance, and substitutes the term "adherence" because "it suggests a partnership between the patient and provider, and a sharing of responsibility for treatment outcomes."

5. See "Developing a System for Tuberculosis Prevention and Care in New York City," in *The Tuberculosis Revival: Individual Rights and Societal Obligations in a Time of AIDS,* a report by the United Hospital Fund of New York, written by New York City Tuberculosis Working Group, 1992, pp. 51–58.

Conclusion

1. Public health then comes to resemble Paulo Freire's description of a monologic model of education, that suffers from "narrative sickness": "The teacher talks about reality as though it were motionless, static, compartmentalized and predictable. . . . Words are emptied of their concreteness and become a hollow, alienated and alienating verbosity" (Freire 57). For Freire, this "banking" style of education, where teachers are the depositors and students are the receptacles, is inherently oppressive. It can only be solved by reconciling the student-teacher relationship, so that "both are simultaneously teachers and students" (Freire 59). In order for this to happen, the teacher has to meet the students where they are, in the "here and now." The "fatalism" so often perceived among historically oppressed populations can only be confronted within the concrete situation, which is posed as a problem to be solved rather than an unchangeable condition. "Reality" thus loses its necessity; it ceases to be fated, magical, and inevitable, and becomes a domain of choice and action. In order to do this, however, we have to be honest about the situation that confronts us. "Reality" may not be a matter of fate, but it is nonetheless real.

Works Cited

Abel, Emily K. "Taking the Cure to the Poor: Patients' Responses to New York City's Tuberculosis Control Program, 1894 to 1918." *American Journal of Public Health* 87, no. 11 (1997): 1808–1815.

Abraham, Laurie Kaye. *Mama Might Be Better Off Dead: The Failure of Health Care in Urban America*. Chicago: University of Chicago Press, 1993.

Acevedo-Garcia, Dolores. "Residential Segregation and the Epidemiology of Infectious Diseases." *Social Science and Medicine* 51, no. 8 (2000): 1143–1161.

Adorno, Theodor. *Minima Moralia*. London: Verso, 1974.

———. *Negative Dialectics*. New York: Continuum, 1973.

Agee, James, and Walker Evans. *Let Us Now Praise Famous Men*. New York: Houghton Mifflin, 1941.

Aldrich, Howard. "The Origins and Persistence of Social Networks." In *Advances in Social Network Analysis*, 283–293. Edited by Stanley Wasserman and Joseph Galaskiewicz. Thousand Oaks, Calif.: Sage, 1994.

Algren, Nelson. *Chicago: City on the Make*. Oakland: Angel Island, 1961.

Allen, Robert L. *Black Awakening in Capitalist America*. Trenton, N.J.: Africa World Press, 1990.

Altman, Lawrence K. "As TB Surges, Drug Producers Face Criticism." *New York Times*, 18 September 1995, A1.

Anderson, Elijah. *A Place on the Corner*. Chicago: University of Chicago Press, 1976.

———. *Streetwise: Race, Class and Change in an Urban Community*. Chicago: University of Chicago Press, 1990.

———. "The Code of the Streets." *Atlantic Monthly* 273 (1994): 80–92.

Asturias, Miguel Angel. *Strong Wind*. New York: Delacorte Press, 1968.

Bahr, Howard. *Skid Row: An Introduction to Disaffiliation*. New York: Oxford University Press, 1973.

Bagley, Cherie, and Juanitaelisabeth Carroll. "Healing Forces in African-American Families." In *Resiliency in African-American Families*, 117–142. Edited by Hamilton I. McCubbin et al. London: Sage, 1998.

Bailey, George, ed. *West Side Stories*. Chicago: City Stoop Press, 1992.

Bates, Barbara. *Bargaining for Life: A Social History of Tuberculosis, 1876–1938*. Philadelphia: University of Pennsylvania Press, 1992.

Bayer, Ronald, and David Wilkinson. "Directly Observed Therapy for Tuberculosis: History of an Idea." *The Lancet* 345 (1995): 1545–1548.

Becker, Howard. *Boys in White: Student Culture in Medical School*. Chicago: University of Chicago Press, 1961.

Bhavaraju, R., D. J. Kantor, B. T. Mangura, and L. B. Reichman. "Implications of Print Media Portrayal of Tuberculosis." Poster presented at American Lung Association/American Thoracic Society Annual Conference, San Diego, 1999.

Blendon, Robert J., et al. "How White and African Americans View Their Health and Social Problems: Different Experiences, Different Expectations." *JAMA* 273, no. 4 (1995): 341.

Bock, Naomi N., John P. Mallory, Nell Mobley, Beverly DeVoe, and B. Brooks Taylor. "Outbreak of Tuberculosis Associated with a Floating Card Game in the Rural South: Lessons for Tuberculosis Contact Investigation." *Clinical Infectious Diseases* 27 (1998): 1221–1226.

Booker, Michael J. "Compliance, Coercion, and Compassion: Moral Dimensions of the Return of Tuberculosis." *Journal of Medical Humanities,* 17 (1996): 91–102.

Bowden, Charles, and Lew Kreinberg. *Street Signs Chicago: Neighborhood and Other Illusions of Big City Life.* Chicago: Chicago Review Press, 1981.

Bowditch, Henry I. "Is Consumption Ever Contagious, or Communicated by One Person to Another in Any Manner?" In *From Consumption to Tuberculosis: A Documentary History,* 43–56. Edited by Barbara Rosenkrantz. New York: Garland, 1994.

Brody, Howard. *Stories of Sickness.* New Haven: Yale University Press, 1987.

Brooks, Durado D., et al. "Medical Apartheid: An American Perspective." *JAMA* 266, no. 19 (1991).

Brown, Phil. "Naming and Framing: The Social Construction of Disease and Illness." *Journal of Health and Social Behavior,* Extra Issue (1995): 34–52.

Brown, Phyllida. "The Return of the Big Killer." *New Scientist,* 10 October 1992, 30–37.

Brudney, Karen, and Jay Dobkin. "Resurgent Tuberculosis in New York City." *American Review of Respiratory Disease* 144 (1991):745–749.

Butler, Judith. *The Psychic Life of Power.* Stanford: Stanford University Press, 1997.

Canada, Geoffrey. *fist stick knife gun.* Boston: Beacon Press, 1995.

Cappetti, Carla. *Writing Chicago: Modernism, Ethnography and the Novel.* New York: Columbia University Press, 1993.

Castells, Manuel. *The City and the Grassroots.* Berkeley: University of California Press, 1985.

Caudill, Chris, Paul Draus, James McAuley, and William Paul. "Investigation of a Tuberculosis Outbreak in an Inner-City Car Wash." Poster presented at American Lung Association/American Thoracic Society Annual Conference, San Diego, 1999.

Chambliss, Daniel. *Beyond Caring: Hospitals, Nurses and the Social Organization of Ethics.* Chicago: University of Chicago Press, 1996.

Charmaz, Kathy. *Good Days, Bad Days: The Self in Chronic Illness and Time.* New Brunswick, N.J.: Rutgers University Press, 1991.

———. "The Grounded Theory Method: An Explication and Interpretation." In *Contemporary Field Research,* 109–126. Edited by Robert Emerson. Prospect Heights, Ill.: Waveland Press, 1983.

Charmaz, Kathy, and Richard G. Mitchell. "Telling Tales, Writing Stories: Post-modernist Visions and Realist Images in Ethnographic Writing." *Journal of Contemporary Ethnography* 25, no. 1 (1996): 144–166.

Chicago Department of Public Health (CDPH). 2001 Annual Tuberculosis Morbidity Report.

Clark, Kenneth B. *Dark Ghetto*. New York: Harper and Row, 1965.

Coker, Richard. "Tuberculosis, Non-Compliance and Detention for the Public Health." *Journal of Medical Ethics* 26 (2000): 157–159.

Coles, Robert. *Times of Surrender*. Iowa City: University of Iowa Press, 1988.

Connors, Margaret. "Sex, Drugs and Structural Violence." In *Women, Poverty and AIDS*, 91–124. Edited by Paul Farmer, Margaret Connors, and Janie Simmons. Monroe, Me.: Common Courage Press, 1996.

Cornwell, Jocelyn. *Hard-Earned Lives: Accounts of Health and Illness from East London*. London: Tavistock, 1984.

Crawford, Robert. "A Cultural Account of 'Health': Control, Release and the Social Body." In *Issues in the Political Economy of Health Care*, 60–103. Edited by John McKinlay. London: Tavistock, 1984.

Curtis, Sarah, and Ann Taket. *Health and Societies: Changing Perspectives*. London: Arnold, 1996.

Dawley, David. *A Nation of Lords*. Prospect Heights, Ill.: Waveland Press, 1973.

Denzin, Norman K., and Yvonna S. Lincoln, eds. *Handbook of Qualitative Research*. Thousand Oaks, Calif.: Sage, 1994.

Diamond, Timothy. *Making Gray Gold: Narratives of Nursing Home Care*. Chicago: University of Chicago Press, 1992.

Dievler, Ann. "Fighting Tuberculosis in the 1990s: How Effective Is Planning in Policy Making?" *Journal of Public Health Policy* 18, no. 2 (1997): 167–187.

DiFazio, William. "Soup Kitchen Blues: Postindustrial Poverty in Brooklyn." In *The Other City: People and Politics in New York and London*, 40–60. Edited by Susanne MacGregor and Arthur Lipow. N.J.: Humanities Press, 1995.

Dobkin, Jay and Karen Brudney. "Resurgent Tuberculosis in New York City." *American Review of Respiratory Disease* 144 (1991): 745–749.

Donaldson, Gregory. *The Ville: Cops and Kids in Urban America*. New York: Doubleday, 1993.

Donovan, Jenny, and David Blake. "Patient Non-Compliance: Deviance or Reasoned Decision Making?" *Social Science and Medicine* 34, no. 5 (1992): 507–513.

Drake, St. Clair, and Horace Cayton. *Black Metropolis: A Study of Negro Life in a Northern City*. New York: Harcourt, Brace, 1945.

Drucker, Ernest. "Communities at Risk: The Social Epidemiology of AIDS in New York City." In *AIDS and the Social Sciences: Common Threads*, 45–63. Edited by Richard Ulack and William F. Skinner. Lexington: University Press of Kentucky, 1991.

Dubignon, Anne. "The Doctor's Dilemma: A Story of Tuberculosis." In *From Consumption to Tuberculosis: A Documentary History*. Edited by Barbara Gutman Rosenkrantz. New York: Garland, 1994.

Dubos, Rene. *Louis Pasteur: Free Lance of Science*. New York: Da Capo Press, 1960.

————. *Mirage of Health: Utopias, Progress and Biological Change.* New York: Harper and Row, 1959.

Duff, Kat. *The Alchemy of Illness.* New York: Pantheon Books, 1993.

Duneier, Mitchell. *Slim's Table.* Chicago: University of Chicago Press, 1992.

Dunlap, Eloise. "Inner-City Crisis and Drug Dealing: Portrait of a New York Drug Dealer and His Household." In *The Other City: People and Politics in New York and London,* 114–131. Edited by Susanne MacGregor and Arthur Lipow. Atlantic Highlands, N.J.: Humanities Press, 1995.

Dyck, Isabel. "Using Qualitative Methods in Medical Geography: Deconstructive Moments in a Subdiscipline?" *Professional Geographer* 51, no. 2 (1999): 243–253.

The Economist, 20 May 1995, 81.

Esposito, Luigi, and John W. Murphy. "Another Step in the Study of Race Relations." *The Sociological Quarterly* 41, no. 2 (Spring 2000): 171–187.

Eyles, John, and Jenny Donovan. *The Social Effects of Health Policy.* Aldershot, England: Avebury, 1990.

Fanon, Frantz. *The Wretched of the Earth.* New York: Grove Press, 1963.

Farmer, Paul. *AIDS and Accusation: Haiti and the Geography of Blame.* Berkeley: University of California Press, 1992.

————. "On Suffering and Structural Violence: A View from Below." *Daedalus* (Winter 1996): 261–283.

————. "Social Scientists and the New Tuberculosis." *Social Science and Medicine* 44, no. 3 (1997): 347–358.

Farmer, Paul, Margaret Connors, and Janie Simmons, eds. *Women, Poverty and AIDS.* Monroe, Me.: Common Courage Press, 1996.

Farrell, James T. *Studs Lonigan: A Trilogy.* New York: Vanguard, 1935.

Fay, Brian. *Social Theory and Political Practice.* London: Edwin Hyman, 1975.

Fee, Elizabeth, and Barbara Greene. "Science and Social Reform: Women in Public Health." *Journal of Public Health Policy* (Summer 1989): 161–177.

Fee, Elizabeth, and Nancy Krieger. "Thinking and Rethinking AIDS: Implications for Health Policy." *International Journal of Health Services* 23 (1993): 323–346.

Feldberg, Georgina. *Disease and Class: Tuberculosis and the Shaping of Modern North American Society.* New Brunswick, N.J.: Rutgers University Press, 1995.

Fife, Betsy L., and Eric R. Wright. "The Dimensionality of Stigma: A Comparison of Its Impact on the Self of Persons with HIV/AIDS and Cancer." *Journal of Health and Social Behavior* 41 (2000): 50–67.

Foucault, Michel. *The Birth of the Clinic: An Archaeology of Medical Perception.* New York: Pantheon, 1973.

————. *Discipline and Punish.* New York: Pantheon, 1977.

————. *Power/Knowledge: Selected Interviews and Other Writings.* Translated by Colin Gordon et al. New York: Pantheon, 1980.

Frake, Charles. "Ethnography." In *Contemporary Field Research,* 60–67. Edited by Robert Emerson. Prospect Heights, Ill.: Waveland Press, 1983.

Frank, Arthur. *The Wounded Storyteller: Body, Illness and Ethics.* Chicago: University of Chicago Press, 1995.

————. "Illness as Moral Occasion: Restoring Agency to Ill People." *Health* 1, no. 2 (1997): 131–148.

————. "Stories of Illness as Care of the Self: A Foucauldian Dialogue." *Health* 2, no. 3 (1998): 329–348.

————. "Foucault or Not Foucault? Commonwealth and American Perspectives on Health in the Neo-Liberal State." *Health* 2, no. 2 (1998): 233–243.

Frieden, Thomas, and Margaret Hamburg. "TB Transmission in the 1990s." *New England Journal of Medicine* 330, no. 24 (1994): 1750–1751.

Frieden, Thomas R., Paula Fujiwara, Rita Washko, and Margaret Hamburg. "Tuberculosis in New York City–Turning the Tide." *New England Journal of Medicine* 333, no. 4 (July 27, 1995): 229–233.

Friedman, Emily. "The All-Frills Yuppie Health Care Boutique." In *Where Medicine Fails*, 333–345. Edited by Carolyn L. Wiener and Anselm Strauss. New Brunswick, N.J.: Transaction, 1997.

Freire, Paulo. *Pedagogy of the Oppressed.* New York: Herder and Herder, 1970.

Freund, Peter E. S., and Meredith B. McGuire. *Health, Illness and the Social Body: A Critical Sociology.* Englewood Cliffs, N.J.: Prentice Hall, 1991.

Gaitley, Roger and Phillip Seed. *HIV and AIDS: A Social Network Approach.* New York: St. Martin's Press, 1989.

Gallagher, Eugene B. "The Medical Dignity of the Individual: A Cultural Exploration." In *Society, Health and Disease: Transcultural Perspectives*, 217–232. Edited by Janardan Subedi and Eugene Gallagher. Upper Saddle River, N.J.: Prentice-Hall, 1996.

Gandy, Matthew, and Alimuddin Zumla. "The Resurgence of Disease: Social and Historical Perspectives on the 'New' Tuberculosis." *Social Science and Medicine* 55 (2002): 387–398.

————. "Theorizing Tuberculosis: A Reply to Porter and Ogden." *Social Science and Medicine* 55 (2002): 399–401.

Gardiner, Michael. "Foucault, Ethics and Dialogue." *History of the Human Sciences* 9, no. 3 (1996): 27–46.

Gerhardt, Uta. *Ideas About Illness: An Intellectual and Political History of Medical Sociology.* New York: New York University Press, 1989.

Geronimus, Aldine. "To Mitigate, Resist or Undo: Addressing Structural Influences on the Health of Populations." *American Journal of Public Health* 90, no. 6 (2000): 867–872.

Ginzberg, Eli. "A Century of Health Reform." In *Where Medicine Fails.* Edited by Carolyn Weiner and Anselm Strauss. New Brunswick, N.J.: Transaction, 1997.

Garrett, Laurie. *The Coming Plague: Newly Emerging Diseases in a World Out of Balance.* New York: Farrar, Straus and Giroux, 1994.

Glaser, Barney, and Anselm Strauss. *The Discovery of Grounded Theory.* Chicago: Aldine, 1967.

————. *Time for Dying.* Chicago: Aldine, 1968.

Glasgow, Douglas G. *The Black Underclass.* San Francisco: Jossey-Bass, 1980.

Goffman, Erving. *Stigma: Notes on the Management of Spoiled Identity.* New York: Simon and Schuster, 1963.

Goldfield, Michael. *The Color of Politics: Race and the Mainsprings of American Politics*. New York: The New Press, 1997.

Granovetter, Mark. "The Strength of Weak Ties: A Network Theory Revisited." In *Social Structure and Network Analysis*, 105–130. Edited by Peter V. Marsden and Nan Lin. London: Sage, 1982.

Gray, Alastair. *World Health and Disease*. Buckingham, England: Open University Press, 1993.

Hall, Stuart, Chas Critcher, Tony Jefferson, John Clarke, and Brian Roberts. *Policing the Crisis: Mugging, the State and Law and Order*. New York: Holmes and Meier, 1978.

Hamsun, Knut. *Hunger*. New York: Farrar, Straus and Giroux, 1967.

Harris, Shanette. "Black Male Masculinity and Same Sex Friendships." In *The Black Family: Essays and Studies*, 82–90. Edited by Robert Staples. Belmont, Calif.: Wadsworth, 1994.

Harrison, Paul. *Inside the Third World: The Anatomy of Poverty*. New York: Penguin, 1979.

———. *Inside the Inner City: Life Under the Cutting Edge*. New York: Penguin, 1983.

Hawkins, John. *Inverse Images: The Meaning of Culture, Ethnicity and Family in Postcolonial Guatemala*. Albuquerque: University of New Mexico Press, 1984.

Haymes, Stephen Nathan. *Race, Culture and the City: A Pedagogy for Black Urban Struggle*. Albany: SUNY Press, 1995.

Herzlich, Claudine, and Janine Pierret. *Illness and Self in Society*. Baltimore: Johns Hopkins University Press, 1987.

Hill, Richard Child. "Race, Class and the State: The Metropolitan Enclave System in the United States." *The Insurgent Sociologist* 10, no. 2 (1980): 45–59.

Hoch, Charles, and Robert A. Slayton. *New Homeless and Old: Community and the Skid Row Hotel*. Philadelphia: Temple University Press, 1989.

Illich, Ivan. *Tools for Conviviality*. New York: Harper and Row, 1973.

———. *Medical Nemesis*. London: Marion Boyars, 1976.

Jaramillo, Ernesto. "Encompassing Treatment with Prevention: The Path for a Lasting Control of Tuberculosis." *Social Science and Medicine* 49 (1999): 393–404.

Jencks, Christopher. *Rethinking Social Policy*. Cambridge: Harvard, 1992.

Jouellet, Pierre. "Images of Health in America." Unpublished manuscript, presented at Annual Conference of the Society for the Interdisciplinary Study of Social Imagery, March 1999.

Jones, James H. *Bad Blood: The Tuskegee Syphilis Experiment*. New York: The Free Press, 1993.

Kaplan, Mark S. "AIDS and the Psycho-Social Disciplines: The Social Control of 'Dangerous' Behavior." *The Journal of Mind and Behavior* 11, nos. 3 and 4 (1990): 337–352.

Katz, Michael. *The Undeserving Poor: From the War on Poverty to the War on Welfare*. New York: Pantheon, 1989.

Kearns, R. A., and A. Joseph. "Space in Its Place: Developing the Link in Medical Geography." *Social Science and Medicine* 37, no. 4 (1993): 711–717.

Kellner, Douglas, and Steven Best. *Postmodern Theory: Critical Interrogations.* New York: Guilford, 1991.

Kleinman, Arthur. *The Illness Narratives: Suffering, Healing and the Human Condition.* New York: Basic Books, 1988.

——. "Pain and Resistance: The Delegitimation and Relegitimation of Local Worlds." In *Pain as Human Experience: An Anthropological Perspective,* 169–207. Edited by Mary-Jo DelVecchio Good et al. Berkeley: University of California Press, 1992.

Koch, Robert. "Aetiology of Tuberculosis." In *From Consumption to Tuberculosis: A Documentary History,* 197–224. Edited by Barbara Rosenkrantz. New York: Garland Publishing.

Kotlowitz, Alex. "Breaking the Silence." In *Resiliency in African-American Families,* 3–16. Edited by Hamilton I. McCubbin et al. London: Sage, 1998.

Krieger, Nancy. "Epidemiology and the Web of Causation: Has Anyone Seen the Spider?" *Social Science and Medicine* 39, no. 7 (1994): 887–903.

Lantz, Paula, James S. House, James M. Lepkowski, David R. Williams, Richard P. Mero, and Jieming Chen. "Socioeconomic Factors, Health Behaviors and Mortality." *JAMA* 279 (1998): 1703–1708.

Latour, Bruno, and Steve Woolgar. *Laboratory Life: The Construction of Scientific Facts.* Princeton: Princeton University Press, 1986.

Leclere, Felicia, Richard G. Rogers, and Kimberly Peters. "Neighborhood Social Context and Racial Differences in Women's Heart Disease Mortality." *Journal of Health and Social Behavior* 39, no. 2 (1998): 91–107.

Ledeneva, Alena. *Russia's Economy of Favors: Blat, Networking and Informal Exchange.* Cambridge: Cambridge University Press, 1998.

Lerner, Barron. "New York City's Tuberculosis Control Efforts: The Historical Limits of the 'War on Consumption.'" *American Journal of Public Health* 83, no. 5 (1993): 758–767.

——. "From Careless Consumptives to Recalcitrant Patients: The Historical Construction of Noncompliance." *Social Science and Medicine* 45, no. 9 (1997): 1423–1431.

——. "Catching Patients: Tuberculosis and Detention in the 1990s." *Chest* 115 (1999): 236–241.

Lemann, Nicholas. *The Promised Land: The Great Black Migration and How It Changed America.* New York: Vintage Books, 1991.

Lewis, Oscar. *Five Families: Mexican Case Studies in the Culture of Poverty.* New York: Basic Books, 1959.

——. *La Vida: A Puerto Rican Family in the Culture of Poverty—San Juan and New York.* New York: Random House, 1968.

Lewis, Sydney. *Hospital: An Oral History of Cook County Hospital.* New York: The New Press, 1994.

Lichtenstein, Edward, and Michael Kroll. "The Fortress Economy: The Economic Role of the U.S. Prison System." Pamphlet published by American Friend Service Committee, 1990.

Link, Bruce G., and Jo Phelan. "Social Conditions as Fundamental Causes of Disease." *Journal of Health and Social Behavior,* Extra Issue (1995): 80–94.

Lipsky, Michael. *Street-level Bureaucracy: Dilemmas of the Individual in Public Services.* New York: Russell Sage, 1980.

Lupton, Deborah. "Foucault and the Medicalisation Critique." In *Foucault, Health and Medicine,* 94–110. Edited by Alan Peterson and Robin Bunton. London: Routledge, 1997.

Mann, Thomas. *The Magic Mountain.* New York: Alfred A. Knopf, 1927.

Martin, Emily. *The Woman in the Body.* Boston: Beacon Press, 1987.

Massey, Douglas, and Nancy Denton. *American Apartheid.* Cambridge: Harvard, 1993.

Mendolsohn, Robert S. *Confessions of a Medical Heretic.* New York: Warner Books, 1979.

Merton, Thomas. *On Theoretical Sociology.* New York: The Free Press, 1967.

McBride, David. *From TB to AIDS: Epidemics Among Urban Blacks since 1900.* Albany: SUNY Press, 1991.

McKeown, Thomas. *The Role of Medicine: Dream, Mirage, or Nemesis?* Princeton: Princeton University Press, 1979.

McKinlay, John, and Sonja M. McKinlay. "Medical Measures and the Decline of Mortality." In *The Sociology of Health and Illness: Critical Perspectives,* 10–23. Edited by Peter Conrad and Rochelle Kern. New York: St. Martin's Press, 1986.

Mills, C. Wright. *The Sociological Imagination.* Oxford: Oxford University Press, 1959.

Morris, Martina. "Epidemiology and Social Networks." In *Advances in Social Network Analysis,* 26–52. Edited by Stanley Wasserman and Joseph Galaskiewicz. Thousand Oaks, Calif.: Sage, 1994.

Morse, Janice M., and Joy L. Johnson. *The Illness Experience: Dimensions of Suffering.* London: Sage, 1991.

Morse, Michelle. "Through the Opera Glass: A Critical Analysis of Tuberculosis as Presented in Opera." *The Pharos* (Fall 1998): 11–14.

Muntaner, Carles, F., Javier Nieto, and Patricia O'Campo. "Race, Class and Epidemiologic Research." *Journal of Public Health Policy* 18, no. 3 (1996): 261–274.

Naing, Nyi Nyi, Catherine D'Este, and Abdul Rahman. "Factors Contributing to Poor Compliance with Anti-TB Treatment Among Tuberculosis Patients." *Southeast Asian J Trop Med Public Health* 32 (2001): 369–382.

Nettleton, Sarah. *The Sociology of Health and Illness.* Cambridge: Polity Press, 1995.

New York City Department of Health, Bureau of Tuberculosis Control. *Tuberculosis in New York City, 1992: Information Summary.* New York, 1992.

Oehlsen, Nadia. "Caught in the Machinery." *The Chicago Reader,* 4 April 1997, 1, 12–25.

Ott, Katherine. *Fevered Lives: Tuberculosis in American Culture since 1870.* Cambridge, Mass.: Harvard University Press, 1996.

Pablos-Mendez, Ariel, Charles A. Knirsch, and R. Graham Barr. "Nonadherence in Tuberculosis Treatment: Predictors and Consequences in New York City." *The American Journal of Medicine* 102 (1997): 164–170.

Parkhurst, Michael. "Adorno and the Practice of Theory." *Rethinking Marxism* 8, no. 3 (1996): 38–58.

Patton, Cindy. *Inventing AIDS.* London: Routledge, 1991.

Peck, Jamie. *Work-Place: The Social Regulation of Labor Markets.* New York: Guilford Press, 1996.

Pérez-Peña, Richard. "An Everyday Struggle for Breath: Childhood Asthma Project Reaches Out in Harlem." *New York Times,* 1 May 2003, B-12.

Piven, Frances Fox, and Richard Cloward. *Regulating the Poor: The Functions of Public Welfare.* 1971. New York: Random House, 1971.

———. *The New Class War.* New York: Pantheon, 1982.

Polanyi, Karl. *The Great Transformation.* New York: Rinehart and Company, 1994.

Rainwater, Lee. *Behind Ghetto Walls.* Chicago: Aldine, 1970.

Richie, Beth E. "The Social Construction of the 'Immoral' Black Mother: Social Policy, Community Policing, and Effects on Youth Violence." In *Revisioning Women, Health and Healing,* 283–299. Edited by Adele E. Clark and Virginia L. Olesen. New York: Routledge, 1999.

Rosenberg, Charles. "Community and Communities: The Evolution of the American Hospital." In *The American General Hospital: Communities and Social Contexts,* 3–17. Edited by Diana Elizabeth Long and Janet Golden. Ithaca, N.Y.: Cornell University Press, 1989.

Rosenkrantz, Barbara Gutmann, ed. *From Consumption to Tuberculosis: A Documentary History.* New York: Garland, 1994.

Roth, Julius A. *Timetables: Structuring the Passage of Time in Hospital Treatment and Other Careers.* Indianapolis: Bobbs-Merrill, 1963.

Rothman, Sheila. "The Sanatorium Experience: Myths and Realities." In *The Tuberculosis Revival: Individual Rights and Societal Obligations in a Time of AIDS,* 72–73. New York: The United Hospital Fund of New York, 1992.

———. *Living in the Shadow of Death: Tuberculosis and the Social Experience of Illness in American History.* New York: Basic Books, 1994.

Roy, Ranjan. "Tuberculosis Epidemic Threatens 16 Nations." *San Francisco Chronicle,* 21 March 1998.

Sbarbaro, John A. 1990. "The Patient-Physician Relationship: Compliance Revisited." *Annals of Allergy* 64 (4): 325–331.

Schluger, Neil, Carlo Ciotoli, and David Cohen. "Comprehensive Tuberculosis Control for Patients at High Risk for Noncompliance." *American Journal of Respiratory and Critical Care Medicine* 151 (1995): 1486–1490.

Scully, Diana. *Men Who Control Women's Health: The Miseducation of Obstetrician-Gynecologists.* New York: Houghton Mifflin, 1980.

Simmel, Georg. *On Individuality and Social Forms.* Chicago: University of Chicago Press, 1971.

Simon, David, and Edward Burns. *The Corner.* New York: Broadway Books, 1997.

Singer, Merrill. "AIDS and the Health Crisis of the U.S. Urban Poor: The Perspective of Critical Medical Anthropology." *Social Science and Medicine* 39, no. 7 (1994): 931–948.

Smith, Dorothy. *The Everyday World as Problematic: A Feminist Sociology.* Boston: Northeastern University Press, 1987.

———. *Texts, Facts and Feminity: Exploring the Relations of Ruling.* London: Routledge, 1990.

Snow, Loudell. *Walkin' Over Medicine.* San Francisco: Westview Press, 1993.

Sontag, Susan. *Illness as Metaphor and AIDS and Its Metaphors.* New York: Anchor Books, 1990.

Specter, Michael. "Neglected for Years, TB Is Back with Strains that Are Deadlier." *New York Times,* 11 October 1992, 1.

Stack, Carol. *All Our Kin.* New York: Harper and Row, 1974.

Star, Susan Leigh, and Geoffrey Bowker. "Of Lungs and Lungers: The Classified Story of Tuberculosis." Unpublished manuscript, 1999.

Stern, Mark J. "The Emergence of the Homeless as a Public Problem." *Social Service Review* (June 1984): 291–301.

Strauss, Anselm. "Medical Ghettos." In *Where Medicine Fails,* 263–275. Edited by Carolyn Wiener and Anselm Strauss. New Brunswick, N.J.: Transaction, 1997.

Sumartojo, Esther. "When Tuberculosis Treatment Fails: A Social Behavioral Account of Patient Adherence." *American Review of Respiratory Disease* 47 (1993): 1311–1320.

Susser, Mervyn. *Epidemiology, Health and Society: Selected Papers.* Oxford: Oxford University Press, 1987.

Suttles, Gerald. *The Social Order of the Slum.* Chicago: University of Chicago Press, 1968.

Syme, Leonard. "Strategies for Health Promotion." *Preventive Medicine* (1986): 499.

Thomasma, David. "The Goals of Medicine and Society." In *The Culture of Biomedicine,* 34–54. Newark, Del.: University of Delaware Press, 1984.

Todd, Alexandra Dundas. *Intimate Adversaries: Cultural Conflict Between Doctors and Women Patients.* Philadelphia: University of Pennsylvania Press, 1989.

Tomes, Nancy. "Moralizing the Microbe: The Germ Theory and the Moral Construction of Behavior in the Late-Nineteenth-Century Antituberculosis Movement." In *Morality and Health.* Edited by Allan Brandt and Paul Rozin. London: Routledge, 1997.

Tönnies, Ferdinand. *Community and Society.* New York: Harper and Row, 1963.

Torchia, Marion M. "Tuberculosis among American Negroes: Medical Research on a Racial Disease." *In From Consumption to Tuberculosis: A Documentary History,* 495–523. Edited by Barbara G. Rosenkrantz. New York: Garland, 1994.

Trattner, Walter I. *From Poor Law to Welfare State: A History of Social Welfare in America.* New York: The Free Press, 1974.

U.S. Public Health Service. *The Cook County Health Survey.* New York: Columbia University Press, 1949.

Van DeBurg, William. *New Day in Babylon.* Chicago: University of Chicago Press, 1992.

Van Maanen, John. *Tales of the Field: On Writing Ethnography*. Chicago: University of Chicago Press, 1988.

Waitzkin, Howard. "A Critical Theory of Medical Discourse: Ideology, Social Control, and the Processing of Social Context in Medical Encounters." *Journal of Health and Social Behavior* 30 (1989): 220–239.

———. *The Politics of Medical Encounters: How Patients and Doctors Deal with Social Problems*. New Haven: Yale University Press, 1991.

———. "Is Our Work Dangerous? Should It Be?" *Journal of Health and Social Behavior* 39 (1998): 7–17.

Wallace, Rodrick. "Urban Desertification, Public Health and Public Order: 'Planned Shrinkage,' Violent Death, Substance Abuse and AIDS in the Bronx." *Social Science and Medicine* 31, no. 7 (1990): 801–881.

Warren, Khey B. *The Symbolism of Subordination: Indian Identity in a Guatemalan Town*. Austin: University of Texas Press, 1979.

Watson, Sidney D. "Health Care in the Inner City: Asking the Right Question." *North Carolina Law Review* 71 (1993): 1647.

Whyte, William Foote. *Street Corner Society*. Chicago: University of Chicago Press, 1943.

Wideman, John Edgar. *Brothers and Keepers*. New York: Penguin, 1984.

Wilson, William J. *When Work Disappears*. New York: Knopf, 1996.

Wright, Talmadge. *Out of Place*. Albany: SUNY, 1997.

Wright, Will. *Wild Knowledge: Science, Language and Social Life in a Fragile Environment*. Minneapolis: University of Minnesota Press, 1992.

Wuest, Judith. "Feminist Grounded Theory: An Exploration of the Congruency and Tension Between Two Traditions in Knowledge Discovery." *Qualitative Health Research* 5, no. 1 (1995): 125–137.

Zola, Irving K. "Medicine as an Institution of Social Control." In *The Sociology of Health and Illness,* 379–390. Edited by Peter Conrad and Rochelle Kern. New York: St. Martin's Press, 1986.

Zorbaugh, Harvey Warren. *The Gold Coast and the Slum*. Chicago: University of Chicago Press, 1929.

Index

Abel, Emily K., 40–41
Abraham, Laurie, 65, 68–69, 170, 271n2
Acevedo-Garcia, Dolores, 91, 260
acquired immune deficiency syndrome. *See* HIV/AIDS
African Americans, 39; County General Hospital and, 72; expectations regarding medical care, 65; health self-assessment by, 203–204; loss of jobs among, 145; lupus in, 65; northward migration of, 122–123; segregation in inner city neighborhoods, 120–121; storytelling tradition and, 84
Agee, James, 186
AIDS. *See* HIV/AIDS
air circulation system, suspect, 106
The Alchemy of Illness (Duff), 8
alcoholism, 94–95, 186; addict's indulgence in, 207–208; and noncompliance, 28; susceptibility to disease and, 94–95; in tuberculosis patients, 152–153;
Aldrich, Howard, 100
Algren, Nelson, 35
Allen, Robert, 121
Altman, Lawrence K., 55, 102
American Apartheid (Massey and Denton), 120–121
Anderson, Elijah, 126
anti-tuberculosis movement, 39
antibiotics: development of, 53; limitations of, 71; in post–WW II era, 90
antibodies, skin test reactions and, 105
arrogance: health and wealth accompanying, 8–9; of physicians, 8–9
asthma, in New York City, 261
audiotaping, of interviews, 9; with field-workers, 238–254
authority, field-workers and police representing, 156

Bailey, George, 122
Bargaining for Life (Bates), 72
Bates, Barbara, 5, 39, 53, 54, 72
Bayer, Ronald, 189
Becker, Howard, 65
Bethune, Norman, 11

Beyond Caring (Chambliss), 66
Bhavaraju, R., 42, 43
biomedicine: limitations of, 4–5, model of, 258; women and, 195
Black Metropolis (Drake and Cayton), 120
Black Panther Party, 121
Black Power movement, 120, 121–122
Blake, David, 189, 190, 191, 195
blat (social network), 96
Blendon, Robert J., 65
Bock, Naomi N., 102
bodily awareness, 8
Booker, Michael J., 189
Bowden, Charles, 118, 136, 149
Bowditch, Henry I., 37
"bribery." *See* negotiation
Brody, Howard, 7, 151
Brooks, Durado D., 65
Brown, Phil, 268n1
Brown, Phyllida, 14
Brudney, Karen, 42–43, 44–45
bureaucracy: interaction with, 9; street-level, 235
Burns, Edward, 171, 271n1
Butler, Judith, 48, 172

car wash, network example involving, 100–109
care: and coercion, 20, 237; inadequate, and disease recurrence, 189
Carlton Arms, Chicago, 109–114
Carmichael, Stokely, 121
Castells, Manuel, 121
Caudill, Chris, 105, 106, 107
causal webs, concept of, 93
Cayton, Horace, 120
Centers for Disease Control (CDC), 14, 34; publications from, 272n4
Chambliss, Daniel, 66, 68
"chart lore," 224
Chicago: DOT in, 90, 92; morbidity rates in, 118; racial spatialization in, 89; rates of tuberculosis in (1949), 89–90; resurgence of tuberculosis in (late 1980s), 90–91; riots of 1968 in, 118;

factors affecting, 84; time disrupted by, 151. *See also* illness narratives
illness experience: in medicine, 5; as underworld, 8
illness narratives, 151–152; impact on illness of, 7–8
illness narratives (female patients): Claudia, 211–228; Linda, 197–211; Ms. May, 191–196
illness narratives (male patients): Isaiah, 153–163; Jeremiah, 173–184; Stormy, 164–173
immigrants, tuberculosis among, 39, 71; distribution of services and, 90; resurgence of, 50
impersonalization, of institutions, 68, 70
income gap, 52–53
industrialization, tuberculosis and, 71
inner city: African American segregation in, 120–121; catch-22 of life in, 136, 149; depopulation in, 91–92; poor in, 136
institutions: doctors in, 75; impersonalization of, 68, 70; interaction with, 8–9; language employed by, 156; police and field-workers as representatives of, 155–156; street life and, examples of, 95–96
interview methods, 9; audiotaping fieldworkers, 238–254
Interview Unit, hospital-based, 19
intimacy, paradox of, 143–144
Inventing AIDS (Patton), 48
isolation, 134; moral, 130
isolation rooms, 1, 59, 73–74

Jackson, George, 122
Jones, James H., 63
Joseph, A., 268n4, 270n3
Joseph, Dr. Stephen, 52
Jouellet, Pierre, 66

Katz, Michael, 49, 50
Kearns, R. A., 268n3, 270n3
King, Martin Luther, Jr., 121–122, 142
Kleinman, Arthur, 7, 151, 271n1
Koch, Robert, 37, 38, 40, 271n1
Kreinberg, Lew, 118, 136, 149
Krieger, Nancy, 47

La Boheme (Puccini opera), 39
La Traviata (Verdi opera), 39
labor market: and homeless, 97–98; subsistence, 98, 137
language: of health institutions, 156; of professionalism, 69

Lantz, Paula, 51–52
Latour, Bruno, 60
Ledeneva, Alena, 96
Lerner, Barron, 35–36, 39, 41, 190, 269n4
Lewis, Oscar, 72, 79
Link, Bruce G., 84
listening, importance of, 82
literacy, 53
"local social world," 271n1
Los Angeles Times, 44
Lungs at Work, 44
Lupton, Deborah, 268n3
lupus, in African Americans, 65

Making Gray Gold (Diamond), 69
Malcolm X, 121, 122
Mama Might Be Better Off Dead (Abraham), 170, 271n2
Maple Grove Hospital, 61, 80; and County General Hospital compared, 78–79; reputation of, 165–166, 170
Martin, Emily, 194
mass screening, at Carlton Arms, Chicago, 109; at car wash, 105
Massey, Douglas, 120–121
McBride, David, 69
McCauley, James, 106, 107
McGuire, Meredith B., 50
McKeown, Thomas, 5
McKinlay, John, 5
McKinlay, Sonja M., 5
McMurphy, R. P., 32
MDR. *See* multi-drug-resistant tuberculosis
medical charts, notations in, 15
"medical dignity" concept, 70
Medical Nemesis (Illich), 267n1
medical system, denial in, 172
medicalization, 267n1; isolation and, 73–79
medication. *See* treatment regimens
medicine: defining people, 172; free market aspect of, 70; goals of, 77; and government, relationship between, 6–7; holistic, 258; and human community relationship, 70; illness experience position in, 5; sociological critique of, 5; tuberculosis paradigm, 4
Mendelsohn, Robert, 267n1
Merton, Thomas, 101
Mexican neighborhood, in Chicago, 144
microbacteriology, 106
microeconomics, 9
Moby Dick (Melville), 18, 20, 268n2
money, role on street, 143–144
moral isolation, 130
morality, 128